Strong, Beautiful and Modern

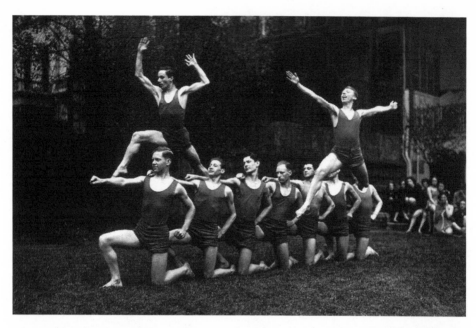

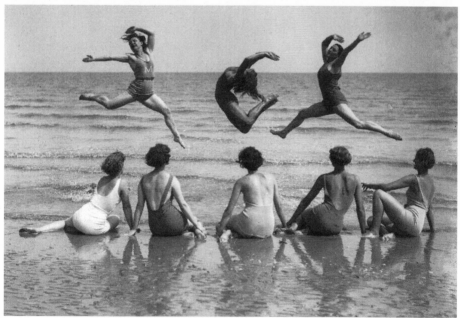

Strong, Beautiful and Modern

National Fitness in Britain, New Zealand, Australia and Canada, 1935–1960

Charlotte Macdonald

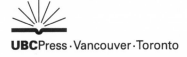

UBCPress · Vancouver · Toronto

21 20 19 18 17 16 15 14 13   5 4 3 2 1

First published in 2011 by Bridget Williams Books Limited, www.bwb.co.nz, P O Box 12 474, Wellington, New Zealand. Published with the support of the Bridget Williams Books Publishing Trust.

Published in 2013 by UBC Press. UBC Press gratefully acknowledges the financial support for our publishing program of the Government of Canada (through the Canada Book Fund) and the British Columbia Arts Council.

Strong, Beautiful and Modern is available in New Zealand (print and e-book) from Bridget Williams Books and in the rest of the world (print and e-book) from UBC Press.

Printed in Canada on FSC-certified ancient-forest-free paper (100% post-consumer recycled) that is processed chlorine- and acid-free.

ISBN 978-0-7748-2528-3 (cloth); ISBN 978-0-7748-2529-0 (pbk.)

Cataloguing-in-publication data for this book is available from Library and Archives Canada.

Front cover: Physical Welfare Branch women officers, during a break in a training course, Hutt Valley, March 1944. Photographer John Pascoe. John Pascoe Collection, F-977-1/4, Alexander Turnbull Library.
Frontispiece: Two groups performing Margaret Morris exercises, 1930s. Topical Press Agency, Hulton Archive; Reg Speller, Hulton Archive, Getty Images.

Cover and page design by Neil Pardington at Base Two
Edited by Ginny Sullivan
Typeset by Tina Delceg
Printed and bound in Canada by Friesens

UBC Press
The University of British Columbia
2029 West Mall
Vancouver, BC V6T 1Z2
www.ubcpress.ca

Contents

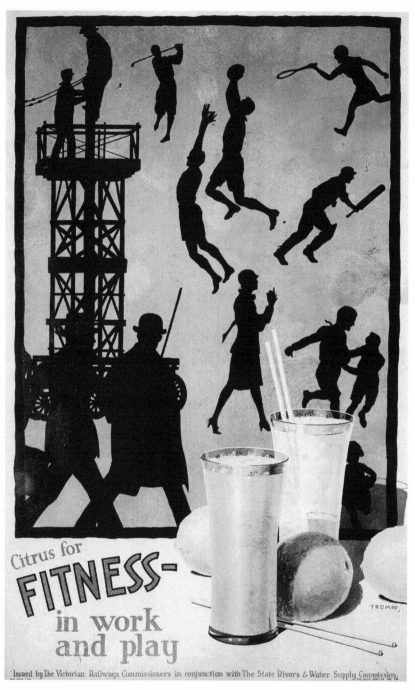

Railways were major players in public education in the mid-twentieth century. At the Victorian Railways Harold Clapp supported campaigns such as national fitness, and ran sport and recreation programmes for employees. The nutritional value of citrus as a supply of Vitamin C, and milk for child development were especially strong messages in this period. VPRS 12903 P1, Box P 504-14, Public Record Office, State Archives of Victoria

Preface and Acknowledgements

To identify the precise origins of this project would be to invent a history. The questions I have been pursuing have remained consistent but the answers have proved elusive and the archives dispersed. Throughout, the underlying research pulse has been insistent, driven by a curiosity sparked by provocation as much as by discovery. That provocation has come in various guises, all of them derived from the paradoxical position sport and physical pursuits occupy in modern culture. Ubiquitous, contentious, at times weighted with symbolism (at others delightfully purposeless), sport and physical pursuits largely inhabit a zone outside critical thinking. Whether that is explained by a lingering hierarchy that rates mind over body; or by a distinction drawn between things that endure over those which are ephemeral and popular, or simply a matter of aesthetics, it remains a central feature of modern life. Otherwise predictable conversations amongst those sharing common interests, spaces, political and social views can falter when the subject of sport and physical pursuits come up – branching either into spirited engagement or falling away into silence. It remains what I have come to call the missing binary: a divider cutting across the familiar lines of class, ethnicity, generation, centre and periphery, public and private. There are ways in which it adheres to contours of gender, but even here, there is not a neat correspondence.

Within the world of historical research it is particularly puzzling. More than half a century's work in a historical canvas massively expanded by an interest in telling a history of ordinary people and events, as well as a history of elites and exceptional moments, has paid slight attention to the history of sport, people at play or leisure in general. These things have not been completely ignored, but they occupy much less space in historians' interests than they do in the pasts they seek to understand.

These knots have sat in my mind for some time. Three things turned them from abstract reflection to active research, though it has taken me awhile to realise their significance. The earliest was W. H. (Bill) Oliver's encouraging interest in the central project of social history (in which sport had a place), and in which the local was no more nor less important to historical argument, than was the evidence from afar. In discussions around a seminar table a long time ago, and in debates with my fellow students that continued, heatedly, beyond that realm, lie some of the important foundations of this work. I think it was at that time that I first read C. L. R. James' *Beyond a Boundary* (1963), a work of continuing inspiration. New Zealand's painful engagement with sporting politics through the 1960s–80s controversies over sporting contacts with South Africa provided the second stimulus. Connections that deserved revisiting were prompted by one of Winifred Davin's stories. Southland-born but living in Oxford in the late 1940s, Winnie recalled Dylan and Caitlin Thomas as house guests appearing garbed in New Zealand rugby jerseys in lieu of pyjamas.

Strong, Beautiful and Modern is, inevitably, a product of the tensions generated by the enigmas of sport and fitness in contemporary society. Many of those who have assisted with this project share an interest in these provocations; others remain mystified by the conversations they generate. All contributions have been valuable, and I would like to acknowledge them here.

For all manner of generosity extended to me over the years engaged in writing this book – practical, intellectual and convivial – I would like to thank the following institutions and individuals: Victoria University of Wellington has provided a place for historical work, both in the company of students, and of colleagues. Students in my HIST 235 Terrible Wonder of Modernity, HIST 427 Empire and Desire courses, and those undertaking postgraduate degrees, have taught me much. Financial support from the School of History, Philosophy, Political Science and International Relations under head Ken Perszyk; the Faculty of Humanities and Social Sciences under Dean Deborah Willis and Deputy Dean Sekhar Bandyopadhyay; and the University Research Committee convened by Neil Quigley, has been vital to seeing the project through. I received warm hospitality while on periods of research leave at the Women's Research and Resources Centre at the Ontario Institute for Studies in Education, Toronto, under director Paula Bourne, and at the International Centre for the Study of the History of Sport at De Montfort University, Leicester, under director Wray Vamplew.

Historians Kate Hunter, Bronwyn Labrum and Margaret Tennant have provided critical company of the best possible kind through the main writing phase. Jane Kominik and Megan Simpson gave crucial monitoring and research assistance, providing what Charlotte Brontë's Shirley would have recognised as 'something real, cool, and solid' when it mattered most. David Colquhoun, Patricia Vertinsky,

Judith Smart and the publishers' anonymous readers offered highly constructive comments on the manuscript.

Librarians and archivists across the world have been unfailingly helpful, often ransacking sections of their collections for less orthodox items. For all kinds of other help I warmly acknowledge Meg Bailey, Rona Bailey (1914–2005), Rachel Barrowman, Michael Bassett, Barbara Brookes, Anna Brown, Hayley Brown, Amanda Beauchamp, Rebecca Burke, Yvette Butcher, Richard Cashman, the Ciochetto Family, Miriam Clark, Derek Clear, Hera Cook, Anna Davin and Henry Tillotson, Amy Davis, Gerry Dowse, Jane Fogden, Pennie Gapes, Nadia Gush, Susan Foley, Bruce Kidd, Manying Ip, Susie Johnston, Graham Langton, Susann Liebich, Noel Lynch (1924–2010), Jim McAloon, Malcolm McKinnon, arch-modernists Evelyn M. H. Macdonald/Mathieson (1918–2003) and G. Jim Macdonald (1921–1982), Judith McKoy, Owen Mann, Jill Matthews, Kate Murphy, Erik Olssen, Trevor Richards and Patti O'Neill, one-time members of both the Onslow Rowing Club and the anti-Rowing Club; Aislinn Ryan, Ben Schrader, Tim Shoebridge, Debbie Stowe, Rosemary Swindells and Noeline Thomson (1908–2001).

The publishing team at BWB, and in particular Ginny Sullivan, Jo Scully and Philip Rainer have seen the book through the press with care and exactitude. To Bridget Williams, whose publishing continues to go beyond the boundaries, a special thanks. Craig Cherrie has read and listened, and, most importantly, kept the mountains of Tongariro in sight.

CM, Wellington, 2011

Introduction

Facing the mantelpiece from which the radio voice spoke in warm and spritely tone, listeners tuning in to the BBC in December 1939 followed instructions to stand up, stretch tall, breathe in, bend slowly, rise up and relax. Repeat again. Now, raise the arms above the head, bend to the left and back to the centre. Bend to the right and back to the centre. And relax. Ten minutes of exercise at the beginning of the day – simple, regular, done at home or at work – the announcer promised, would make all the difference to feeling good and keeping healthy.[1]

The BBC fitness programmes, small items in the daily schedule, were a novelty in 1939. Similar programmes were broadcast on New Zealand radio in 1939–40, scripted and presented by Noeline Thomson. In Sydney, listeners to the ABC heard the Canadian accent of Gordon Young guiding them through the 'daily dozen'.[2] Across Toronto, Montreal, Vancouver and homes throughout Canada, the same set of stretch, bend and breathe exercises came down the wireless. All these broadcasts were part of national fitness campaigns launched across Britain and the 'white Dominions' between 1937 and 1943. Designed to persuade people that 'exercise is good for you', they represent a convergence in the history of states, bodies and modernity. To be strong, beautiful and modern became a collective as well as a personal endeavour.

Campaigns to encourage greater physical activity by men and women beyond their school years were the products of legislation passed in Britain in July 1937, New Zealand in November 1937, New South Wales (Australia) in 1938, the Commonwealth of Australia in 1941 and Canada in 1943.[3] The legislation established schemes to raise public awareness, to distribute funds to existing sporting and recreation associations, to encourage local authorities to provide sports grounds and swimming pools, and to foster the professional development of physical education. Although the

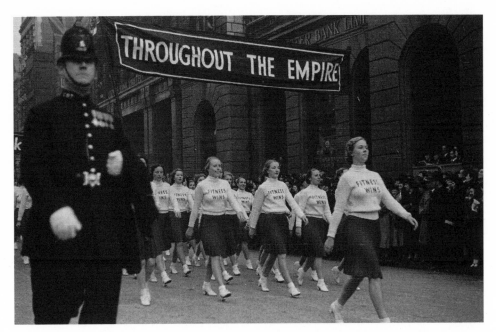

National Fitness was the theme for the Lord Mayor's Parade through the streets of London in November 1937. The women were followed by a group of men in black tops and white trousers parading under two further banners carrying the words 'In work or play' 'Fitness Wins'. Topical Press Agency, Gamma Keystone Collection, Getty Images

formal names given to the programmes varied – Physical Training and Recreation in Britain, Physical Welfare and Recreation in New Zealand, National Fitness in Australia and Canada – the schemes were popularly referred to as 'national fitness' or, in New Zealand, 'physical welfare'. Introduced by governments of the right and the left with widespread support across the political spectrum, the campaigns flared brightly but briefly. Attracting high-profile and sometimes glamorous endorsement, they foundered on the difficulty of reconciling state initiative with the freedom defined in voluntarism: the right of healthy adults to pursue fitness in games, sport and recreation at their own behest and for their own ends. In all but Australia, the campaigns lasted only a few years. However, their limited success served as a curtain-raiser for later and more sustained involvement by governments in promoting sport and physical exercise, towards the end of the twentieth century.

Strong, Beautiful and Modern tells the story of the national fitness campaigns as a movement spanning the 'British world' in the 1930s and 1940s. They were a product of the tumultuous uncertainty of the pre-World War II era. The history is discomfiting in its origins, significant in the dilemmas it exposes of the limits governments faced in urging people into sport and exercise, and interesting for what it reveals about 'being modern' in the mid-century decades. But if living in modern times meant being strong and beautiful, making better bodies was not just a project of government: the political initiatives came on the crest of a contemporary wave. A key theme running through the book is the widespread and diverse 'healthy body culture' that was a novel feature of the 1930s.[4] It was evident in the burgeoning popularity of sport, in fitness 'fads' and in the fashion for sports clothes and outdoor pursuits such as hiking. 'Movement is Life', the slogan of the immensely popular Women's League of Health and Beauty, founded in 1930, captured the mood of the time. From many quarters – medical, educational, commercial and popular – came the message that it was possible, and desirable, to have a better body. And this was the way to a better life.

The schemes brought into existence by the national fitness legislation across all four countries between 1937 and 1943 encompassed a wide array of activities. They ranged from organised, competitive sport, played at levels from the local to national and international, to more participation-based recreation and outdoor pursuits. In urging people to be more active, the schemes were deliberately broad in scope, seeking to provide as wide a stimulus as possible to the greatest number of people. At this time the sharp distinctions that would later come to be made between elite sport and other levels of competition and activity did not exist. Much more significant at the time was the line drawn between professional and amateur sports.[5]

What it meant to have 'a modern body', the empire-wide character of the national fitness movement, and the difficult political questions of government in sport and fitness form the principal themes of *Strong, Beautiful and Modern*. The introduction sets those three themes in context, and signals what is elaborated in the chapters to follow. The particular histories of the schemes in Britain, New Zealand, Australia and Canada are explored in Chapters 1–4. The final chapter draws together the thematic strands, in a discussion of the connecting and comparative lines that emerge from the local histories.

Modern Bodies, Modern Times

In 1938 the British company HMV employed Hungarian Edit Mezey, the star of a newsreel item 'A little slimming a day – keeps the avoirdupois away', to make records providing instructions for exercises to be done at home. The company saw an opportunity in the massive popularity of the culture of the healthy body.[6] So central had the pursuit of the 'better body' become by the 1930s that it seemed almost to define the modern condition. New norms in behaviour and appearance marked the post-World War I world so that it became unmistakably and irreversibly a different place from what had been before. Those novelties were everywhere visible – in the shortened skirts and bobbed hair of women, or the new habit of men smoking cigarettes and keeping their chins clean-shaven. The ever-expanding world of cinema soon added the wonder of the human voice to the delightful sight of bodies walking, running and leaping on screen. Highly successful commercial promotion of soaps, creams, lotions and lipsticks democratised the pursuit of beauty.[7] What was portrayed as new-found freedom for the body was celebrated in enthusiasm for 'natural' places and pursuits. Exercising with bare feet; exposing skin to fresh air and sunlight; walking, hiking, camping and cycling in the outdoors were all taken up with gusto. The suntanned hiker is a motif for the era some have termed 'the long week-end', a figure capturing both the outdoor body culture and a greater access to leisure for working people.[8]

In advertising, popular culture, education and medicine, the message that physical activity was the key to health and happiness was pervasive. In the 1930s it was also novel. Celebration of the active body was premised on the new notion that constant replenishment of the body's powers was necessary to human health and functioning. It replaced an older understanding of the body as a closed system, born with a finite quantum of energy that was gradually expended over the course of a lifetime. Constraints on women's physical activity, where vital energies were supposed to be saved for maternity, were fundamentally challenged by the modern approach. Female figures dancing, leaping and running – in actuality and in the iconography of the time – spoke strongly of the contemporary.[9] Bodily freedom amplified the political emancipation achieved by British and North American women in winning the vote at the end of World War I (New Zealand and Australian women had won the vote in 1893 and 1902, respectively).

But the making of better bodies also points to the profound awareness amongst people during the 1920s and 1930s of the fragility of human life. World War I had demonstrated that the nineteenth-century achievement of industrial production could become the uniquely twentieth-century horror of industrial death, mutilation and destruction. The 1918 influenza pandemic reinforced a perception of the vulnerability of populations even in the so-called 'advanced' world. As Ana Carden-Coyne has recently argued, the interwar decades were powerfully consumed by the project of reconstructing bodies. The impetus was both remedial and regenerative – seeking to mend actually and symbolically the broken bodies of the war years, while also looking for new vitality. Health and fitness were central to this reconstruction.[10] The idea that the body was malleable – that it could be reconstructed, made fit and made healthy – was true insofar as medical science was making such transformative miracles more possible than ever before. It also underpinned the wide array of attentions to which the body became subject in these years. The belief that social improvement could be facilitated through improving bodies was one that, from this point forth, became a major goal for states and for individuals.

There were, however, some darker aspects to these ideas, which in their extreme form surfaced as theories about 'race purity' and symbols of totalitarian power. These connections form part of the disquieting context for the early national fitness movements. But while these elements have understandably come

New Zealander Jack Lovelock shortly after winning the 1500 metre glamour race in the Olympic Stadium, Berlin, 6 August 1936. Lovelock ran a perfect race, keeping close in the first laps and sprinting out to a commanding lead and record-setting time of 3:47.8 minutes. *Berliner Illustrite Zeitung*, 1936, Ullstein A. G. Berlin, p.88

to dominate historical imagination of the period, the 1920s–1930s world of sports and body culture was much broader and more diverse. Sport and physical culture movements offered forms of political engagement for progressives as well as fascists in this period. In Britain, those who first argued for a national fitness scheme believed that the country risked 'falling behind' the model being set in continental Europe. Envious and admiring glances were cast toward the well-organised groups performing physical exercises and participating in feats of strength and skill on the Continent. In addition, the holiday schemes, playgrounds and cultural programmes providing mass leisure through Germany's Kraft durch Freude (Strength through Joy) and Italy's Dopolavoro (after-work) movements spoke of populations that were better provided-for, more successful and more vibrant than those in Britain. Competitive fixtures between British and empire sports representatives extended far beyond participation at the Olympic Games held in Berlin in August 1936. Officials, politicians and ordinary citizens from Britain and the Dominions visited Germany, and reported in complimentary terms on what they observed of sporting and recreation programmes.

Sport, fitness and dance movements, and leisure in many forms, provided places of mixing and exchange through these years of polarising politics and international tension.[11] It is a proximity that subsequently proved discomforting. National fitness in Britain and the Dominions was the product of a period in which the promotion of greater fitness and physical activity amongst adult populations was not the monopoly of any single political ideology or party. In this study an effort is made to see those years from the perspective of contemporaries who were unaware, even as they became increasingly apprehensive, of how events would unfold. The huge disjuncture that the events of 1939–45 cut through the midst of twentieth-century history make it extraordinarily difficult to see the 1930s, and especially the years 1936–39, except through the lens of the impending catastrophe.

Today, the phrase 'national fitness' inevitably raises the spectre of eugenics. The term itself draws on the common language of social improvement pervasive through many parts of the world in the first half of the twentieth century. As recent commentators have noted, eugenics was 'not simply the sinister pro-Nazi precursor it looks like today', but 'rather, a broad church with confidence in its own scientific standing'.[12] The archives consulted for the current project yield little evidence of attempts to advance a specific eugenic agenda. Encouraging greater physical activity and levels of fitness among the existing adult population was the overriding goal. The focus was, in this sense, a limited one. Nowhere is there any indication of an attempt to distinguish 'fit' from 'unfit' portions of the population. Promoters of national fitness through physical exercise believed it was possible to improve physique, but there is no sign they sought to 'improve' national populations through the eugenic science of selective breeding. The shadow now carried by the term provides another reason why the campaigns have fallen out of view. It might be fairly argued that the question remains open, on the basis that historians work within limits of evidence. Is it the silence that speaks?

National fitness finds a place within Ina Zweiniger-Bargielowska's recent *Managing the Body: Beauty, Health and Fitness in Britain 1880–1939* (2010), and Caroline Daley's *Leisure and Pleasure: Reshaping and Revealing the New Zealand Body 1900–1960* (2003). Both works feature the fitness schemes as notable episodes in national histories of ideas and government-initiated policies around the body. For Zweiniger-Bargielowska, Britain's physical training and recreation initiative serves as the end point in a history charting the transformation from late Victorian anxieties over urban degeneration, the state of the nation and empire, and the effects of such decline on masculinity, to the modern mass phenomena of the 1920s–30s where femininity was to the fore. In Daley's discussion, New Zealand's physical welfare scheme is a 'state experiment' in a story tracing the impact of physical culture and recreation from Eugen Sandow's 1903 visit through the dynamics of restriction and emancipation, concealment and uncovering, in a society often characterised in this period as one of provincial puritanism. Together with Carden-Coyne's *Reconstructing the Body: Classicism, Modernism, and the First World War* (2009), a comparative and interdisciplinary study of England, the United States and Australia, these works provide a rich account of the contest of ideas and circumstances in which the 'modern body' came to be imagined, treated, described, regulated and also, indeed, enjoyed.

These three studies form part of a much larger field. Thinking about 'the body' has proved a lively area of interest for scholars in recent years. While topics, questions and approach vary hugely, an underlying thread is the idea that human bodies are made as much as they are born. Historical, cultural and political circumstances, in other words, have a direct bearing on people's physical lives, both individually and collectively. While early work in the field had a tendency to concentrate either on the ways in which bodies were regulated or idealised (Bryan Turner's *Regulating Bodies*, and Kenneth Dutton's *The Perfectible Body* point to these directions), later work has produced more multi-dimensioned accounts of changing meanings, uses and forms of the human body.[13]

Nonetheless, there remains some tension between 'the body' as a conceptual object of critique and analysis, and the unique, variable and ever-changing forms of living bodies. In part, this is a response to an earlier presumption that the human body, as a biological entity, lay beyond the realm of explanation afforded by history, politics or culture. A critical insistence has been important but has, perhaps, left 'the body' at some distance from a fuller historical explanation and imagining – an evocation of historical actors as living breathing people. Admittedly, this can be difficult given the limits and partiality of the archival traces.

In *Strong, Beautiful and Modern* some attempt has been made to address these tensions, or at least to acknowledge the difficulties they pose. While the book focuses on 'the body' as the subject of government attention through the national fitness schemes, the history is framed by wider questions. The dominant view may be offered by archives created and maintained by states, but other vantage points can be found – in contemporary advertising, entertainment, radio broadcasting (commercial and public), photographs and personal papers. These offer a fuller sense of what it was to be active, to enjoy physical exertion, to run onto a field, to plunge into the cool water of pool or river, to feel sun on bare skin, to sweat and shiver. The young women who appear on the front cover, photographed by John Pascoe as they pause in their training as physical welfare officers, and those from the Waipawa workplace team who posed formally for their group portrait (page 19), may offer more vivid evidence than the formal written record.

The discussion also pays attention to those for whom sport, exercise and fitness were matters of indifference, hostility or even dread. Many failed to heed injunctions to get up and begin the day with 'the daily dozen'; some were prevented by illness, disability or age. For significant parts of the population the unceasing and expanding stream of sports reporting in newspapers, radio and newsreel was a matter of boredom, banality or incomprehension. Within the world of radio broadcasting, too, there were sharply differing views as to the pros and cons of sports and fitness as subjects to put 'to air', the BBC adopting a particularly vehement stance. Some of these voices, less enamoured of the fit body enterprise, will also feature in the chapters that follow.

Understanding the contrary nature of attempts to make bodies modern takes us to the broader context of modernity. A sense of living in times that were new and different, at once exciting and frightening, gave contemporaries their identity as 'modern'. They felt and spoke of themselves as living in a world in sharp contrast to that of their parents, let alone of their grandparents. Dressing in a short black skirt to perform in Hyde Park with the Women's League of Health and Beauty before a watching public and movie cameras, for example, was to be modern. Physically fit and active young women such as the members of the League were highly conspicuous forms of the new modernity.

Marshall Berman's classic elaboration of modernity in *All That is Solid Melts into Air* (1982) presents it as a maelstrom: a time and state of being simultaneously alive to wonder and terror, excitement and monotony, hope and despair.[14] Berman identifies the period from the late nineteenth century to the 1930s as one of profound and constant change: technological, social, political. For others the interwar decades represent the epitome of modernity, when the aesthetic currents of modernism in architecture, design, typography and art make 'the modern' most manifest. Whether the temporal boundaries are drawn broadly or more narrowly, the period is characterised by rapid innovation, advancing technology, a shift from production to consumption, urbanism and, above all, constant novelty. The pace and rate of change, the speed and exhilaration of modern life, the revolutions in material life linked to those in politics and culture, the much-vaunted and decried 'death' of religion – all coexist with shadowier features. On the dark side lie the alienation and anonymity of city living, the capacity of speed to numb rather than thrill, the power of technology to destroy as well as to create. The diverse meanings of modernity, and its symbolic moments, radiate from these common points – as described by the work of writers such as Christopher Wilk, Martin Daunton and Bernhard Rieger, Jill Julius Matthews, Roger Griffin, Becky Conekin, Frank Mort and Chris Waters.[15] Modernity remains one of those concepts that are constantly recognised and regularly debated, but always elude neat capture.

Contrasts between city and country living were, in many ways, more important to a sense of living in modern times than was the matter of being a resident in Australia, Canada, New Zealand or Britain. Urban living was central to modernity in its material and imagined forms. Living in cities, listening to jazz, walking on footpaths and pavements rather than fields and tracks, conveyed what it was to be modern. Dance halls and picture palaces were the quintessential places where Matthews tells us the 'romance of modernity' came to life for Sydneysiders. That story is not unique. In cities and metropolises throughout the world in the early decades of the twentieth century, from London to Toronto to Buenos Aires to Sydney to Wellington, the same was true.[16] The city was exciting and welcoming, but also a source of anxiety and even danger. In the national fitness story, cities were depicted, at times, as sources of energy enlivening physical exercise. But they were also imagined in contrary tones as places that constrained and inhibited freedom of body and mind. Ways to offset the ills of city living – whether in urban parks and playgrounds, or in access to countryside and open spaces for walking, hiking, camping, swimming and cycling – were a major focus of many national fitness programmes. For Australians the space of 'the bush' took on particular significance in the continuing national fitness story of the 1950s and 1960s.

If the outer world was made new by the conditions of modernity, so too was the inner world. A new language of 'the self' came into popular currency from increasingly influential 'sciences of the mind'.[17] Anthony Giddens defines self-identity as the central problem of modernity in his *Modernity and Self-identity* (1991).[18] Compared with societies in which status, function and daily practice are ascribed (and therefore provide identity), in modern societies, he argues, the task of establishing identity becomes the job of the individual. 'What to do? How to act? Who to be?' become questions answered in behaviour and words. New languages of self, along with new experiences of embodiment, were part of what it was to be modern by the 1920s and 1930s. Discussion of the 'modern self' has largely been

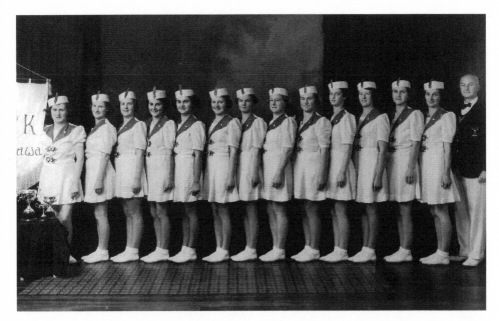

Workers at the Williams & Kettle stock and station agents competed as an interhouse sports team in the late 1930s. From the provincial town of Waipawa (New Zealand) they travelled to Napier and to Wellington to compete with other workplace teams. Left to right: Jean Milne (Captain), Mrs Turner, Pat McQilkan, Barbara Pederson, Claire Hawke, Hazel Hutt, P. Logan, Vida Knobloch, May Harris, Joyce Bishop, Barbara Moore, Mrs Mary McIntosh, Mrs Ivy Dick, Cyril Woods (coach). Central Hawke's Bay Settlers Museum, Waipawa

pursued in terms other than those concerning the body – through, for example, biography and autobiography, writing, the popularisation of psychological ideas, the place of education in instilling a 'social selfhood'. Here, however, it is here connected to the popularity of sports and physical activity.[19] This orientation is in keeping with the strong contemporary idea that described physical activity as the vital key to 'a healthy mind and human happiness'.[20]

An Empire-wide Movement

Telling the history of national fitness as an empire-wide movement acknowledges the reach of empire well into the mid-twentieth century alongside current historical questioning of the concept of empire in relation to the 'British world' (as Britain, Canada, Australia and New Zealand are sometimes collectively described).[21] The national fitness campaigns comprised a strand in interwar imperial relations, specifically those tight bonds between Britain and what was termed by most contemporaries, with pride, 'the Dominions'. When the newly crowned King George VI launched the national fitness publicity campaign at London's Guildhall in February 1938, his speech was broadcast on the national service and widely reported across the Dominions.[22] While each country acted independently, the close links are apparent at all levels. Through sport and recreation, cultural ties of empire were being reinforced even at a time when (it is often argued) political and constitutional ties were holding less firmly.[23] *Strong, Beautiful and Modern* contends that national fitness movements inaugurated in Britain and the Dominions between 1937 and 1943 were part of a connected whole, one that can be fully understood only by reference to its empire-wide frame.

Connections between the histories set out in Chapters 1–4 abound: in people who travelled from one place to another, in the frequent reference to events from one to the other, in the exchange of ideas, and in the circulation of correspondence and information at both official and informal levels. Professional networks – including the powerful arms of the British Medical Association, educational and university links, sporting and youth organisations – and popular movements such as the Women's League of Health and Beauty all saw the wider British world as their 'natural' sphere of operation. Most crucially, there was a common understanding of what the 'British tradition of games' meant, shared in tangible and symbolic terms.

The British Empire Games were staged first in the Canadian city of Hamilton, Ontario, in August 1930. Opening the Games the Governor-General, Lord Willingdon, remarked that the 'greatness of the Empire is owing to the fact that every citizen has inborn in him the love of games and sports'.[24] Subsequent Empire Games were held in London in 1934 and Sydney in 1938. They signified both a new importance of links within the empire *and* a desire amongst 'British' peoples to declare a common set of values against those being promulgated by others. That distinction survives in the identification of the Commonwealth Games as the 'Friendly Games'.[25] (The Commonwealth Games were originally called the British Empire Games, renamed as the British Empire and Commonwealth Games in 1954, the British Commonwealth Games in 1970, and the Commonwealth Games in 1978.)

In other games, the identification implies, friendship is less apparent. And to many in the British world, the increasingly global world of competitive sport, so richly portrayed in Barbara Keys' *Globalizing Sport: National Rivalry and International Community in the 1930s* (2006), seemed to be endangering the true culture of sport. There were fears that the British 'games ethic' was being surpassed by a science of winning; rising stakes and a ruthless pursuit of victory was more important than 'playing the game'. The Hollywood-produced Olympic Games held in Los Angeles in 1932 only reinforced such attitudes. Turning what had been a club-like festival dominated by elites into a global spectacle, the 1932 Games marked the beginning of the modern Olympics as a mass event.

It is relevant to note here that while the 'British world' and the United States shared much common ground in terms of sport, leisure and recreation, there were also important differences in this period. Sporting culture in the United States had developed along different tracks, both in regard to popular codes (baseball rather than cricket, basketball rather than netball, American football rather than soccer or rugby union) and in its structures of playing and watching. By the 1920s and 1930s, a strong collegiate sports system co-existed with professional leagues and amateur associations. This tripartite sporting world was the product of a different political as well as cultural and economic system. The strong and politically dominant associational basis for sport and recreation in Britain fostered a culture of voluntarism. That 'right to play the game' was also a kind of underlying synonym for the freedom enjoyed under 'British law', and for a constitution that existed by way of a set of arrangements shaped by the evolution of conventions. In the United States, the traditions were very different. Freedom, in political terms, was defined in the republican forms of a written constitution and bill of rights.

Strong, Beautiful and Modern takes as its geographical scope the four 'British' domains that introduced legislative initiatives supporting sport and adult physical exercise between 1937 and 1943: the UK, New Zealand, Australia and Canada. South Africa sits at the edge of this discussion. Although there was some correspondence between officials in Pretoria, London and the Dominions' capitals, as far as can be ascertained no legislative initiative to encourage sport and physical exercise among adults was ever taken in South Africa. The African Broadcasting Company was, however, an eager leader in coaxing listeners into daily exercise routines and broadcast early morning exercises each day.[26]

The four countries at the centre of *Strong, Beautiful and Modern* allow an international exploration of the history of the body, providing a comparative context for existing local research. In particular, making a study of the empire-wide span of campaigns enables a fresh perspective to be brought to the appraisal of the success and failure of the schemes. Australia apart, the programmes set in motion by the Physical Training and Recreation, Physical Welfare and Recreation, and National Fitness Acts in Britain, New Zealand, Australia and Canada have generally been regarded as disappointing failures. (See studies by Justin Evans, Mariel Grant and Stephen Jones for England and Wales; Donald MacIntosh et al., Don Morrow et al., Barbara Schrodt and Bruce Kidd for Canada; and Hugh Buchanan, Janet Alexander and Caroline Daley for New Zealand.[27]) Failure is seen in terms of national histories, with insufficient funding, too general and diverse goals, confused or confusing machinery, and a lack of professional leadership in each place. While this study does not offer a rehabilitative reinterpretation, it does explore the broader context for an assessment of effectiveness and achievements.

Empire has come back on to the historical agenda in recent years. That is part of the legacy of an imperial and colonial past that has demanded attention in each of these places. An era of national-history writing in New Zealand, Australia and Canada, important as this is, has not offered sufficient answers to the problems the empire created for history as it is lived and as it is told. How bonds of empire operated

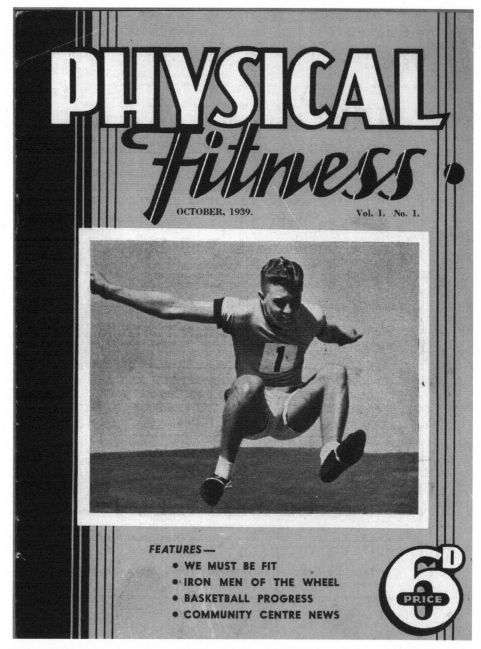

One of Gordon Young's many initiatives in Australia was to start a magazine. The first three issues of *Physical Fitness* appeared in late 1939 before war precluded continued publication. IA 1 139/104/25, Archives New Zealand, Wellington within and beyond the formal machinery of power has become a key question. So too has the vexed problem of how imperial bonds, so long occupying a central place in these societies, evaporated at some point in the post-1945 period. How did these bonds loosen? Outside of the processes of decolonisation, revolution or war, those old links changed fundamentally. Or was it a case of Britain relinquishing them?

As empire has returned to the historical foreground, the place of popular culture (including games and sport) in the shaping of imperial bonds has gained new prominence.[28] The interwar period is often thought of as a time when the links between Britain and 'the Dominions' were becoming more attenuated. The 1926 Balfour declaration (that Britain and the settler Dominions were autonomous communities 'equal in status') and the 1931 Statute of Westminster served as markers of a loosening of political ties. At the same time the inauguration of new and popular bonds, such as those in sport and through radio, can be seen as moving in the opposite direction. Along with the Empire Games, there was an escalation in the number and frequency of sporting fixtures between national teams. Cheaper and faster travel made sporting tours by national sides regular rather than rare events. Even New Zealand, a minnow in the world of cricket, hosted visiting national (or MCC) teams almost every summer throughout the 1930s, with tours by the national side to other places occurring a little less frequently.[29] With visiting sports teams came greater press coverage. Simon Potter has reminded us of the closely networked nature of the imperial press system well into the twentieth century.[30] That network of communication was given new life by the advent of the BBC Empire Service bringing radio broadcast into households across the world. The stream of British-made film, including newsreel, also provided a substantial portion of the cultural diet consumed in the settler Dominions. Against this background, the British government's inauguration of a physical fitness campaign, while provided for in an Act that was domestic rather than imperial in reach, was seen to be relevant throughout the 'British world'.

In this story, sport and games occupy an uneasy position, exemplifying both connection and disconnection. Sporting victories over imperial teams represent important moments in the emergence of a sense of national feeling – first within an imperial setting, and then in marking the substitution of nation for empire. For Australians, it is the first 'Test' cricket victory over England in 1882; for New Zealand, the 1905 tour to England by the all-conquering 'All Black' rugby team. Successive contests in which colonial teams won, inverting the hierarchy between metropolitan and colonial powers, reinforced the significance of sport in the trajectory from colony to nation. Lacking moments of revolutionary upheaval, such contests have taken on greater significance in stories of national becoming. Yet the continued popularity of the sports themselves and their centrality to ever more marked 'national' cultures serve to reinforce the long reach of imperial influence. Cricket, rugby and netball (known as basketball in New Zealand and Australia until the early 1970s), for all their adaptation in the world of modern sports, are still played almost exclusively within the old boundaries of the British Empire.[31]

From the Dominions' points of view, the interwar period has come to occupy an uncomfortable phase in their national histories: uncomfortable because it is seen as a time in which those societies lingered in a kind of limbo between colonial and independent status. The principal machinery and responsibilities of self-government were in place, yet they were still tied constitutionally to Britain, and old habits of deference lingered. In histories written from the 1950s onward, works prompted by and instrumental in shaping national cultures, there is a barely contained impatience at the continued hanging on to British apron strings through the 1920s and 1930s.

In their recent discussion of the long-lasting British affiliation in Australian society and its recession from the 1960s, James Curran and Stuart Ward in *The Unknown Nation: Australia After Empire* search for the factors that led to the sudden, even dramatic, falling away from the sense of Britishness that had dominated Australian 'European' society for such a long time, and the awkward search for a new identity in the post-imperial age.[32] Similar processes were at work in New Zealand and in Canada. There are important differences across the three former settler colonies, but the overall pattern of separation, mild repudiation and burgeoning cultural nationalism is evident from the 1960s. It runs in parallel with the intellectual work of nation-building: a new generation of national histories were produced by W. H. Oliver and Keith Sinclair for New Zealand and by Manning Clark and Russel Ward for Australia, with regional and thematic histories emerging in Canada. Somewhere between '1945 and now' is when this process of separation and national 'maturation' is thought to have taken place. But exactly how and where is at issue. And as Curran and Ward remind us, no matter how sure these societies have become about their independence, their 'mature' state, their difference from Britain and their casting off of the old dependency, the surprising thing is just how long British affiliations lasted – before being rather abruptly set aside.

Governments and Healthy Bodies

The third strand in this history concerns the role of governments in national fitness. This theme sits within the longer-term pattern of expansion and subsequent retreat of the state throughout the twentieth century, a period when the umbrella of 'big government' spread widely over social life from roughly the 1940s to the 1970s, to be withdrawn sharply under the neoliberal challenge in the 1980s–90s. But the national fitness programmes of 1937–43 and the initiatives that succeeded them followed a path at odds with the dominant trend. Behind this story lies a strong civic culture underpinning sport and physical activity, compounded by the difficulty in funding 'health' rather than sickness.[33] The history set out in *Strong, Beautiful*

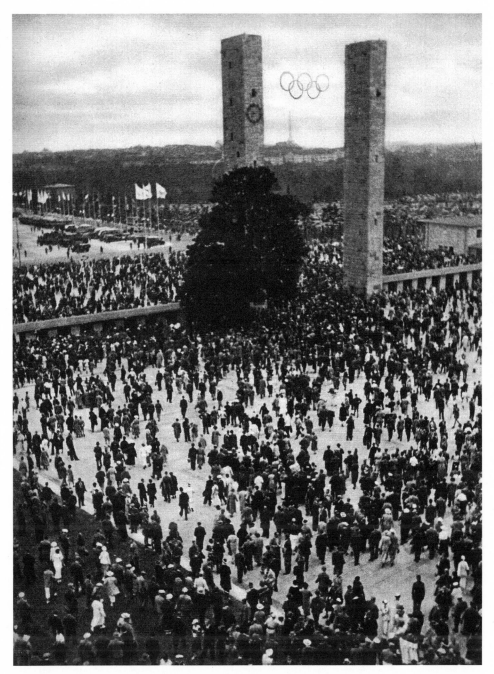

Up to 100,000 people packed in to the Olympic Stadium to watch events through the 16 days of competition in Berlin in August 1936. They came from across the world. From high in the stadium the photographer has caught the crowd heading towards the avenue and the U-Bahn station. In the souvenir booklet published by the popular weekly, *Berliner Illustrite Zeitung*, the end-of-day spectacle is described as a flood heading to the sea. *Berliner Illustrite Zeitung*, 1936, Ullstein A. G. Berlin, p.41

and Modern shows how adult fitness and sport became the subject of government attention in Britain, New Zealand, Australia and Canada. But in how this theme played out lie some of the strongest contrasts in the study. In this introduction to the theme, Britain is in the foreground as the place in which a legislative scheme was first devised and as the fount of the sporting spirit – the phrase used to invoke the shared culture.

By the 1930s, it was widely accepted that children's health and fitness should be fostered by medical inspections, health camps, milk-in-schools schemes, well-equipped school playgrounds and the like (even if the reality often lagged behind the promise). But the Physical Training and Recreation Act, passed by the British Parliament in July 1937, was remarkable as the first engagement by central government in adult sport and recreation. This was a domain that, in a British context, traditionally lay outside the purview of government; it was pursued on a voluntary basis and staunchly preserved by independent associations. Professional sports, on the other hand, were run by private organisations. Neither the loosely run world of sport and recreation nor the more rigorous world of professional sports had formal links to government. In the mid-1930s this pattern was broken, in part because sport had become too powerful and too attractive for politicians to ignore, and in part because healthy adult citizens now demanded more of governments in the form of leisure time and health. Governments in turn demanded more of citizens in maintaining health and fitness for social as well as individual benefit. The dilemmas and arguments around these issues remain part of political debate. In this theme the contrasts between the histories of national fitness in each place are most pronounced.

The 'Nazi Olympics' held in Berlin in 1936 exposed most conspicuously the powerful stage provided by sport for the conducting of international relations. Whether as a force for good or bad, sport had become part of the way in which populations imagined themselves as nations. Contests between national teams took on symbolic power in the highly volatile international circumstances of the 1930s. Less well remembered were the struggles between national and international interests that were also part of the sporting world of the pre-1939 years. The 1936 Olympic Games was only the largest and most famous of many sporting occasions of the decade. The first football (soccer) World Cup was played in Uruguay in July 1930, a month before the first British Empire Games were held in Hamilton, Ontario. Four Women's World Games were held between 1922 and 1934, organised by the Fédération Sportive Feminine Internationale, to provide an arena of competition for women largely excluded from Pierre de Courbetin's modern Olympics. Tel Aviv was the city where athletes and supporters gathered to compete in the first Maccabiah Games (the 'Jewish Olympics') in 1932, just a few weeks before Los Angeles became the first non-European city to host the modern Olympic Games.

Major fixtures such as the Joe Louis v Max Schmeling heavyweight boxing match at New York's Yankee Stadium in June 1938 were broadcast to radio audiences in America and Germany. (When it was clear Schmeling was going to lose, the German broadcast went dead.) In December 1935 the British Trade Union Congress had called on Prime Minister Stanley Baldwin to intervene to stop the German football team from playing against England at London's White Hart Lane for fear of the rightwing sympathies the team's supporters would drum up in the East End. In such contexts, politicians could not ignore sport.

It was not a matter, as some would insistently argue later in the twentieth century, of whether sport and politics mixed. Rather, it was what kind of politics were being conducted through sport. Prominent Labour MP, Philip Noel Baker was a key figure in the British national fitness movement. A former athlete and disarmament advocate, Noel Baker believed fervently in sport as a means to secure international understanding, and of its value in enhancing citizenship. While the events of 1939–45 only confirmed the views of those who felt, with George Orwell, that sport was as likely to exacerbate as bridge international divisions, Noel Baker believed in its power to transcend and indeed to mend differences. It was his work, as a minister in the Attlee government, that did much to make London the host of the first postwar Olympics, the so-called 'austerity games' of July–August 1948. All this points to the impossibility of governments and politicians escaping matters of sport in the 1930s, and to the attractions that sporting success and popular athletes had for politicians. Being associated with such success was irresistible, while national failure brought international embarrassment. The glow of athletic glory became a powerful currency on the world stage. Medal ceremonies such as those instituted at Berlin in 1936 with flags, anthems, and the tiered winners' dais, provided a highly dramatic spectacle of success. The presence – and absence – of athletes wearing national colours, spoke of wider narratives of success and decline. Maintaining national prestige through sporting success had political value. That lesson, first learned in the 1930s, has carried forward. Government funding (whether direct or indirect) for sport and physical activity became almost inevitable. The increasing dominance of American, German, Italian and even 'Dominion' athletes put Britain's record as the first and best sporting nation under pressure. But how to secure greater success (and offset the appearance of being a people in decline) while maintaining the games-playing voluntarism that defined 'British' habits of sport and leisure became the problem. In a 'land which has been the cradle of games and sport', the British had a traditional 'love of exercise', according to England's National Fitness Council in 1939.[34] But the National Fitness Council, as its name implied, was a government-funded body, tasked with urging Britons to exercise and play more than they were doing, and distributing significant public monies for the purpose. There was nothing 'traditional' in the Council's role, or indeed in its very existence.

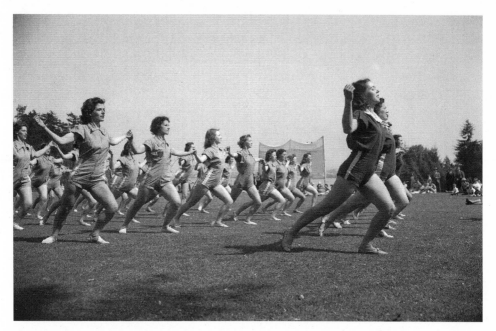

'Pro-Rec' exercise programmes in Vancouver were particularly popular amongst women in the city. Whether in work, or at home, the low fees and attractive activities drew large numbers of participants. The one-piece uniform was cheap to make and worn proudly by 'Pro-Rec' members. CVA 1184-2355, Vancouver City Archives

By the mid-1930s there was widespread apprehension that 'playing games' might not be enough for Britain to 'keep up' in either sporting or wider national contests for power. Government action was prompted by a recognition that physical fitness beyond people's school years could not be left to the discretionary realm of voluntary effort. Politicians were signalling a desire for physical fitness to be acknowledged as a national as well as personal benefit, a kind of duty or component of citizenship. But this purpose sat uneasily with another government message, promulgated initially in Britain and later in New Zealand, Australia and Canada – that participation in sport and physical activity urged by fitness campaigns was only ever to be on a voluntary basis. The tension between government coaxing and reiteration of voluntary participation determined the shape of the national fitness schemes. It was akin to applying the accelerator and the brake simultaneously to an already highly uneven and, in Britain especially, class- and gender-contoured set of sporting and recreation activities and opportunities. Grants, subsidies and tentative steps towards systematic physical education made little impact. In contrast to European initiatives, no new organisations were established, no large-scale public investment made in facilities, no uniforms were designed and, beyond an ill-fated suggestion of a National Fitness badge, no insignia adopted. From a post-1945 perspective, these failures were a relief rather than a disappointment.

Questions about the place of governments in urging people to play were part of the contentious origins of the national fitness schemes. For some the doubts arose from suspicion that the schemes were no more than the soft end of conscription. In England in 1937 and Canada in 1943, in particular, the local circumstances were such as to feed doubts of this kind. But while defence was a factor in prompting the schemes, it was by no means the only or even the leading one, and it did little to shape the character of the schemes as they were devised or as they unfolded. To view the national fitness measures across the four nations only in these terms is to mistake their full context. Louder and more persistent voices questioned the paradox contained in the very rationale for the national fitness schemes: if sport and physical recreation were activities pursued for fun, as ends in themselves, why was there a need for government to urge people to take them up? In doing so, was there not a danger of killing the very spirit that made such activities enjoyable? The third reservation came from the very, even deliberately, vague goal that the Physical Training and Recreation, Physical Welfare and Recreation, and National Fitness Acts set out. The general aim of making people more active, fitter and more successful at sports was all very well, but fitter or more active *for* what and *than* what? How much was enough? Herein lay a problem that was encountered first in this period, and that has continued to bedevil campaigns in later times.

Whether justified in terms of national prestige, health, social cohesion or simply because games and activity are part of national culture, politicians face two problems. First, it is hard, especially in health care, to defend spending on keeping healthy people well, when urgent demands exist for funds to treat those already ill. Whatever might be the argument on cost efficiency, the compassionate appeal is likely to be stronger. Secondly, how fit, healthy or happy do people have to be to be healthy 'enough'? General measures of good health, fitness and athleticism, let alone general happiness, are very difficult to make. Without such baselines to measure the effectiveness of publicly funded programmes, they become vulnerable to critiques of unknown impact.

These considerations point to the overlapping debates in the 1930s–40s between national fitness and health. The basis and extent of public provision was to become a major feature of 'welfare states' thereafter. But the definition of what constituted a healthy life was also a subject of debate. The innovative Peckham Health Centre, established in south London in the 1930s, was an attempt to build a centre for a healthy community rather than a medical practice serving a roster of patients; a health rather than medical centre.[35] The inspiration behind the Peckham Centre was the same as that which lay behind the World Health Organization's 1940s definition of health not simply in terms of the absence of disease, but more positively as the ability of individuals to participate in society (later, the formulation would become one of well-being, variously described).

All of these factors served to complicate the work of national fitness programmes. By far the most powerful constraint, however, arose from a growing awareness of the use of national fitness programmes by Nazi and fascist regimes' in the 1930s and 1940s. Compulsory recruitment into the Hitler Youth movement, military service, and into home and motherhood functions for women, were all means to build strong and aggressive states through subordinating individual will to collective goals. Such regimes turned power against their own citizens. And then used the power of a militarized state to establish supremacy over other peoples, and to attempt to annihilate those who threatened the deeply repugnant notion of 'race purity'. A reaction against state involvement in the healthy bodies of adult citizens was a strong feature of the post-1945 world. In the years after World War II, the voluntarist basis for sports and leisure was vigorously reasserted, and a line was drawn between the responsibility of government (on the one hand) and the role of civic society (on the other). Support for central government involvement in sports and leisure fell away. 'Social citizenship' denoted the era of a 'welfare state' but not a 'leisure state'.

Greater time for leisure was one of the factors that made sport and physical activity a matter of government policy. By the late 1930s, long-standing pressure from workers for reduced working hours and paid holidays saw some people for the first time enjoying a working week that ended at midday on Saturday, with a week's summer holiday taken without loss of wages.[36] Such benefits were uneven. Leisure existed only in contrast to work. For those without jobs, or whose work fell in the unbounded realm of the home rather than within the limits of workplace (including most married women), such aspirations lay beyond reach. But the growing array of dance halls, greyhound tracks, movie theatres, youth hostels, illustrated magazines, weekend cycle trips and gramophone records testified to new concept of 'time off'. Waiting for the weekend, as Witold Rybczynski suggests, became modern workers' salvation.[37]

For some people this new-found time for leisure ushered in delights; for others it was another sign of one of the novelties of modern times, 'the problem of leisure'.[38] Concern grew in some quarters, at the perception that people were watching rather than doing, and buying fun rather than making it. Young people, women and those unaccustomed to 'free time' were seen as requiring protection from the predations of commercial exploiters, from their own gullibility and from the temptations of hedonism. Efforts to urge 'democratic leisure' varied from the Recreation and Leadership Movement in Australia, to international organisations such as the World Congress for Joy and Leisure (formed in 1930), which was a concerted attempt to address the novel prospect of leisure time and activity by large numbers of working people. Many of its leaders were drawn from totalitarian states and its meetings were held in Hamburg (1936), Rome (1938) and Tokyo (1940).[39] Representatives from Britain and the Dominions were amongst those attending the Congress. State provision for worker leisure in the German Kraft durch Freude and Italian Dopolavoro movements was more fervently nationalistic. Political organisation of mass leisure contributed, in the Italian context, to what Victoria de Grazia describes as 'a culture of consent'. The political hold achieved by Mussolini's party was not a simple imposition of authoritarianism but a crafted mesh of inducement and coercion. By the 1930s many Italians had become accustomed to the pleasures of 'the fascist Saturday'.[40]

When governments re-engaged in the areas of sport and physical exercise for adults from the 1960s onwards, they did so in changed circumstances, and generally with more specific goals. The Fitness and Amateur Sport Act passed in Canada in 1961 and the Advisory Council on Sport established by the British government in 1964 had a narrower remit on organised sport than earlier legislation. Nonetheless, these and subsequent measures have continued to wrestle with various questions: whether governments should support competitive sport (for reasons of national prestige, models of excellence or international exposure in a global marketplace) or participation sport (as a generally good thing, for reasons of social cohesion and preventive health); and to what extent governments should take responsibility for adults' organised sport and recreation activities (for general purposes or solely for public health, as in the case of the 'obesity epidemic').

Such questions about how far the state should go in securing social improvement were raised by the 'exercise is good for you' schemes launched across Britain, New Zealand, Australia and Canada in the late 1930s. The history of national fitness has much to tell us of the dilemmas governments faced in becoming involved in the bodies of adult citizens, and in what is generally regarded as the autonomous sphere of sport, recreation and fun. As the first steps toward direct government involvement in sport and physical recreation in the adult population, the national fitness campaigns occupied an uneasy place in the broader expansion of government–citizen relations marked by the advent of 'welfare states'. Instead of becoming a part of that extended realm of public entitlement and responsibility through the classic era of 'social citizenship' from the late 1930s to the 1980s, the areas of sport and physical recreation were largely cast beyond the reach of central government. *Strong, Beautiful and Modern* tells the story of national fitness campaigns within the longer-term rise and retreat of 'big government' in Britain and the former settler Dominions, across the twentieth century.

Strong, Beautiful and Modern traces the themes of modern bodies, political dilemmas and the connections of empire through chapters that focus on the principal characteristics of the national fitness campaigns in each of the places in which they were introduced. The emphasis in each chapter varies. This reflects both the

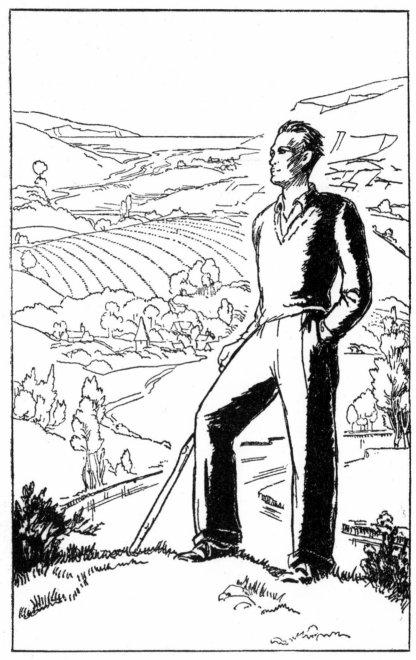

Standing in the open air on the landscape, the hiker was a quintessential figure of the 1930s. Hiking was not only hugely popular but the ideal antidote to city living. In Harry Roberts' guide to good living the hiker encapsulated the virtues of physical activity, nature, open air and freedom. Philip Smithells gave a copy of Roberts' book to the University of Otago Medical School Library. Hiking in Britain had close but not exact parallels with Australian bushwalking and New Zealand tramping. Harry Roberts, *The Practical Way to Keep Fit*, Odhams, London, 1939, frontispiece contrasting national contexts and the inflection given to the scheme in each place by political circumstances, key protagonists and its varying duration. Contrasts in focus also provide a means to illuminate different dimensions to the schemes, and the archive they have left. The chapters follow the chronological sequence in which legislation providing for the schemes was passed in each parliament.

Beginning in Britain, the first chapter, examines the origins and implementation of the Physical Training and Recreation Act, the concern with 'British physiques' falling behind those in Europe, and the popular fitness and sporting activities characteristic of the mid-1930s. A feature of the British history was the strong public endorsement given to the national fitness campaign in its early phase by figures ranging from the King to the stars of popular comedy. However, the shadow of totalitarianism that adhered to notions of national fitness could never be dispelled, and the effective end to the scheme came when war was declared in September 1939. Some of the functions of the National Fitness Council continued through the war years, but it was not until the early 1960s that the Labour government of Harold Wilson once again made sport and adult physical activity a matter of state concern.

While New Zealand passed its Physical Welfare and Recreation measure within five months of the British Act, the political context was starkly different. As set out in Chapter 2, it was the reform-minded Labour administration, renowned for building a comprehensive welfare state, that sponsored government provision for sports and active recreation. A former miners' leader, Bill Parry, championed the legislation at the Cabinet table. It sat alongside labour reforms such as a reduction in the length of the working week, providing the means for workers to use their leisure constructively. Notable features of the New Zealand scheme were the work of public servants employed in what became known as the Physical Welfare Branch, the prominence of efforts to foster women's sport and recreation, the brief postwar flourish in activity including the extension of physical welfare activities in Māori communities, and the influence of several key protagonists for whom modern body culture was part of a wider politically progressive agenda. The New Zealand national fitness scheme faded quickly in the 1950s: the conservative National government that came to power in 1949 saw no rationale for extending state support to the 'private' realm of sport and recreation.

In Australia, national fitness schemes had their longest and arguably most effective existence. Chapter 3 discusses the development of national fitness schemes in a country where an active outdoors life and success at sport were seen as part of national identity by the 1930s. The origins of the campaign in Australia owed much to the lobbying of leaders of civic progressive movements of the 1930s. These advocates of democratic leisure and urban reform, who included C. E. W. Bean and Edith Swain, did much to press the government into action. Federal legislation was passed in 1941 but state action preceded it in New South Wales and Victoria. Gordon

Young, the Canadian appointed to head the New South Wales programme in 1938, was amongst those who subsequently transformed national fitness into a young adult movement suited for the postwar world. Outdoor camps were a distinctive feature in the New South Wales national fitness story, an idea that owed a good deal to models developed in Ontario. A tension between state and federal initiatives saw the schemes in Australia shaped by the vying interests of proponents of education on the one hand and health on the other. The Australian schemes evolved into later programmes and departments variously labelled sport, community development, health and tourism.

Although the Canadian story comes fourth in the sequence (with federal legislation passed only in 1943), the antecedents of the scheme date from the early 1930s. In the recreation programmes developed as a response to widespread unemployment in the Pro-Rec scheme in British Columbia and the Ontario Athletic Commission lies the longer story of government action in the realm of sport and fitness. The Liberal government led by Mackenzie King was finally persuaded to introduce the National Fitness Act in 1943 under pressure from leftwing parties for more substantial postwar reconstruction promises, and specifically around debates for a public health programme. The impact of the Cold War was particularly pronounced in bringing the Canadian scheme to an end, and in determining the fate of its most prominent figure, Jan Eisenhardt.

A common thread through Chapters 2, 3 and 4 concerns the ways in which national fitness programmes became part of postwar policies for the 'advancement' of indigenous minorities – Māori, Aboriginal and First Nations people in New Zealand, Australia and Canada respectively.

The final chapter, 'Healthy Bodies, State and Modernity: A Twentieth-century Dilemma', draws together the strands of connection and comparison. It also provides a further elaboration of the themes and arguments outlined here and developed through the geographically organised chapters. The origins of the schemes in the circumstances of the mid-1930s provide the starting point for the discussion. The end point is less easy to fix, as the schemes had contrasting lives. Only in Australia did the national fitness initiatives last into the 1960s, but the end of the 1950s serves as a cusp to a new era of thinking and action in these places around sport and recreation as public responsibilities. Some observations are made regarding the new initiatives governments took from the 1960s in supporting sport, recreation and healthy bodies. Very different circumstances shaped these efforts. The message that 'exercise is good for you' and the appeal of successful national athletes continue to be important and sometimes contentious parts of contemporary life.

1 Movement is Life

National Fitness in England and Scotland[1]

Neville Chamberlain had been Prime Minister for just a few weeks when the Physical Training and Recreation Bill was finally debated in the House of Commons. Speaking in its support on 11 June 1937, Conservative MP Wavell Wakefield,[2] a member of the National Fitness Council (NFC) and former England rugby captain, explained that 'our aim is to try to make the great mass of the people, young and old, physically fit, and to provide facilities for improving their general physical fitness and well-being'.[3] For a brief time the government's highly novel campaign glittered in the light of popular public attention. Cinema audiences were drawn into the joke of Cabinet ministers performing press-ups and touching their toes. Local authorities and sporting associations leapt at the chance to fund swimming pools and build new boatsheds. Wembley stadium hosted spectacular mass displays of exercising men and women. The message was simple: being fit was good for you and good for the country.

If the message was simple, the government's action in taking up the role of cheerleader and funder of sport and recreation for adults was certainly not. It ran against the strong civic culture articulated in notions of 'fair play' and of 'playing the game for the game's sake' – things that defined what it was to be British, or even more specifically, English.[4] But by the mid-1930s neither games nor freedom were as they had been. A fear that Britain was being left behind in a world where games and sport were pursued for state rather than athletic glory was one concern. Beyond that, the mobilisation of populations along militarist lines – as was occurring in Europe – presented a model of citizenship that was impressive even as it was disparaged in references to what was going on in 'robot countries'.[5] Was it necessary to rely on something more than games to be modern?

The disappointing performance of British athletes at the Berlin Olympics in

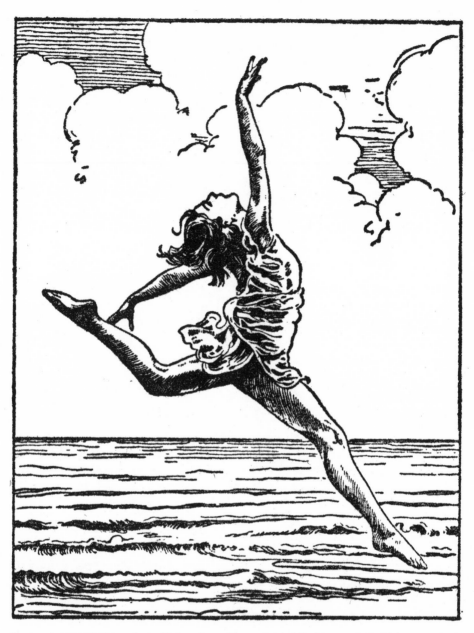

The leaping female figure beneath the slogan Movement is Life became the widely recognised symbol of the Women's League of Health and Beauty. Formed in London in 1930, the League became hugely popular on the promises of outward beauty from inner vitality and the charismatic charm of founders Mollie Bagot Stack and her daughter, Prunella, 'Britain's perfect girl'. A. J. Cruickshank and Prunella Stack, *Movement is Life. The Intimate History of the Founder of the Women's League of Health and Beauty and of its Origin, Growth, Achievements and Hopes for the Future*, Bell, London, 1937, title page.

1936 was also deflating. And it was disconcerting to look across Europe only to cast increasingly envious glances at the well-organised and impressively fit young people in Germany and elsewhere.[6] The prospect of a better drilled, and better prepared, population in the event of war was also a consideration, but it was only one in a series of catalysts driving action.[7] Something needed to be done.

Some suspected the Physical Training and Recreation Act of being the wolf of conscription dressed in the innocence of sport as sheep's clothing. It was hard to dispel entirely the impression that the coaxing of strong, fit bodies was a sign of a desire for a stronger, even authoritarian politics. Edward Cadogan, deputy chairman of the National Fitness Council, was forced to dismiss this with an indignant protest: 'Was it necessary ... for us to encourage men and women and children to be lazy, obese and malformed in order to convince the world that we did not want to fight?'[8] The contradictions within the scheme gave rise to such suspicions, to its exuberant beginnings and deflated hopes, to the fizz and fizzle of its short life, and to its perplexing yet influential history.

Britain's Physical Training and Recreation Act, designed to encourage more people to take up – or keep up – physical exercise through publicity campaigns and funding sports and recreation activities and facilities, provided the model for legislation passed in other parts of the British world. Yet the national fitness movement it inaugurated was, in most respects, the least successful and shortest lived.[9] Ross McKibbin described it as 'small beer' and Tony Mason as 'feeble'.[10] Making adult physical fitness a government policy, and allocating funds to sporting and recreational activities, marked a radical departure in British history. While the ideal of more physical exercise was generally thought a good thing, turning it into a practical scheme proved more difficult. The level of demand for grants vastly exceeded the funds available. But what became more problematic was the resilience of the notion that sport and recreation belonged firmly in the realm of individual choice. People were free to participate, or not, as they chose, in games that were played as ends in themselves. The game for the game's sake was a statement not only of an amateur ideal but, even more, of the voluntary principle. Reconciling government action with this principle, which was a palpable expression of a uniquely British freedom guaranteed in law and politics and lived out in the social autonomy and civic culture of local sports and leisure clubs, proved insurmountable. By 1939 the initiative had faded; by 1945 the attempt to make state activism in sport and leisure something acceptable had been thoroughly discredited by revelations of the horrors inflicted by Nazi and fascist governments on the bodies of their citizens. The national fitness experiment in Great Britain, suspended at the outbreak of war, was quietly buried.

Political Fitness

By the mid-1930s it was hard for governments, even if they so wished, to avoid the issues of sport and recreation. Against a background of polarising international politics, matches between national teams took on larger and often dangerous dimensions. In December 1935 British fears that 'a large and carefully organized Nazi contingent' of fans accompanying the German football team would provoke street disorder led the Trade Union Congress to call for the scheduled match against England to be cancelled. The game was to be played at London's White Hart Lane. Sir John Simon, the Foreign Secretary, was reassured by the German ambassador that the game would be regarded 'purely as a sporting event'[11] and the match went ahead, with England beating Germany 3–0. The German government's assurance of athletic contest purely for sporting ends was less credible following the August 1936 Olympic Games in Berlin. Those who had been involved in efforts to stop participation in the Games on the basis of the Nazi government's racist policies, including the British Workers' Sports Association, had their misgivings confirmed.[12] The old faith in Britain's political battles being won on the playing fields of Eton was further eroded by the events of the mid-1930s. Against the impressive Americans, Germans and Italians, some in Britain began to question whether leaving sport and physical fitness in the hands of schools and voluntary associations was adequate.

At the same time, the new-found interwar popularity of sun and fresh air fired the demand of hikers, ramblers, campers and cyclists for the 'right to roam' and greater access to the countryside. Around half a million people were regular walkers by the late 1930s, with membership of the Youth Hostel Association at around 83,000 in 1939, up from 6,000 in 1934.[14] The Mass Trespass at Kinder Scout in the Peak District in 1932 (organised to break the shackles of private land ownership) was only the most notable event in a sustained campaign. Enjoyment of the outdoors was paralleled by a rapidly burgeoning 'keep-fit' movement, chiefly conducted in halls and indoor spaces. Derived loosely from Swedish and Danish forms of gymnastics, classes such as those run by Norah Reed in Sunderland typically lasted for around an hour, with participants working through a sequence of exercises to music.[13]

Nowhere was this movement more popular than in the Women's League of Health and Beauty. Founded in 1930 by Mollie Bagot Stack, a trained physical culturist and skilful publicist, the League had grown to a membership of 120,000 in 220 branches by 1937. In the weekly exercise classes offered at an affordable sixpence a session, the League offered participants the chance to combine personal improvement with a wider purpose, and to belong to a larger movement that was characterised by pageantry, drama, excitement and glamorous leadership. Mollie Bagot Stack and her daughter Prunella, dubbed Britain's 'perfect girl', presented an attractive message of inner health and outer radiance. The League's annual demonstrations in Hyde Park and the Royal Albert Hall were major events that

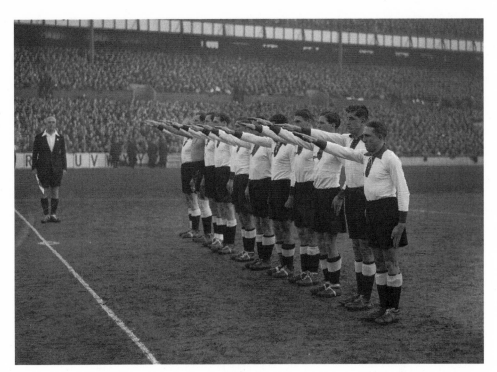

The German football team give the Nazi salute before playing England at White Hart Lane, London, 4 December 1935. Appeals from the left for the match to be called off on the grounds that travelling fans were political activists intent on drumming up far-right sympathies in London's East End, were brushed off. England won 3-0. PNA Rota, Hulton Archive, Getty Images

commanded wide attention. In white blouses and black satin shorts or velvet skirts, League members performed to large live audiences and even larger film and press consumers. 'Movement is Life', the League's motto, captured the zeitgeist of the era.[15] It was one that was widely embraced. Sabra Milligan, a Birmingham University representative swimmer, summarised the approach in her 1934 book *The Body and How to Keep Fit*: 'Life is change, and change is brought about by movement. This, therefore, implies that one should lead an active life and never be idle and incapable of vigorous movement.'[16]

These prominent manifestations of 'healthy body culture'[17] cast into even greater relief the abiding preoccupations of the decade: unemployment and its associated poverty and ill-health. The spectre of the 'hungry thirties' was given all the more certitude by John Boyd Orr's 1935 survey results which revealed that up to half the population lacked an adequate diet. Economic failure was lived out in sick mothers, idle men and the bodies of children who were slow to develop. Who was responsible and what was to be done fired political debate. Government action emerged from political anxiety as well as from the popular momentum behind better health, sports and fitness 'fads'.

The Conservative Party's manifesto for the general election in 1935 signalled intentions for a physical training scheme. Three developments ramped up the impetus in 1936. The first was an emphatic and widely cited report on physical education released by the British Medical Association (BMA), which found that Britons needed to be more physically active and concluded that more facilities were required to enable them to become so. It made 65 recommendations for change, an indictment on the health of the British population. The second was the growing profile of the newly founded Central Council for Recreative Physical Training, which brought many organisations running programmes in physical recreation, including the influential National Playing Fields Association and the King George V Jubilee Trust, under a national umbrella. The third was the August Olympic Games exposing Britain to international embarrassment as a nation in decline.[18] A scheme was proposed and set eagerly before public and politicians by Chamberlain at the Conservative Party Conference, with details under discussion in Cabinet by the end of the year.[19]

In November 1936, less than a month after the Conservative Party conference, Sir Kingsley Wood, Minister of Education, stood self-consciously in front of the Pathé movie cameras in formal suit, while a group of Battersea boys, clad only in shorts, performed a series of tumbling and vaulting exercises. The newsreel carried the message of the government's commendation of such physical activity. Appealing to the cinema audience, Wood made a joke of the incongruity of his own and his colleague Minister of Health Oliver Stanley's middle-aged, stockier and well-clad frames next to the lithe, bare-chested, barefoot boys. Turning with a smile to his fellow minister, he remarked, 'Oliver, you have made the suggestion that you and I should do this physical exercise ourselves – why not extend it to the whole Cabinet or even the House of Commons. How much fitter and better we should all be!'[20]

A scheme for everyone, not just ministers or MPs, was what was proposed in the White Paper released in January 1937. Its goals were simple, if ambitious. It was not

> ... to secure that between certain ages every boy and girl practises certain physical exercises or achieves a certain standard of physical development, but to inculcate a wider realisation that physical fitness has a vital part to play in promoting a healthy mind and human happiness. It is a way of life and an attitude of mind, the importance of which is continuous and not limited to certain years in early youth. The ultimate aim is 'a healthy mind and human happiness': the immediate aim is to convince all who need to be convinced that in the achievement of health and happiness physical fitness has 'a vital part to play'.[21]

Rejecting a dualism of mind and body in favour of a broader notion of 'human happiness' was a theme emphasised in the BMA's report. 'The mind and body are so essentially one', it noted, 'that the divorce between them in what is commonly

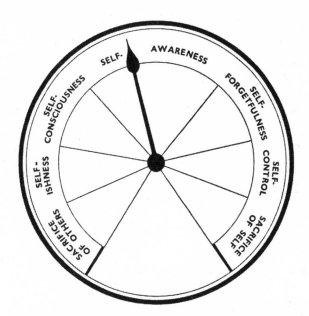

The Barometer of Self. 'Used carefully, and with the reasoned doubt which should temper all intelligence', R. E. Roper argued that 'both self-sacrifice and selfishness develop out of self-awareness... they represent changes in a single condition...not opposites but relatives.' The barometer appeared in his 1938 *Movement and Thought*. New ways to talk about individuality, and the self, were part of what it was to be modern, not all of which were derived from Freud's notion of the unconscious and practice of psychoanalysis. R. E. Roper, *Movement and Thought*, Blackie, London, 1938, pp.112, 116

called education appears as unscientific as it is pronounced.'[22] The inseparability of mind and body was insisted on by a modern science of health. It also formed part of a new language of self, a sense of the individual that encompassed a distinctive inner life more connected to mental and physical states than the religious notion of the soul. Individuality had come to be thought of more in terms of a 'psyche', a concept not necessarily explicable in terms of a single creed of psychology or psychoanalysis, but as an entity that gave unique shape to identity and experience. Popular works, often written by doctors and other experts, were commissioned by publishers to meet demand. They included Harry Roberts' *The Practical Way to Keep Fit*, Bengamin Gayelord Hauser's *Eat and Grow Beautiful*, John F. Lucy's *Be Fit and Cheerful* and R. E. Roper's *Movement and Thought*. As Winston Churchill noted in one of his Sunday columns, 'Sport is the Stimulant': 'The business girl of today carries a book with her handbag, and thinks the one as necessary as the other.'[23]

Such works reached a wide readership within Britain and across the English-speaking world. Books carrying the official endorsement of government-approved experts were also part of prolific publishing in the area. *Recreation and Physical Fitness for Girls and Women*, and *Recreation and Physical Fitness for Youths and Men* were released by the HMSO in early 1937. The publishing and book distribution

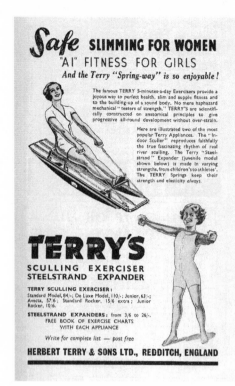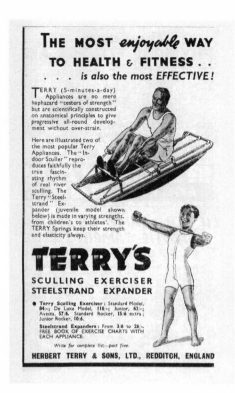

Equipment and clothing makers were quick to seize on the fitness fad. The sculling exerciser promised 'safe slimming for women' and an enjoyable and effective way 'to health and fitness' for men. The advertisements appeared in the endpapers to the widely-used official exercise guides. *Recreation and Physical Fitness for Girls and Women; Recreation and Physical Fitness for Youths and Men*, HMSO, London, 1937, endpapers

network linking the empire (but not the United States) was part of, and in turn helped sustain, a common 'British' culture. The modernist goal of a better body was given different emphases in the endpapers of the HMSO volumes, both of which carried advertisements for the same piece of equipment, the 'sculling exerciser'. For women, Herbert Terry & Sons' machine appeared under the heading 'Safe slimming for women. A1 fitness for girls', while for men it was presented as 'The most enjoyable way to health & fitness ... [and] also the most effective!'[24] A healthy and modern body were to be maintained by effort. For women that goal was also about sustaining a good appearance. But, additionally, in the language of health and beauty there was a broader guide to being modern and living in the stream of something new. Even the BBC, in October 1937, was prepared to begin a series presented by popular columnist Mary Embrey on 'Making the Most of Your Looks'. The 'attitude of most sensible women', Embrey suggested, 'is a realization that artificial conditions of modern life call for artificial aids and that just as they visit their dentist to preserve their teeth so they must give their skins, hair and figures expert care to keep them in good condition'.[25] Government action came on the crest of a wave in which active bodies, sport, leisure and games enjoyed a popularity and novelty that were unprecedented.

Appropriately, it was Oliver Stanley, a relatively youthful 41 years old, and member of the Tory ginger group dubbed the 'YMCA' of a few years earlier, who introduced the second reading of the Physical Training and Recreation Bill in the House of Commons on 7 April 1937. [26] Stanley had taken over the education portfolio, where responsibility for the statutory bodies set up by the Bill would fall. Declining to give a demonstration of the front bench's physical fitness, on the grounds that 'it would enable the House to see us trying to touch those toes which from some of us for years have been concealed', Stanley invited his parliamentary colleagues to regard the measure as one of national rather than party interest. 'The scheme, after all, raises no issue of party politics. It is one of those rare, but for that reason all the more welcome, occasions when we can all co-operate without any sacrifice of principle.' [27]

The legislation followed the government's White Paper, giving statutory authority to two organisations: the National Advisory Council and the Grants Committee. Together, they would be responsible for distributing the £2 million voted for the scheme, and extending powers of local authorities to provide recreation and sporting facilities for those over the age of eighteen. Bracketing 'physical training' with 'recreation' in the Bill's title broadened its appeal – downplaying the military associations of 'physical training', while signifying the scheme's goal of providing for greater leisure and fitness as a matter of health and national duty. It is a measure of the political significance attached to the initiative that the government did not simply extend the powers and grant-aid of the newly established Central Council for Recreative Physical Training (CCRPT). The CCRPT was an independent national co-ordinating organisation whose purposes in promoting the shared interests of recreation, youth and physical education efforts were akin to the National Council of Social Service. Led by its energetic secretary, Phyllis Colson, it served as a clearing house and lobby group for disparate organisations, and was particularly important in securing influence in government policy extending into new areas and in raising a profile as a national charity. Many of the key people supporting the CCRPT were also invited to become involved in the national fitness campaign. In launching its own scheme, the government brought fit bodies, sporting associations and healthy recreation clearly under the purview of central government while avoiding too close an association with the physical education profession's 'knee bending and arm swinging'. [28]

Deflecting criticism that the scheme was 'totalitarian in character', Stanley pointed to the Swedish and Czechoslovakian origins of the physical training that he had in mind, distancing this training from that practised under the extreme regimes. The problem with the British focus on games, Stanley noted, was that 'the participant tends to degenerate into a spectator until you come to a period when too large a number, after spending an afternoon at Goodison Park or an evening at the Oval, pleasantly feel that they have done their bit to make a fitter Britain'. Stanley reassured the House, and the public, that what the government was intending to do was not 'to substitute physical training for games', but 'to supplement games by physical training'.[29] In other words, there would be no loss to a national tradition and disposition, only an extension of it. In a final flourish, Stanley quoted Bertrand Russell: 'To be able to fill leisure intelligently is the last product of civilization.' In doing so he pointed to the Bill's broader purpose of providing for constructive use of modern leisure. Success in this goal would be no less than a triumph for the 'greater Empire'.[30]

MPs across the House welcomed the Bill. Opposition criticism generally focused on whether all sections of society would benefit equally from its provisions, rather than on its overall purpose. The long hours worked by miners, mill girls and factory operatives, and the arduous nature of such work, raised the question of whether the promotion of greater physical exercise was a message appropriate to all. Debate on the second reading came a few days after the annual Oxford–Cambridge boat race. Ede (Labour, Tyneside) raised the uncomfortable question of the continuing class basis of some of the major national sports. Was it true, he asked, that men who earned a living 'by their hands' were still ineligible to compete in races organised by the Amateur Rowing Association?[31] Defending the crowds of mostly 'middle aged people' who attended football on Saturday afternoons from the Minister's 'rather superior remark' about spectator non-participation, Lees-Smith (Labour, Northampton) suggested that what these people wanted at the end of the working week was 'restful occupation', 'not more physical exercise'.[32]

Captain Elliston (Conservative, Blackburn) pointed to the recent success of the 'keep-fit' movement amongst Lancashire factory workers. Welcoming the Bill, he noted, approvingly, that the scheme had nothing to do with 'the production of cannon fodder', but was a useful 'antidote to the deadly monotony of mechanized industry'. He was only partly in jest in remarking that on passing the Bill the government would make Stanley its Minister of Leisure (or even of Pleasure, as Lord Horder had remarked outside the House) to go alongside its Minister of Labour.[33] Facetious as it may have been, Elliston's colleagues, and the wider public in 1937, were very aware that across Europe there were precisely such departments. In France the Blum government appointed Léo Lagrange as Under-Secretary of State for Sport and the Organisation of Leisure, Italy had the well-established Dopolavoro leisure and sport organisation, while Germany's highly organised sport and youth movements were renowned. Most speakers were at pains to stress the distance between what Britain was doing and what went on in 'robot countries'.[34] Only

Richard Pilkington, Tory MP for Widnes, regretted that by 'keeping this scheme voluntary there will be a certain percentage, as there would be in any country, of slackers who will remain slackers.'[35]

Views of leisure, sport and fit bodies were not necessarily divided across party lines. Saturday afternoon crowds attending football games were, to one MP, an indication of healthy worker recreation, whereas to others they were a sign of the sedentary nature of modern recreation, and, in particular, a place where working men got colds and influenza, and threw away their money. Sporting and non-sporting Tories found their match among similarly divided Liberal and Labour camps. Some believed in the power of sport and recreation to surmount social, educational and regional differences, while others pointed to the gulf between Ascot and the local dog track, and the distinction between the gentlemen's and professionals' entrances in cricket.[36] Not in office at the time but wielding influence through his widely syndicated newspaper columns, Winston Churchill recognised sport as 'the stimulant' of modern society and its centrality in the life of British people, but was agnostic on the part government should take in its prosecution.[37]

By far the most original speech in the debate was given by Aneurin (Nye) Bevan, Labour member for Ebbw Vale and later Minister of Health in the 1945–51 Attlee government.[38] Speaking from the libertarian left, he took a characteristically iconoclastic torch to orthodoxies of the left as well as to those of his Tory opponents. Bevan condemned the idea of competition in sport and the Bill's aim of fostering 'enthusiasm' for fitness. 'I do not desire to see any enthusiasm for physical recreation. I desire to see physical recreation indulged in as a normal aspect of everyday life.' There should be no other rationale for playing games than the wish to play, he argued. He supported the Bill's desire to provide better facilities for those who wanted to play, but asserted that it should be up to the individual whether they did so or not. 'The idea that you must borrow some justification for playing is one of the worst legacies of the Puritan revolution.' The last thing he wanted to see was 'all the boys and girls in rows, like chocolate soldiers'[39] – 'a miserable substitute for giving them sufficient playgrounds in which they can play their own games in their own ways'. He urged the President of the Board of Education, Oliver Stanley, not to 'try to set us all goose-stepping from John o'Groat's to Land's End, putting us, like robots, through evolutions which are entirely unnecessary in themselves and by no means pleasing to look at'. With reference to his Labour colleague Philip Noel Baker and the Tory MP David Burghley, both former Olympic medalists and ardent supporters of the measure, Bevan warned: 'whilst I congratulate them upon their prowess I believe that, sometimes, they are the most dangerous members of the community, because nothing has a more unfortunate influence upon the man who wants to practise virtue than the spectacle of perfection'.[40]

Get Fit – Keep Fit: Taking the Message to the People

Posters carrying the national fitness message began to appear in April. Urging people to 'Get Fit – Keep Fit', they were the first in a series to make their mark through spring and early summer.[41] The text may have been imperative in tone but it was the imagery that spoke more loudly. In a world dense with visual culture, images of active bodies were particularly strong symbols of modernity. Promoting awareness 'of the value of physical fitness for its own sake' was the first priority for the newly established National Advisory Council.[42] As anticipated, the Council and Grants Committee were conflated with the campaign, both by name and face (from the outset it was referred to as the National Fitness Council). Cabinet discussions over membership of the Council recognised that credible heads – and bodies – were vital to its success. Men 'whose names would make wide public appeal', and 'if possible, … comparatively young men' were sought out. So too were the right women.[43]

The charming and stylish Lord Aberdare, better known as Clarence N. Bruce – at 52 years old still competing in, and winning, tennis championships against younger opponents – was chosen as chairman. An outstanding cricketer (Middlesex) and member of the International Olympic Committee Executive, Aberdare gave the Council an attractive and contemporary profile of sporting success.[44] Among its other 30 members were 23-year-old Prunella Stack of the Women's League of Health and Beauty;[45] Stanley Rous, secretary of the Football Association; Wavell Wakefield, former cricket and rugby player; fellow MPs and former Olympic medal winners, the aristocratic Lord David Burghley (Conservative) and Quaker Philip Noel Baker, who were part of the enchanted generation of Cambridge athletes that inspired Hugh Hudson's 1981 film *Chariots of Fire;*[46] the reigning English tennis champion, 28-year-old Dorothy Round, who won her second Wimbledon title in 1937;[47] and movement exponent and bohemian Margaret Morris;[48] Major Sir Edward Cadogan, long involved in the work of Boys' Clubs;[49] and a number of others drawn from national organisations including the YMCA and YWCA, the Industrial Welfare Society and Girls' Clubs.[50] President of the BMA E. Le Kaye Fleming, and Lord Dawson of Penn, physician to the royal family, represented the medical profession.[51] The Board of Education officer who recommended the 'very good looking' Dr Woods, a well-known Cambridge athlete (a weightlifter), was disappointed his man did not make the final cut.[52] Sir Henry Pelham, a highly experienced public servant, retired from heading the Board of Education to chair the three-person Grants Committee. Mildred Assheton, prominent in Lancashire education and women's guilds, was selected as a result of a search for a woman and someone outside London;[53] and J. C. Fuller, Ealing mayor and businessman, were the other two members. It was a remarkable, if incongruous, group to gather around a table, especially one in a Whitehall office. Secretary to both committees was Captain Lionel Ellis, who took up the position after eighteen years with the

National Council of Social Service.[54] A separate Scottish Fitness Council chaired by Sir Iain Colquhoun existed alongside its counterpart for England and Wales, in recognition of the distinct nature of education and local government on each side of the border.[55] It also recognised the strong role sport played in maintaining separate national cultures and identities *within* the United Kingdom as well as in the empire-at-large.

There was some truth to Hastings Lees-Smith's (Labour, Keighley) accusation that the Council was unduly representative 'of middle-class athletes ... sprinters, sloggers, pugilists and tennis stars', people unlikely to appreciate 'the problem of the anaemic mill girl'.[56] The hint of the Oxbridge 'hearty', with its class overlay and even sinister whiff of sympathy for the pursuit of 'strong politics' through 'strong bodies', could never entirely be dispelled. Oswald Mosley's British Union of Fascists had been discredited and the wearing of blackshirts outlawed by the Public Order Act of 1936, but there remained an association of physical prowess with political extremism. Mosley was the most forthright proponent of a government-backed sports policy, proposing construction of large national stadia.[57]

Membership of the Council and Grants Committee was announced on 1 March 1937. There was warm public response to the government's plans that was made clear to the press: around a hundred letters per day had been flowing in. These contained a great many constructive suggestions including some from those eager to assist the scheme 'with songs of their own composition to be sung by those engaging in the movement for a fitter Britain'.[58] Transforming the enthusiasm of those already convinced of the value of the scheme into a mass campaign was the next goal. It was a task that fell to some of the most creative contemporary talent, for whom government publicity offered a source of patronage and worthwhile purpose. John Grierson, in film, is perhaps the best known. But staking an official interest in the popular world of sport and the high-profile activities of groups such as the Women's League of Health and Beauty carried its dangers. As BBC producer Janet Quigley warned, there was a danger that 'as soon as anything becomes the object of a national campaign it becomes, in the same instant, suspect'.[59]

The publicity campaign relied on suggestion rather than direction, volition rather than compulsion. The government was entering into a realm founded on the arts of persuasion and the politics of culture, and was attempting to build a political culture that promoted fitness through encouragement, idealism and consent rather than inducement, direction and coercion. There was already a popular movement in existence: what the government had to do, if it was to succeed, was to turn the already present goodwill and interest into a broad public campaign and to signal its support and encouragement carefully.

Using the powerful medium of radio to get the fitness message across was an early focus. Morning exercise programmes were particularly favoured in encouraging

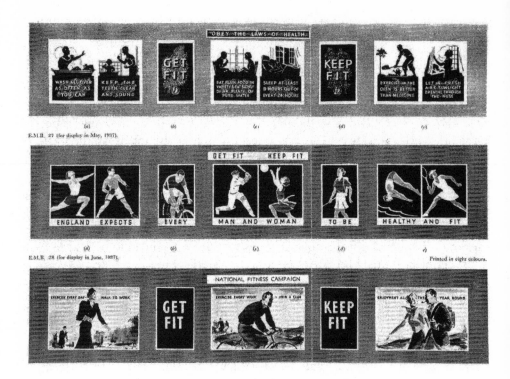

Daily habits, sporting games and holiday pleasures were portrayed as progressive steps in the National Fitness Council's posters released in April, May and June 1937. The first two strips were printed in black and white, the third showing holiday pursuits released in June, appeared in colour. At the time the posters went on display at least a third of houses in Britain had no bath. A quarter of Birmingham houses had no bathroom at all in 1946. ED136/91, The National Archives, London

people to make exercise part of a daily routine at home, a place where they were likely to feel at ease. Chairman of the NFC's Publicity and Propaganda Committee, the high-profile David Burghley, was surprised to find the BBC unreceptive to the idea at their first meeting on 23 March 1937.[60] It quickly became clear that, far from being a simple matter, persuading the BBC to run such programmes would prove difficult. The BBC's opposition led to a stand off and questions in the House of Commons as the Physical Training and Recreation Bill went through its final stages.[61] A number of MPs commented favourably on such broadcasts in other parts of the world, including Sweden, Norway and the United States, while acknowledging that the effectiveness of such programmes was less easily established. Listening and acting could be different things, as William Astor (Conservative, Fulham East) was honest enough to admit. Reflecting on listening to morning exercise programmes on American radio, he observed, 'I do not say that one always did them [the exercises], for sometimes one sat in one's bath and thought of other people doing them. But the wireless did keep the subject of physical fitness in one's mind.' Astor went on to make the point that broadcasting in America was commercial and advertisers would not be supporting such programmes if there was no public demand for them.[62]

Keeping fitness in mind was exactly what Burghley, Aberdare and the National Fitness Council hoped to do. Over the next two years their approaches to the BBC met steady resistance. Only late in 1939 did it finally give way, early morning exercise broadcasts beginning on a trial basis in Scotland as 'Up in the Morning Early'. Burghley's request for national broadcasts was rebuffed on a series of specific grounds: lack of confidence in the medical safety of those following the instructions given during the broadcasts, lack of transmission capacity at that time of the day, and cost. But the BBC's opposition ran deeper and was of longer standing. As early as 1929, 'psychological' and practical problems were identified as standing in the way of such programmes. 'Psychologically, I doubt whether we are a nation which likes to be dragooned in intimate matters of personal habit', was the view of the Talks Director. The audience, the exercises and the early hour presented the practical difficulties.[63] Stronger sentiments were shared between BBC directors a few years later. The 'broadcasting of any instructions about physical exercise would only be achieved over the dead bodies of a large proportion of the senior members of Head Office Staff', one BBC director told another in December 1933. Confident in his colleague's view, he went on to applaud his solidarity: 'I am glad to see you will join them in committing hari-kari in defence of our corporational honour.'[64]

Early morning fitness broadcasts were everything that the BBC, at its Reithian zenith, was not.[65] They were American, and commercial; they were European, and smelt of dictatorship; they were old fashioned, and carried the echo of military parade grounds; perhaps also, they were championed by sporty types who were perceived as wanting to carry the games culture (and their own success) from schooldays into the adult world; they were anti-modern and in all ways out of line with the BBC culture. By 1937, the BBC's desire to maintain its independent stance by preserving some distance from the government's political programme may also have stiffened resolve. The National Fitness Council's view was that running such broadcasts in the clear public interest was part of the BBC's responsibility. Nonetheless, in frustration they agreed to carry the cost of a series of programmes if this was the only option. In the end even those plans came to nothing.[66]

Talking about health and fitness was something the BBC was prepared to do, even if instructing in it was not. Janet Quigley's twelve-week 'What's all this talk about health' evening series, which ran through the spring of 1937, drew a large audience and has come to be recognised as a landmark in the advent of 'social action broadcasting'.[67] In the blurb for the series, comprising six talks on nutrition and five on physical culture, Quigley set out some of the questions provoked by recent public debate:

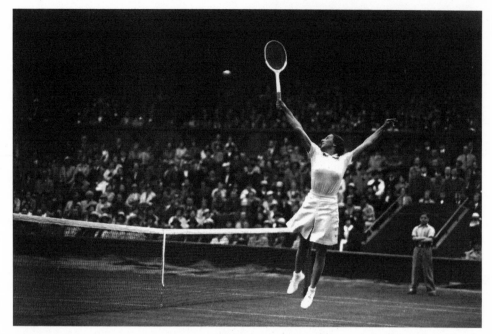

Dorothy Round, England's ladies tennis champion, competing at Wimbledon, 13 June 1936. She lost in the quarters but won the mixed doubles with Fred Perry. The following year, she won the Wimbledon title, defeating her Polish opponent 6-2, 2-6, 7-5. She had become a member of the National Fitness Council in March of the same year, one of youthful faces for the campaign. Topical Press Agency, Hulton Archive, Getty Images

> Why, for instance, should so many people conclude that nations are only made healthy for war, and never for peace – for death, in fact, and not for life? Why, again, should some contradiction be suggested between health from the inside, i.e. nutrition, and health from the outside, i.e. physical culture? Again, why should nutrition – which means adequate nourishment and is therefore the serious concern of everyone, poor or rich – be confused with fancy diets, which are the passing hobbies of the fashionable rich and the serious concern of none?[68]

Two talks on 'Fitness for Housewives' providing some descriptions of simple exercises as 'relaxation from stooping, polishing, etc' were also broadcast in 1937.[69]

In 1937 the BBC could 'talk the walk', but it was only in 1939 that it took the plunge to walk the talk. When morning broadcasts began in December 1939, listeners were invited to tune in at 'the unearthly hour of 7.35'; the accompanying music 'will set you stretching and bending – though you must remember not to overdo that bit through an excess of zeal'. If listeners had any misgivings, these were to be put aside: 'don't feel you are making a lone fool of yourself. Take what inspiration you can from the thought that a nation, hidden in the sanctity of countless homes, is right along with you'.[70] Coleman Smith, the announcer for the men's exercises (Monday, Wednesday and Friday), was a hit with many listeners. His signature injunction, 'Down with a bounce and a bounce and up again', soon flowed into general circulation. One woman inscribed the cigarette case she sent as a Christmas gift to her husband serving with the British forces in the Middle East with her personalised greeting: 'Down with a bounce and a bounce'.[71] Another listener wrote with eagerness bordering on rapture:

> Six weeks ago I went into my sitting room to hear 'Lift Up Your Hearts' [the 7.55 a.m. programme]. I was early, tuned in, and heard a voice – and what a voice! Asking us to lift our right legs higher, higher. It is a wonder the tables and chairs didn't join in. I did, clumsily, but with delight, and went on. Some days after that, the women's exercises came on. I hadn't known the others were for men. Since then I've done both. No one can resist Coleman Smith, he's a master-piece, he ought to take men and women. I cannot tell you what they have done for me. I seemed to have hints of rheumatism everywhere, I was very tired, my home not fit to live in, I'd had a great sorrow. Here was something to help life practically, the music is life giving too.[72]

In-house surveys after three months suggested that about half a million women and slightly fewer men were doing the exercises, around 40 per cent of those who listened to them. Initially designed for the 'under 40s', a complementary set of programmes for the 'over 40s' was recommended to run from 7.45 to 7.55 a.m., starting on 1 May.[73]

The actual age range of listeners was wide. Six-year old Margaret Ball wrote to Coleman Smith telling him she did the exercises every morning with her sister, with her kitten watching on.[74] Other listeners were in their 70s and even over 90. Over time, factors that detracted from listeners doing the exercises included cold weather and lack of sleep, and a lack of conviction, greater amongst working class people, as to whether the exercises did them any good.[75]

If the BBC was slow in coming to the party, there were plenty of others keen to take part in major public events. The Festival of Youth at Wembley in July 1937 offered a more satisfactory public occasion than the ongoing ruckus with the BBC. Ten thousand young people from Boys and Girls' Clubs, the Royal Lifesaving Society, Girl Guides, Boy Scouts and other youth organisations performed a series of physical exercises before a crowd of 60,000. At the centre of the stadium stood a figure symbolising youth, flaming torch in hand, while the King and Queen attended bestowing the royal grace of patronage. In the filmed newsreel of the event, the commentator was careful to point out the difference between this display where 'the legions of peace are on the march' and those seen 'in other parts of the world'. The 'magnificent' Wembley display was presented as an example where 'Britain shows what she's doing to give her youth a body splendid and the mind born free'.[76]

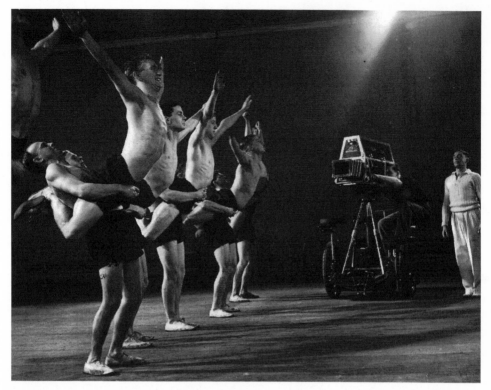

Fit bodies and making fitness films were newsworthy subjects in the late 1930s. This shot of men from the Carnegie Institute of February 1939 was published under the title 'Perfect Men'. They were making a promotional film for the National Fitness Council. Fred Morely, Hulton Archive, Getty Images

The large-scale drama and synchronous movements created a mass spectacle on a model that was popular through the 1930s.

Film was the most powerful medium for popular communication, and was particularly suited to convey the active body. Getting the message of fitness across through film was also an early part of the NFC's work. Popular actors Barbara Allen and Don Stannard, 'England's perfect couple', played the starring roles in four short films made by Gaumont–British Instructional for the NFC in mid-1937 in a series entitled *Strength and Beauty*. Screened for the first time in late October, the films showed a 'refreshingly normal' couple going through the routine of an ordinary day – gulping down their food, nearly missing a train, being not very good at games and showing 'a very understandable reluctance to get up in the morning'. The films were designed to 'open our eyes to the haphazard way in which most of us look after our health' and to suggest 'how simple it is to keep fit'. Directed primarily at people in their early working years, it was also hoped it would appeal to 'those who were on the borderland of becoming old fogeys'.[77] The films came across with what one reviewer described as 'a pleasant air of informality'.[78] *Health of the Nation*, made in April 1937 with support from the Pearl Assurance Company, was one of a number of other promotional films.[79]

Publicity under the slogan of 'Fitter Britain' emphasised national unity over political difference. 'Fitter Britain' was the goal that Prime Minister Neville Chamberlain identified in launching a major publicity initiative in September 1937. Sharing a podium with Arthur Greenwood, MP for Wakefield and Minister of Health in the previous Labour government,[80] and Sir Percy Harris, a prominent Liberal, the Prime Minister's speech emphasised that health and fitness were matters too important to reside within party politics. Deliberately intermingling the government's physical training and recreation initiative with the National Campaign to Encourage Wider Use of the Health Services took some of the political heat out of the health debates, while reassuring skeptics that fitness goals were linked with attention to the core needs of diet and medicine.[81]

'The great national campaign towards a fitter Britain', as *The Times* described it, was accompanied by lavish publicity. The Prime Minister's speech was broadcast on national and empire radio, while the major daily papers ran extensive coverage. *The Times* devoted several pages to comprehensive features, including Lord Aberdare's 'Building a Healthier Nation', an illustrated two-page spread; Prunella Stack's 'Physical Culture for Women'; an article on trends in physical culture 'in other lands'; Minister of Health Kingsley Wood's advocacy for the health campaign; as well as items on the campaign in Scotland and the work of Area Committees.[82] If the terms 'national fitness' and 'Fitter Britain' shared a common language with eugenics, there was nothing in the policies that leaned in that direction. In 1930s Britain, understanding of eugenics was vague. As C. P. Blacker, general secretary of the Eugenic Society, complained in 1932, 'for many people "eugenics" is confused with "eurythmics"'.[83] 'Fitter Britain' became the title of the Health and Fitness exhibit in the Government Court at the Glasgow Empire Exhibition in 1938.

A further big publicity splash came with the Lord Mayor's Parade in November 1937 where the theme of the procession was 'Physical Fitness'. Floats featuring golf players, a boxing ring, Elizabethan bowls, rowing, cycling, mountain climbing and 'How to keep fit in a hundred ways' passed before crowds and cameras along London streets behind the mayor's golden coach.[84] Under a large banner, 'Fitness Wins', were two groups, one of men from the Lucas-Tooth Club (a physical training institute in London's Tooley Street), the other of women from the Women's League of Health and Beauty. Dressed in white trousers and royal blue sweaters (men) and white sweaters and blue skirts (women), they made a striking spectacle, stopping along the route to give demonstrations of simple fitness exercises.[85] Their appearance was also intended to convey the benefits of regular exercise and most of the participants displayed an attractive youthful vigour.[86] Another innovative promotion was demonstrations of fitness exercises staged before football matches.

Stanley Rous, a member of the National Fitness Council and secretary of the Football Association, was instrumental in making these possible.[87]

The level of coverage was an indicator that public interest was running high through the autumn of 1937. Even the Regent Street fashion house Jaeger advertised the season's range of underwear with endorsement of the campaign, while reminding readers that 'Jaeger pure wool underwear sprang up fifty-five years ago as a new Health Movement. In the Autumn of 1884 *The Times* in its leader page said about Jaeger: "A new gospel has reached us," and Jaeger still leads the way to Health, Freedom and Action.'[88] The more middlebrow *Radio Times* carried advertisements for shoes under the heading 'National Foot Service' and with the claim that 'Fitness begins in the feet'.[89] In the popular arena, the call to 'get fit' was so much in the public eye as to provide the title and theme for the 1937 comedy film *Keep Fit*, in which George Formby, starring as a weedy barber, joins the keep-fit campaign to impress his 'girl', a pretty manicurist played by Kay Walsh. Overcoming odds of size and strength, and the corrupt machinations of his middle class rival in the boxing ring, Formby emerges triumphant. Having as its hero an optimistic working class underdog, who is a testament to the benefits of keeping up a fitness regimen, the film embraced the cause while poking gentle fun at its excesses. Formby's three songs from the film became popular hits: 'Biceps, muscles and brawn', 'I don't like' and 'Keep fit'.[90]

Nothing did more to mark the national fitness campaign as a British cause in the broadest sense than the appearance of King George VI and the Queen at the Guildhall in February 1938. Speaking to a live radio audience, as well as to the assembled representatives from national fitness Area Committees, the King lent his weight to the cause. '[N]othing adds more to the pleasure of life and to the joy of work and play than physical fitness', he explained. 'In order to become physically fit we must all have the opportunity for regular exercise.' Outlining the role of the NFC and its Area Committees in making this possible, and calling for support for their work, the speech underlined the voluntarist basis of the movement and the continued importance of the British love of the game for the game's sake. No 'one need take part in any organized training unless he wishes to do so'. 'The decision is left to your free choice. It is for you to make the effort.' But the speech ended with a gentle reminder that national as well as individual interests were at stake: 'There is much leeway to be made up but if we all do our share success is assured and the greater wellbeing of our people will be the supreme reward.'[91] Prominence of the speech was also assured by the *Radio Times* featuring the King's portrait on the cover of that week's issue, drawing listeners' attention to the royal occasion.[92]

Royal patronage lent the campaign prestige, but also linked healthy bodies, sport and fitness to the tradition and sentiment of the monarchy. Launching the campaign with a royal figure underlined the continuity between the fitness movement and

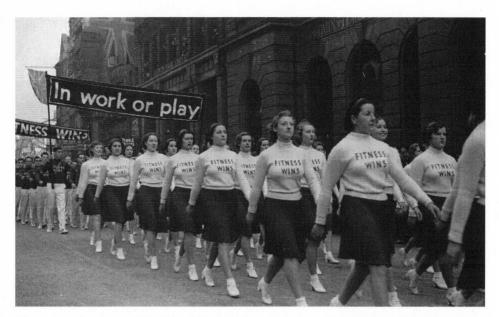

Women from the League of Health and Beauty and men from Lucas-Tooth Club paraded under banners carrying the National Fitness Council's 'Throughout the empire' 'In work or play' 'fitness wins' through the streets of London in the Lord Mayor's Parade, November 1937. Their outfits were made especially for the occasion. Along the route they stopped to perform exercises before the crowds. Newsreel of the Parade was viewed worldwide through Pathé's extensive network. Topical Press Agency, Hulton Archive, Getty Images

the voluntary traditions of sport and independent organisations. Widely reported across the empire, the King's speech also underlined the fact that the campaign was an imperial as much as a domestic project. Nonetheless, it was not without some irony. The former Prince Albert, Duke of York, George VI did not cut the robust sporting figure of his brother, the Prince of Wales, Edward VIII. And the NFC's later attempt to capitalise on the royal patronage by issuing a set of posters featuring the King in a tennis shirt with a personal endorsement of fitness was a bridge too far. The Palace declined.[93]

By the middle of 1938 the campaign's high profile gave new ground to the lingering suspicion in some quarters that fitness was to be made compulsory (a form of conscription), and in others to new criticism that there was not enough happening. The day after the Guildhall event, Lord Stanhope, President of the Board of Education, faced down both charges. He reiterated 'that the Government's policy in this matter is and continues to be that the movement shall be run purely and solely on voluntary lines'; and on the matter of too little action, he acknowledged 'the recent cartoon of a little man with knees bent and arms outstretched in the middle of some movement waiting until a sub-committee had studied the position and decided what the next movement was to be'. Admitting that things had been slower to get going than had been hoped, he reminded his audience that 'the seed which sprang up quickly withered at the first scorching rays of the sun'. Lord Aberdare also reiterated that the Council was adamantly behind a voluntary fitness campaign: 'We stand, four square, for a policy of which free choice and freedom from any kind of compulsion is the fundamental principle ... We have no ulterior motive and no hidden objective. And while it is of course open to every man to think for himself it is in my view impossible that those who advocate compulsion should find a place in our ranks.'[94]

Persuading people that being active was a good thing, both for them and for the country, remained the core of the Council's publicity campaign. The posters displayed on the former Empire Marketing Board frames in the spring of 1937[95] were followed by pamphlets entitled *National Fitness: The First Steps* (1937) and *In Work or Play Fitness Wins: Twenty-four ways of Keeping Fit* (1938).[96] *In Work or Play Fitness Wins* set out a series of activities from 'Morning Exercises' to 'Holiday Games on the Beach' and 'Work'.

Attractive depictions of healthy bodies made for appealing advertising, but whether they worked was harder to gauge. In places, the accompanying text had something of an imperative tone: 'obey the laws of health', 'England expects every man and woman to be healthy and fit', 'Get fit. Keep fit'. Whether the pamphlets achieved the hoped for circulation is doubtful. In June 1938 it appeared that just 30,000 of the 500,000 copies of *In Work or Play Fitness Wins* had left the office.[97] More broadly, the NFC's publicity campaign was an early example of what became the increasingly expansive role of the state as a shaper of citizen behaviour. Mariel Grant suggests that an 'unofficial official' approach to publicity in Whitehall at this time made government personnel wary of publicity campaigns, and set limits on the role of central government as public educators. Providing information to voluntary bodies and local authorities who would then do the 'educating' was the aim. There is more active intent in the NFC campaign than Grant allows. Britain's endeavours to provide for greater recreation and incentives to fitness and physical activity did not go far enough to constitute what de Grazia describes as the 'culture of consent' in Mussolini's Italy.[98] But there was an uneasy line between suggestion and direction (if not compulsion). If freedom to play (or not) defined the essence of a healthy civic culture (a basic British freedom), then government interference in that realm was something that raised suspicions.[99]

Defeating lethargy and inertia remained constant targets for physical fitness publicity campaigns. As the NFC made plain, it was the 'man in the street' who had the most important part to play in the campaign. 'His first task is to conquer his own apathy.' 'No one can make another fit or take exercise for him.'[100] Equally, no one could 'rightly blame the borough council or anyone else' if it wasn't done.[101] For most people, it remained easier not to do exercise, whatever their intentions. The habit of fitness required more effort to instil than handwashing, toothbrushing or bathing, which were more readily absorbed into a daily routine. Fitness required constant urging. And, most difficult of all, the open-ended nature of the goal – being fit or fitter – was indistinct and immeasurable.

Eighty-year-old E. T. Hall, Mayor of Lewes on the Sussex coast, made headlines when he appeared in shirt sleeves joining the bare-armed and bare-legged members of the local Health and Beauty League to inaugurate the town's 'Health and Happiness Week' in November 1937.[102] This was exactly the sort of local initiative the NFC was looking for. The continued vulnerability of the population to infectious disease even as greater fitness was pursued was underlined by the article immediately adjacent to the story of Mayor Hall with a report about a typhoid epidemic spreading from Croydon to Kensington. Tainted watercress was thought to be the cause, but the deeper problem identified was a lack of co-ordination and supervision of the country's water supply.[103] Action at local level was seen as the key to the fitness campaign. While many local authorities took up the opportunity for funding projects made possible by the national fitness initiative, the fact that Area Committees did not coincide with existing local administration and the lugubrious process of applying for grants made progress slow and frustrating. Nonetheless, the NFC advanced what Stephen Jones has identified as the important growth of sport and recreation at municipal level in these years.[104]

Fitness for What? The Campaign on the Ground

By early 1938 all of the Council's 22 Area Committees (21 in England and one in Wales) were finally in place. Applications to the Grants Committee had first to be vetted by one of the Area Committees, and there was no shortage of projects coming forward from 1937 onwards.[105] By 1939 the total funding sought was almost three times what the Council had to distribute: 1,176 projects totalling £6,609,514 in capital costs had been proposed by local authorities and voluntary organisations.[106] The largest of these were for municipal amenities such as swimming pools and social centres, the smallest for equipment sought by local clubs and associations.

The popularity of swimming for recreation, fitness and general leisure was at a high point in the 1930s. Learning to swim and swimming as a form of active recreation had replaced the older, more passive, pre-World War I notion of 'bathing'.[107] Swimming pools were rapidly becoming an amenity that any town or city with pretensions to modernity wanted to have. Swimwear and water-based leisure had also come to comprise one of the glamour sides of physical recreation by the mid-1930s. Municipal and public authorities seeking to encourage physical recreation regarded swimming pools as their best option in coaxing people into action. They also had the attraction, when conceived of as indoor or roofed facilities, of offering a year-round option.

Employing paid organisers to assist in both administration and coaching in major sports was also supported by the National Fitness Council. Charles Tugwell began work with the National Amateur Rowing Association on 1 November 1937 at a salary of £600 per annum. A few months later the talented Marjorie Pollard, a graduate of Bedford College, former member of the national hockey team, and sports writer and broadcaster (writing for *The Times*, and broadcasting for the BBC on the All-England Women's Cricket tour to Australia and New Zealand in 1933–34), began work as the national organiser for the Women's Team Games Board (in charge of hockey, lacrosse and netball) at a salary of £400 per annum.[108] Around twenty organisers were working for national sports bodies on a grant-aid basis by mid-1938.[109] Less successful were plans to establish a National College of Physical Training. This was one of the specific goals of the Council in providing impetus to qualified physical education and fitness leaders. Although a site at Merstham in Surrey was announced in May 1938 as the future home of the College, it was still on the drawing board when everything came to a stop in September 1939.[110]

The Northampton Roadmender Club was one of the successful applicants to the National Fitness Grants Committee. Offering activities every night of the year except through August, the Club gave 'boys who would otherwise get into mischief in the streets' a place to play games and do physical training, 'and a certain amount of moral, mental and physical education'. Sited in a disused factory, the Club looked to improve its premises and was granted £6,000 towards the capital cost and equipment of a new headquarters. Like a number of other 'juvenile organisations', the Roadmender Club saw itself as having a purpose beyond that served by sporting activities on their own. Compared with the man who, when asked why he played golf, replied 'Because it makes me so fit', and when pressed with the further question 'Fit for what?', replied, 'For golf', the Roadmender Boys Club set out its object as 'to make its boys'

> Fit – Fit for what?
> Fit for Life's handicap.
> Fit to earn their living.
> Fit to be good Northampton citizens.
> Fit to maintain their Country as the 'Best Country in the World'.

In its appeal for money and personal help, the Club's chairman, Alan Page, reminded the public that –

> All the British people who were spectators of the recent Olympic Games at Berlin, have returned full of admiration for the physical efficiency of the German boys and young men.
>
> In our Country we believe rightly or wrongly that we can get better results by Voluntary Physical Training, but it is no use shutting our eyes to the fact that failing this Compulsion must come, or as a Nation we shall go under.[111]

The Roadmenders may have answered the lurking question that publicity had left hanging, fit for what? But their answer was one that, in turn, stirred a disquiet that dogged the campaign.

Thirteen men creating a human pyramid in an unnamed Nottinghamshire village were photographed and featured in the *Nottinghamshire Countryside*, the journal of the Nottinghamshire Rural Community Council, alongside acclamation from Lord Aberdare. Another contributor to the magazine suggested that the county embrace the campaign with a 'national rural fitness festival' along the lines of Germany's 'Strength through Joy' movement. Unlike its inspiration, however, the writer noted that: 'While continental countries achieve fitness by discipline imposed from above, Britain plans to succeed with fitness schemes that appeal because they come from a self-imposed discipline generated in the heart of the individual.'[112]

Not all claimants for funding, recognition or offers of assistance to the national fitness campaign were deemed of equal stature. Small organisations such as the Maccabi Sports Club of East London were also applicants for funding. In this case a suspicion that the Club was not getting a fair hearing due to anti-Semitic attitudes led to representations from the Club's officials.[113] The Society of Miniature Rifles' request for recognition of their activities got the firm bureaucratic brush-off: 'no further action taken'. Lengthy deliberations were set off by the Greyhound Racing Board's offer to make tracks available for national fitness activities. Extended discussions took place within the Fitness Council over two meetings. In the end, the offer was politely declined. 'Going to the dogs', with its associated gambling and drink-oiled sociability, had the wrong flavour for national fitness and healthy recreation.[114] Gwen Pemberton, one of the surveyors on Dr John Boyd Orr's systematic and influential 1937–39 nutrition study, noted the comment of a health visitor in the mining town of West Wemyss, Fifeshire. The visitor drew Pemberton's attention to the men's interest in greyhounds, bought often on a syndicate basis, provided with butter and meat and, in her view, 'better fed than the children'.[115]

Scots were urged to join in becoming more physically active by the separate Scottish Fitness Council. Particular national attributes and opportunities were highlighted at the same time as empire was reiterated as a central feature of contemporary life. *Scotland for Fitness* was one of seven films made under the supervision of John Grierson for the Glasgow Empire Exhibition. The Exhibition, staged at Bellahouston Park, in what was considered the British Empire's 'second city' (after London), ran from May to December 1938 and drew 12 million visitors. A successor to the great world exhibitions stemming from the original Great Exhibition of 1851, Glasgow's 1938 event was conceived very much as a project designed to provide economic stimulus to a region hard hit by the Depression.[116] The film featured Sir Iain Colquhoun, chairman of the Scottish Council, exhorting fellow Scots to 'Keep Fit and Raise the Scottish Standard'. Presenting the aim of the

Council as 'improving our Scottish physique' through, among other things, walking in the hills and staying at youth hostels, the film went on to show a kilt-wearing Mr Barr apparently walking straight from the loch country into Colquhoun's office, rucksack slung from his shoulders. Weekend expeditions were described with reference to a map spread over the desk, Barr explaining that he had never spent more than 2/6 per day on camping holidays. Jack Gardner, centre-half in the national football team, described the fitness routine kept up by his club side as being dependent on just two evening training sessions fitted in around his work as a civil engineer and attending evening classes. Mrs Brown, organiser of the national women's 'Keep-Fit' movement, emphasised the importance of 'internal health' to women attending classes, and the beneficial relief that exercise to music achieved for those confined day-to-day by monotonous labour. In a final series of striking shots, viewers were urged to 'get ready and go' when the Saturday 1 p.m. whistle signalled the end of the working week. Walking, footballing, golf, hurdling, camping, pool diving and many more activities were shown in dynamic footage.[117]

In the 'Fitter Britain Exhibit' that occupied a quarter of the space in the Government Court at the Exhibition, a similar message was conveyed in the 'Health at Play' section. The value of regular exercise, especially outdoor exercise, as an antidote to the speed and regimen of modern work routines was one of the reminders conveyed by 'Godfrey', the 11-foot high Mechanical Man who stood at the centre of the pavilion. While the machine age brought its benefits, the human spirit needed refreshment through physical recreation, and just as machines needed regular maintenance to work effectively, so too the human body needed the health-giving benefits of exercise and purposeful movement.

Although the Scottish Council was faced with many of the same problems as its counterpart in England and was similarly short-lived, it was to leave more of an impact. It did so through the people it drew into sports and recreation administration who went on to shape postwar development. And through what Callum Brown suggests was a greater willingness in Scotland to look to sports promotion as part of a wider social development. May Brown was the pivotal figure in this history. In the longer span from the 1920s through to the 1960s, the Fitness Council in Scotland occupied only a short interlude but served as an important catalyst. May Brown began work with the fitness campaign training youth leaders in the Edinburgh area. She had been educated at one of the leading private girls' schools in Edinburgh and at Anstey College of Physical Education in Warwickshire. From her initial work she went on to be employed as one of two permanent staff employed by the Scottish Fitness Council. The other was a retired Army colonel. Her work was largely within the mining communities in Fife where economic depression had left many unemployed. When the Fitness Council was wound up, she worked successfully to establish a separate Scottish section of the Central Council for Physical Recreation

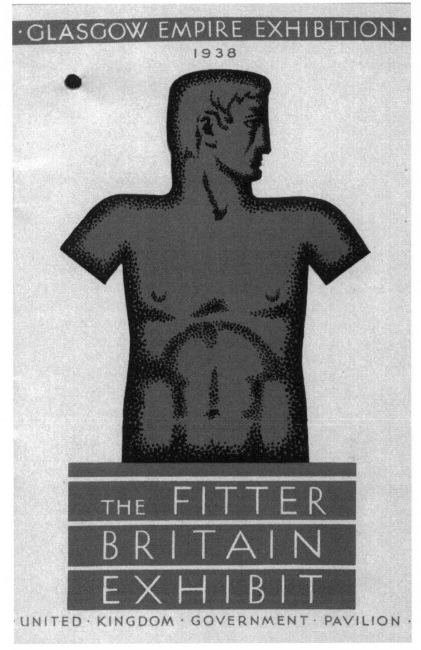

Classical modernism was the style finally adopted for the design of the Fitter Britain Exhibit at the Glasgow Empire Exhibition. Finding the right title for the health and education hall at the exhibition took officials some deliberation. '"Health" was considered a bad word to use'. They toyed instead 'with some variation of the word "Life"'. In the end it became The Fitter Britain Exhibit. 'Godfrey' the nine foot tall mechanical man, moving and 'speaking' healthy messages and three mounted rats as enemies of health proved popular attractions. ED 136/91, The National Archives, London

(CCPR) in 1944, and to create the separate Scottish Office-funded Scottish Council of Physical Recreation from 1953. With others, Brown successfully brought sport and recreation facilities into new housing schemes, providing them with social and community centres, and melding a strong sports structure from volunteer and paid officials. Callum Brown's interpretation was drawn from a critical vantage point but one also illuminated by personal connection to the archive and the subject. More recent, comparative studies have tended to paint the Scottish story less favourably.[118]

Overall, the task of raising public awareness and co-ordinating sport and fitness activities throughout Great Britain was larger than could yield easily measurable results in a short time. Moreover, the rapidly shifting political ground between 1936–37, when the scheme was devised, and mid-1938, when the urgency of the international situation became more pressing exacerbated tensions within the scheme. The NFC became squeezed between pressure from local and central government. It was also caught between expectations that it would primarily play a co-ordinating role, and of those who saw it as more initiating and directive. As a statutory organisation sitting at arm's length from its administrative masters in Whitehall and its political masters in Westminster, it was easy to get snared in varying, and shifting, expectations.

A 'few shillings towards a pair of sculls for a rowing club' and 'a pair of shorts for a hiker' were all that could be seen for the NFC efforts: so claimed Charles de Roemer in a letter to *The Times* in August 1938.[119] De Roemer was a member of the London Area Committee and one-time supporter of the NFC. His was one of a mounting set of disgruntled and disappointed voices, rising in volume by the end of the summer of 1938. Chiding de Roemer for conflating a lack of *local* progress with what had been achieved on a *national* basis, NFC secretary Lionel Ellis pointed to the £700,000 in grants that had been approved for capital expenditure on facilities, none of which had been made for 'shorts for a hiker': £74,000 had gone towards extra playing fields; £144,000 towards swimming baths; and £2,300 towards additional youth hostels. Much had been done to bring rowing 'within the reach of all who have easy access to river or sea', and 'anyone with knowledge of the difficulties in which rowing is carried on by clubs whose members cannot afford any considerable subscription would hardly undervalue the help that is being given to them'. Ellis also pointed to the 20,500 men and 17,750 women and girls 'enrolled voluntarily in physical training classes provided by the London County Council', an indicator of a pattern that could 'be brought from all over the country'. Facilities could not be planned and built in a day, and the fact that some areas were still to develop schemes 'should not blind Major de Roemer or your readers to what is being achieved after little more than six months' active work', he concluded.[120]

But it was clear that the tide of public opinion that was running high a year before was fast on the wane. Major de Roemer's letter to *The Times* was but one sign of a wider mood around the country and further afield.[121] Disappointment about the levels of grants, slowness in getting projects going, and criticism about the purpose and character of some of the activities supported by the NFC (and the way in which they were being instituted) deflated earlier momentum.[122] The high hopes and idealism, if not utopianism, of the fitness campaign of 1937 were hard to sustain, let alone fulfil. While Captain Ellis, secretary to the NFC, endeavoured to reply to the criticisms, he had a difficult task against what had become a much less sympathetic mood.

A sign of the frustrating gap between the early impetus and the actual yield from the campaign was also evident in work of the medical sub-committee of the National Fitness Council. Only in May 1938 was it able to agree on a definition of fitness as 'a state of physical, mental and spiritual well being in which the individual can perform and enjoy the activities of his [sic] leisure and working hours'.[123] The committee's deliberations point to the broader project of 'reconstructing bodies' that Carden-Coyne has most recently highlighted for this period. A wide and powerful project in the interwar period, what it meant to be 'fit' was far from carrying a single or agreed set of meanings; instead, it represented a wide-ranging discussion that included defining and distinguishing disabled and enabled capacities.

Public disappointment voiced in the summer of 1938 was matched a few months later by the disappointment of the Earl de la Warr, the new President of the Board of Education, at the Cabinet table. When Cabinet came to consider de la Warr's bid for an additional £3 million funding at its meeting of 14 December 1938, the President was unable to convince his colleagues. Commitments to capital expenditure (most of them going to local authorities) had already exceeded the sum originally intended. A further £1 million had been committed, while applications for £1.75 million had been lodged. Prime Minister Chamberlain was unimpressed and the Chancellor of the Exchequer, Sir John Simon, unsympathetic. 'It was clear that money had been spent in quite different directions' to those contemplated at the outset of the scheme, the Prime Minister noted. In defence of the NFC, de la Warr 'pointed out that playing fields, swimming baths and gymnasia were the items specifically mentioned on page 6 of the White Paper .... It would not be fair to criticize the Committee for having made grants in aid of those items.'[124] Political realities could be tough. While a further £1,200,000 was offered to the NFC, it was clear that no further funds were likely to be forthcoming for capital expenditure beyond the initial £2,400,000.[125]

The campaign had been successful in stimulating proposed projects, especially those whose impetus came from local authorities.[126] Indeed, the scale of expectation that had been aroused was daunting. But it raised a question of the limits to government responsibility and action: should the government's role be to stimulate interest that would be met largely at a local level through the work of town and city

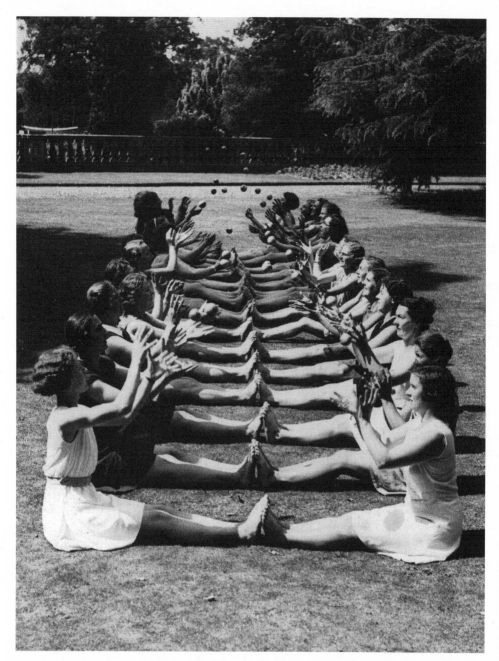

Keep Fit Class, August 1938. 'Keep-fit' classes reached such popularity in the 1930s they were referred to as a 'fad'. Doing exercise in the outdoors was regarded as especially beneficial. Fox Photos, Hulton Archive, Getty Images councils, and voluntary organisations, or to act as the central fount of funds and direction? Criticism of funding and the effectiveness of the NFC came from two levels: the broader top-down one that the level of funding committed by government was too low to get near achieving what was set out,[127] and the narrower criticism from de Roemer et al that the spending they authorised was poorly, unevenly and ineffectively delivered. The debate on this in the leader of *The Times* of 6 August finishes, presciently, with:

> There is every reason, in short, why local enthusiasts should be free to criticize the rate of progress in their own areas, but no justification for any general condemnation; and it may be found in the long run that the chief target of criticism will be not so much alleged slackness as the great cost of intensive activity.[128]

In this context the NFC's proposal to award a badge to those who had completed a course of prescribed fitness activities became a point of contention. To those keen to see fitness activities more rigorously and energetically pursued (that is, for those for whom the NFC was too hesitant, cautious and low key), a badge was neither an adequate incentive nor an appropriate recognition of activities that needed to be taken more seriously. To those who harboured suspicion that the NFC simply supported and surreptitiously backed a government's desire to introduce conscription, the badge proposal smelled of something bad. The badge, in the latter view, hinted at military insignia, a thin end of a wedge that would soon lead to uniforms, salutes, commands and regimentation.

By early 1939 the British government's continued willingness to participate in the totalitarian-led World Congress for Recreation and Leisure was causing division among NFC members.[129] It was the view of Labour MP and NFC member Philip Noel Baker that any common ground between the work being done under the Physical Training and Recreation Act and the state run worker leisure organisations in Germany and Italy had been expunged by the nature of political regimes of which the latter were a part. Baker led the opposition to Britain's continued involvement.[130] But his view did not prevail.

Members of the British government and the NFC welcomed delegates to a meeting of the World Congress for Leisure Time and Recreation in London in February 1939. Most of the leading members came from the totalitarian regimes. In his speech to the Congress, Chamberlain noted that there had never been a time when 'the English people ... had a more international outlook than they have today', and that with their 'increased interest' in the subject of recreation 'there could hardly be a more opportune time than now for your visit'. Among those who 'received' the Prime Minister at the Congress were Gustavus Town Kirby of the United States; Dr Robert Ley, head of the German Labour Front and the 'Strength through Joy' movement;[131] Sir Noel Curtis-Bennett, a member of the NFC; and Commendatore

Corrado Pucetti of Italy. At the Congress banquet at the Savoy Hotel, Walter Elliot, Minister of Health, told his guests that the English view of leisure was simple and summed up in the word 'sport'. He outlined the work of the National Council in increasing spending on sports facilities between 1932–4 and 1937–8.[132]

By May 1939 mounting disquiet about continued British involvement in the World Congress had become even more vociferous and the outright opposition of Noel Baker and others more strident.[133] The centenary festival of Swedish gymnastics founder Per Ling in a Lingiad festival in Stockholm in July 1939 offered a more innocent stage for international collaboration. Among the 7,000 participants were around 250 from Britain. Unlike the uniformly clad national delegations from Denmark, Germany and Sweden, Britain's representatives were variously attired in the outfits of the Women's League of Health and Beauty, the Liverpool Physical Training College team, and other clubs and colleges. Their ill-sorted appearance created some embarrassment at the time. They were put in the centre of the large display so as not to disturb its symmetry and order. In retrospect this lack of conformity in the national group was a source of pride, a signal of Britain's adherence to a deep-seated freedom. There was no single, let alone official, national physical fitness movement to belong to.[134]

An End and No New Postwar Beginning

Within hours of war being declared, Captain Ellis, secretary to the NFC, was instructed to close the office. All NFC activities were frozen 'for the duration'.[135] Officers employed by local committees found that their jobs had disappeared. On 5 September Muriel Cornell of the Women's Amateur Athletic Association was one of many to receive a letter advising, with regret, 'that in view of the National Emergency, it has been necessary to review all grants made under the Physical Training and Recreation Act, 1937, and the offer of grant ... made to your Association in our letter of the 20th May, 1938, must be regarded as withdrawn'.[136]

Activities left in suspension and the residual functions of the NFC as at September 1939, subsequently became the responsibility of the Board of Education through the 1944 Education Act. Here, the work of the NFC was quietly buried. Justin Evans, writing a retirement view history of the period in 1974, noted (but did not reference) a credible report that when the NFC offices closed, 'the order was given for its records and surveys to be destroyed' – the war coming as something of a relief to an effort that had become an embarrassment.[137]

Phyllis Colson at the Central Council of Recreative Physical Training staved off a similar fate with the support of influential Board members. Arguing that their services were all the more needed in wartime, the CCRPT ran a 'Fitness for Service' programme largely for 14–20-year olds and was active in recruiting and training physical education instructors for the armed services and civilian auxiliaries.[138] In

1944 the organisation changed its cumbersome name to the Central Council for Physical Recreation (CCPR). It was more than a cosmetic change. Repugnance at what lay behind the Nazi and fascist governments' encouragement of regimented physical exercise tainted forever the term 'physical training'. [139] Besides, Phyllis Colson appreciated that the peacetime future would bring a very different environment for the Council's work. Education would be a priority; and maintaining a strong foothold at the Board of Education was vital. With the rising school leaving age, the Council became involved in training leaders in youth work, and in supporting the foundation of a more robust physical education profession. The CCPR deftly managed the transition to the now state-led, but still thick undergrowth, of grant-aided associations. The CCPR was an example of what Lord Beveridge was to describe in his largely neglected 1948 report *Voluntary Action*. Set aside by contemporaries, it has become the focus of much renewed interest in recent decades. [140] Asserting, unfashionably at the time of publication, the continued importance of the voluntary principle and associational life, Beveridge was emphatic in defining sport and leisure as existing beyond the boundary of state action. Identifying 'the needs that remain in a social service state', Beveridge made it clear that the 'last stage in totalitarianism would be reached if the use of his leisure were being arranged for each citizen by the State'. [141]

Clement Attlee's Labour government, elected in 1945, was not hostile to sport, but nor did it see sport or physical recreation – beyond more and better provision for young people in schools – as part of its broader project of social reconstruction. An overall improvement in the standard of living would lead, it was expected, to greater opportunities for leisure of all kinds. But those opportunities remained vastly different for rich and poor, in town and country, for old and young, and especially between men and women. What people did at the weekend, what sports they chose to play or watch, was up to them, and as such, the prewar pattern of sharply contrasting class, age and gender leisure cultures was left unaltered. [142] When the Labour government was forced to intervene, in the miserable winter of 1946–7, the gaps between those cultures became very apparent. Bans on midweek sport, imposed as a result of the severe coal shortage, made little difference to cricket or horseracing – where fixtures were simply moved to Saturdays – but led to outbreaks of disorder at dog tracks around London. After several instances of spectator stands, bars and restaurants being destroyed by angry crowds, and widespread scuffles at several London stadia, some action was taken. [143] Deprived of their midweek night out, working people were unimpressed with Labour representatives who had little knowledge of, and even some hostility to, things they enjoyed. Disdained as places of working class fecklessness and tacky commercialism, or worse, they were not part of the brave new world of meritocratic progress. Even Lord Beveridge, the great inspiration of the plan behind Britain's welfare state, was not immune to a judgement that not all ways in which people spent their 'free time' were equal. 'It is difficult to imagine any standard by which transfer of time from even the dullest form of earning by work to the filling in of a football coupon in hope of unearned wealth', he wrote, 'can be regarded as progress.' He called for a review of government policy towards gambling, but again warned, 'the main attack on wasteful or harmful use of leisure cannot, in a free society, be made by direct action of the State'.[144]

Nonetheless, sport could be part of rebuilding the new world order. Philip Noel Baker, holding a ministerial post in both the wartime Cabinet and Attlee's administration, managed to persuade Ernest Bevin that hosting the 1948 Olympics in London was worth the effort, if for no other reason than in attracting overseas funds. But it might also be a place where Britain could recover some international standing.[145] These were pragmatic arguments, but Noel Baker retained a deeply held belief in sport's unique power to bring people together through personal and collective understanding and friendship. From the left and right, George Orwell's charge that international sporting contests were no more than 'war minus the shooting' attracted both support and vehement denial.[146] The 1948 Games (the 'austerity games') were a reasonable success, although hopes of greater international peace and understanding were dashed by the Berlin airlift, which began a few weeks before the Games opened on 29 July.[147]

If Orwell had lived beyond 1950, he would have felt himself vindicated in watching the unfolding world of international sport, a spectacle that was increasingly beamed to television publics around the world. From 1952 at Helsinki when a Soviet team competed at the Olympic Games for the first time, the athletic track, boxing and weightlifting ring, gymnastic and other arenas quickly became platforms not only for the contest for sporting success but also in the struggle for supremacy between capitalist and communist powers. Amateurism was insisted upon, but a multitude of arrangements could support athletes who might still swear honestly that they were not paid to play. By 1956, a group of physical education academics at the University of Birmingham could no longer hold back in critiquing what they regarded as the atrophied arrangements encasing British sport. Their report, together with Lord Wolfenden's 1960 *Sport & the Community*, provided the basis for central government to re-engage with sport and physical recreation.[148]

Both Labour and the Conservatives accepted that Wolfenden's call for greater interaction between government and voluntary bodies, especially in addressing the unevenness that constituted the weakness, even danger, of independent organisations, opened the door to greater government participation in sport and recreation. But it was Harold Wilson's Labour Government that took the first step. In 1964 Denis Howell was appointed as the first Minister Responsible for Sport.[149] An Advisory Sports Council was set up to promote co-ordination among sporting organisations and between sports and recreation activities and broader government policies.

The Council also served as the vehicle for some small distribution of public funds to sports bodies. Strengthened with executive powers in 1970, and two years later by a Conservative government with a royal charter and parallel bodies for Wales, Scotland and Northern Ireland, the Council signalled a larger but still arm's length interest in sport by the state.

The subsequent replacement of the Council in 1996 by new bodies known as UK Sport and Sport England did not change the arm's length status that typified these organisations, including their Welsh, Scottish and Northern Irish equivalents. UK Sport was responsible for high performance or elite sport, and Sport England for the promotion of community participation. Like their predecessors, they also existed by royal charter, but were accountable both to Parliament and independent boards of directors. The 'social good' of sports is recognised in the public nature of these bodies and their funding, yet the distance from central government remains integral to their definition and their identity.[150] For all the differences in context between the early twenty-first century and the mid-1930s, the competing dynamics of political attraction to competitive sport and simultaneous repugnance at state interference in the freedom to play are reflected in the contrasting funding streams for UK Sport, substantially funded by the Exchequer, and Sport England, substantially funded by lottery income.

2   Leisure and Democracy

Physical Welfare as the People's Entitlement in New Zealand

Taking the opportunity of Olympic hero Jack Lovelock's brief visit home in late 1936, railway manager and sports administrator Wallie Ingram surveyed New Zealanders on their levels of fitness. He was dismayed, if not altogether surprised, with what he found. Of twelve people interviewed not one reported that they followed the 10–12 minute exercise regime broadcast on the local radio. They all had good, but differing, reasons for not doing so. 'New Zealanders, like their kin in the Old Land', Ingram observed, 'take sport haphazardly – in other words, purely as a recreation.'[1] But Jack Lovelock's 'perfect race' to win the gold medal in the glamour 1,500-metre race in Berlin's Olympic Stadium on 6 August 1936 was anything but the result of haphazard preparation. By the 1930s, success in international sport required dedicated commitment. Lovelock was at the forefront of a new breed of athletes who trained scientifically, and whose success was the result of highly organised regimes of diet, training, physiological monitoring and mental preparation.[2]

William (Bill) Parry, New Zealand's political champion of government-supported sport and recreation, was equally a harbinger of modernity.[3] Parry was convinced that the enjoyment of leisure could no longer be left to the arbitrary whim of voluntary or private provision. Greater leisure was a sign of modern times, a benefit won from 'scientific development' such as mechanisation and a right guaranteed to working people by politicians such as himself.

Legislation that expanded opportunities and encouraged greater participation in sport and physical recreation became part of the radically reforming agenda of the government in which Parry was a minister, the welfare-state-building Labour administration (1935–49) led by Michael Savage, Peter Fraser and Walter Nash. The Physical Welfare and Recreation Act, a close replica of its British counterpart, but with the important substitution of 'Welfare' for 'Training' in its title, was passed in

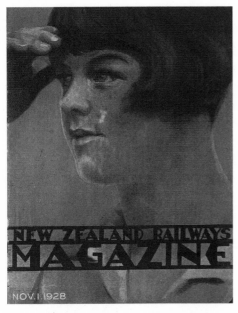

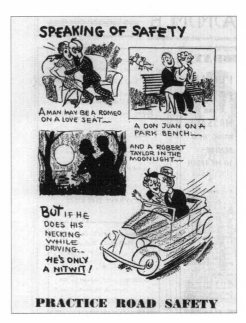

Conquering time and distance with speed was one of the wonders of modern times. For the *Railways Magazine*'s feature on 'the new dawn' of economic revival Stanley Davis chose the symbolic figure of a young woman sporting a modish short hair cut. The *Railways Magazine* at this time enjoyed a huge circulation of 26,000 in the mid-1930s. In the brochure printed to accompany the Easter Saturday demonstration of interhouse women's sports teams at the 1940 Centennial Exhibition it was the dangers of speed, and over-amorous young men, that was pointed to with an advertisement for road safety. *New Zealand Railways Magazine*, November 1928; IA 62 4/38, Archives New Zealand, Wellington

the New Zealand Parliament in November 1937. Part of a tidal wave of legislation enacted in Labour's first term, it was on the New Zealand statute book within five months of the original measure being enacted in the British House of Commons. The Act provided 'for the development of facilities for, and the encouragement of, physical training, exercise, sport, and recreation, and to facilitate the establishment of centres for social activities related thereto'. A National Council and district committees were to oversee grants to local authorities and voluntary organisations, and local authorities were to gain borrowing powers to fulfil the measure's purposes.[4] On 19 August the cover of the popular weekly, the *New Zealand Free Lance*, drew a parallel between Savage and Lovelock, depicting both as 'world beaters' under Hitler's anxious eye.[5]

In New Zealand the physical welfare and recreation scheme took on the imprint of its political sponsors. It was part of a modernist dream. Realising the goal of a five-day, forty-hour week was to be matched by providing opportunities for a constructive use of the newly won leisure time. Parry's advocacy of playing sport, swimming, enjoying the outdoors, singing in a choir or joining a WEA study group was now every citizen's entitlement – as much as an income, housing and medical care.[6] It was part of the overall object – to secure a decent standard of living for all, and to restore a society in which everyone was able to fulfil their potential. It grew more from an expansive notion of the possibilities of body and mind rather than from an anxiety about their inadequacies.

Minister Parry and his energetic administrative head, Joseph Heenan, both passionate sports followers and appreciators of literature, were personal backers of the scheme. A former miners' leader, Parry was a large man who took pride and pleasure in keeping fit throughout his life. Previously a champion cyclist, and a good shot and keen fisherman, he set up a gymnasium in parliament's basement from which colleagues could hear regular thumps from hits on the punchbag. Heenan held office in a range of sports bodies, wrote turf notes as 'The Saint', and literary columns for the Sydney *Bulletin* as 'O'H Aonian', and appalled the scholarly General Assembly Librarian Guy Scholefield by reading the racing columns in the newspaper reading room.[7] The support of key Labour leaders, including Peter Fraser and Heenan in the Department of Internal Affairs (the descendant of the original Colonial Secretary's office) has been recognised for its crucial part in shaping the state as a major patron of cultural life in New Zealand, but Parry and Heenan's partnership in nurturing a local culture of the body has been less acknowledged. It was a creative, if ultimately less enduring, endeavour.[8]

After an exuberant and optimistic start, a diversion into war activities and a brief second wind in the immediate postwar years of 1945–48, the New Zealand physical welfare and recreation scheme faltered, and, after coming under political attack, was left to wither in the early 1950s as voluntarism enjoyed a resurgence. But it was a different kind of failure than that suffered by its British equivalent. Although it failed to find a place in the bi-partisan consensus of the postwar welfare state, it did leave some indent on the independent world of sporting associations dominated by middle class elites and working class masculinity.[9]

A Dream of Free Saturdays

Plans for a 'leisure' policy followed closely on the heels of the government's actions in instituting a forty-hour week. A campaign goal since the 1920s, this was in keeping with the 1935 ILO[10] Convention, as well as an attempt to recapture New Zealand's (and Australia's) earlier reputation as a 'workingman's paradise'. The struggle for the eight-hour day had been won in the nineteenth century, but the old demand for the '3 8s' – eight hours' work, eight hours' rest, eight hours' recreation – had now become one for a reduced working week and an entitlement to paid holidays.[11] Work and workers were increasingly bound by the clock rather than the task. The demand for leisure, or regular time off, was also a response to the pace and nature of modern work. Reduced working hours were first seen in the insistence on the half-day holiday beginning at 12 noon on Saturdays. Factory and industrial workers

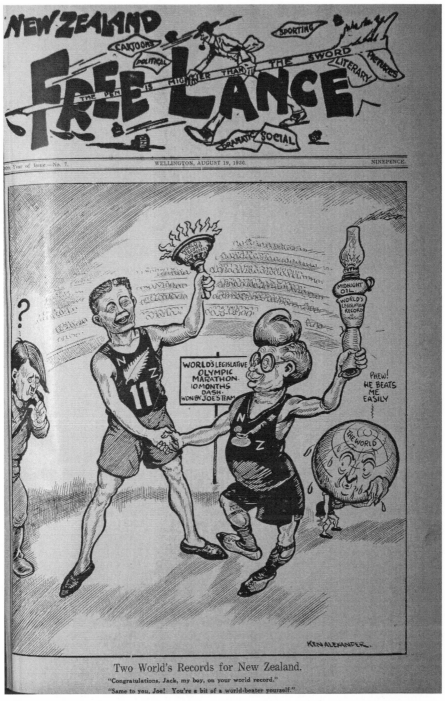

Readers were encouraged to think of their country in flattering terms by the *New Zealand Free Lance*'s cover of 19 August 1936. The national popular weekly paper depicted both Jack Lovelock and Prime Minister Michael Savage as world beaters. *New Zealand Free Lance*, 19 August 1936, Hocken Library celebrated the forty-hour week ahead of shop and office workers, but both had to wait for the demands of war work to recede to see Labour's full commitment realised. From 1944 all workers enjoyed a statutory entitlement to two weeks' paid holiday a year.[12]

A distinctive feature of the New Zealand story was the accompanying reduction in shop trading hours. The New Zealand 'weekend' was one which saw shops close at 9 p.m. on Friday and reopen only at 9 a.m. on Monday, with Saturday and Sunday becoming a non-commercial hiatus in the week. Pubs played a limited role in leisure in both New Zealand and Australia through much of the twentieth century, with restricted numbers of licensed premises and early closing (6 p.m. in New Zealand) being the norm from World War I until 1967. To visitors it was a source of puzzlement or even derision. One was famously to remark that she had come to New Zealand to find 'it was closed'.[13] Time had its own local shape.

Parry's initial ambitions for a 'people's leisure' had been trimmed by the time he introduced the Physical Welfare and Recreation Bill into Parliament in October 1937.[14] Early discussions with sporting associations had drawn reactions requiring some second thoughts. From the Imperial Conference in London in May, Prime Minister Savage (a close friend and political ally of Parry) brought back the latest briefing on the British government's Physical Training and Recreation Bill, then before the House of Commons. As the Department of Internal Affairs' annual report curtly put it, the new local measure was framed 'largely on the lines of a similar Act passed by the British House of Commons but with certain differences to meet the Dominion's requirements'.[15] Under the New Zealand legislation the Minister had executive power as chair of the National Council, with the scheme being the responsibility of Internal Affairs under Joe Heenan. District committees around the country were expected to play advisory roles, and local authorities – city, borough and county councils – were given statutory powers to raise loans for sporting and recreational facilities. However, this provision proved to deliver less than it might have promised, given the traditional, and in this period even more pronounced, inequality between central and local government.[16] Comparing the New Zealand measure with its British original, Wellington's morning paper, the *Dominion*, considered the difference more one of 'presentation' than substance.[17]

Parry had originally proposed a 'National Council of Sport' to the large meeting of sports representatives he called together at Parliament in March 1937. The council's general object would be 'the encouragement and development of all sport with the co-operation of all the different sports bodies and the co-ordination of all their activities'.[18] While he was quick to reassure those present that 'the best forms of leisure and recreation are those which encourage the greatest measure of personal initiative and creative ability', Parry saw the new organisation as having overall oversight of physical education in schools, with its prime responsibility being 'to organize their national sports organisations so as to keep the young people fit during the rest of their lives'. 'For this purpose', Parry argued, 'I feel that the existing sports organisations should be dovetailed into the national physical educational system.' Existing organisations 'need not be interfered with so far as their domestic affairs are concerned', but the job of national organisation and co-ordination 'must' have 'intelligent national direction.' Citing various international examples of just such schemes and making reference to the government's broader plans for social security and health, he headed off the question of cost by setting out the classic health efficiency argument for such measures: money spent on sport and recreation 'will be saved in respect of the building of hospitals'.[19]

Many of his listeners were not convinced. Martin Luckie, representing the New Zealand Cricket Council, noted that the government's action 'in making the whole of Saturday free, a measure likely to become universal, was throwing a new burden on sports bodies'. The shortage of grounds was of particular concern in Wellington.[20] Luckie noted that the problem 'of money for running such grounds was one not looked on with favour by the ratepayers'. This was, indeed, to be a long-running dilemma in which sport was caught in the municipal sandwich – between central government's hands-off approach to providing facilities, and ratepayers' perennial niggardliness. The problem was exacerbated when community facilities such as halls, swimming pools and sports grounds were built using capital raised by major fundraising efforts, but lacked the ongoing income for their adequate maintenance. The vice-president of the Wellington Racing Club, C. W. Tringham, complimented the Minister but thought his plans 'did not go far enough'. Hon Sir William Perry, president of the long-established and powerful New Zealand Bowling Association (also national president of the Returned Services' Association and a member of the Legislative Council), was more challenging, pressing the Minister on how far the proposal was likely to go: was the government proposing a Ministry of Sport, as in France? And would the proposed national council be a government department? The need for intellectual as well as physical leisure was urged by Dr Anson of the Hutt Valley Gun Club.[21] Sounding a greater note of dissent, Harry Amos of the Olympic and Empire Games Council asked whether unanimity would be necessary for the National Council to be established. Adjourning the discussions until later in the year, allowing representatives to consult with executives and members, S. S. Deans, chairman of the New Zealand Rugby Union, concluded the meeting.[22]

The prospect of being brought into a single national council under government control was anathema to established sporting organisations. New Zealand's sporting culture was built on strong associational lines in which local clubs and codes guarded their interests with a fierce and proud independence. Organisations such as the New Zealand Cricket Council, New Zealand Rugby Union, New Zealand Bowling Association, New Zealand Golf Association, and their provincial and club constituents were represented by fervently autonomous self-governing bodies, with strong local interests and affiliations. Co-ordinating with other sports, or giving away powers and interests that had been hard won and were closely guarded were possible outcomes that were not only uninvited but also unwelcome.[23] When Parry's idea was discussed at club level, the suspicion and hostility were less guarded than they were in the precincts of Parliament. At the annual meeting of the Midlands Cricket Club strong objection was raised to the government's proposal. Mr Hatch, a club member, condemned what he saw as government interference in people's 'private life'. The meeting also addressed the problem of a 1.15 p.m. starting time for senior matches. Despite changes in hours of employment, some team members were still working on Saturday mornings and anticipated difficulties reaching their scheduled grounds in time for start of play.[24] Reservations about the Minister's intentions were not necessarily allayed by assurances such as those he gave when speaking to the Royal Life-Saving Society at their season opening night on 1 October 1937: Parry told the meeting that the council his legislation would create would not be 'concerned with making champions. It would be a question of creating physical fitness.'[25]

Perry's question to the Minister in Parliament articulated a suspicion that proved hard to dispel. Parry found himself continuing to have to explain that the government's policy of encouraging greater physical activity was purely voluntary and did not amount, in any way, to an attempt to make sports and recreation an extension of government bureaucracy. In its adoption and introduction of a slightly modified form of the British legislation, the New Zealand government had eventually had to bow to the pressure of the sporting associations, especially those representing the powerful national bodies governing men's sport, for assurances of autonomy and volunteerism. In particular, the National Council established by the Physical Welfare and Recreation Act was nothing like the representative or co-ordinating council for existing sports organisations that Parry had proposed early in 1937.

Work on the physical welfare and recreation scheme got underway in earnest after Parry returned from the Empire Games and celebrations marking Australia's 150th anniversary in Sydney in January 1938.[26] Four meetings of the National Council which were held during the year set up an ambitious programme of work. Perhaps wary of attracting accusations of favouritism, or simply out of conscientiousness, the Council resolved not to distribute any of its modest grant monies to sporting and recreational projects until a national survey of facilities and demands had been undertaken. The survey was never completed.[27] Only at the end of the year, and following Labour's return to office with the biggest electoral mandate in the country's history on the back of its massive social security scheme (due to take effect on 1 April 1939), could Heenan and Parry push forward with the physical welfare and recreation plans.[28] It was, in a sense, the icing on the cake of the government's reformist agenda.

Senior men's and women's officers were appointed to lead the newly created Physical Welfare Branch within the Department of Internal Affairs: C. Ruxton Bach, a graduate of the University of Southern California, at £420 per annum; and Helen Black, from Australia, at £320.[29] It was a sign of the difficulty that would follow and indeed plague the Physical Welfare Branch throughout its life, that the initial officers came from outside New Zealand. Apart from the third-year physical education speciality at Teachers' Training College (an option that had been unavailable since being a casualty of Depression retrenchment), there was no place for advanced training in physical education in the country. Staff with qualifications and experience were either those, like Bach and Black, recruited from outside New Zealand, or the very small number of New Zealanders who had studied overseas and returned, generally to positions in secondary schools or with the YWCA and YMCA.[30]

With a few exceptions, the Physical Welfare Branch had to rely on the general recruitment process into the government service, and the rather vague criteria as to the qualities needed to be a successful officer in what was a completely new field of public service. L. G. McDonald, an employee in the Auckland office of the Government Tourist Bureau, was one of a number of hopefuls who put his qualifications to Ruxton Bach in anticipation of combining his sporting passion with a livelihood. With a photograph as testimony to his letter, McDonald explained he had been a cricket, football and athletic representative at school, was the current New Zealand and Australasian Lightweight Lifting Champion, and was making a 'serious study' of physical culture. Ruxton Bach had to disappoint, but did hold out the prospect of study at his alma mater, the University of Southern California, although this was a costly option.[31] A year or two later, Helen Black commented unfavourably on the merits of Gisborne-born Dorothy Adams' suitability for a position in the Branch. With a certificate from the Sydney Women's League of Health and Beauty, Miss Adams was 'a very nice type of girl, but ... [would] conduct classes under the Bagot Stack System and this is a system open to question in the physical education world'.[32] That world was one in which some qualifications were more equal than others. In the much more developed realm of women's physical education training, which for various reasons had developed as a special field, professional qualifications were based on formal instruction in anatomy, physiology, and systems of exercise and movement such as those set out by the Swedish exponent Per Ling.[33]

In February 1939 a Fitness Week was organised to raise awareness throughout the country and to stimulate district committees into action.[34] A range of exhibitions, events, displays, sports matches and the like took place, attracting some press attention. Reports written at Head Office in Wellington highlighted the enthusiastic response by residents in the South Island town of Fairlie, rather than the surly quiescence of Wairarapa's Greytown.[35] Caroline Daley's discussion of the physical

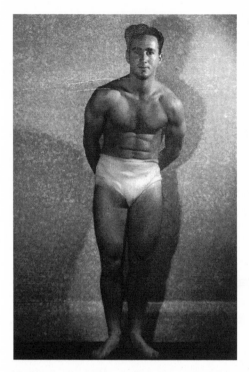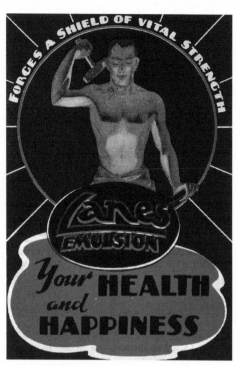

Working in the Auckland office of the New Zealand Government Tourist office L. G. McDonald saw more attractive prospects in the Physical Welfare Branch of the Department of Internal Affairs. He enclosed a photograph to accompany his letter of application for a position to the senior men's officer Ruxton Bach. For those people less dedicated to physical culture Lane's Emulsion offered a quicker path to vitality, strength and happiness. IA 1 139/27, Archives New Zealand, Wellington; Eph-A-Pharmacy-1936-01-front, Alexander Turnbull Library

welfare scheme contains a fuller description of the activities put on through the Fitness Week. These ranged from carnivals and mass demonstrations, hikes and surf lifesaving, to lunchtime and evening events during the week (free swimming, boxing and fencing classes), and radio programmes including a speech by Governor-General Lord Galway and endorsement by popular morning host 'Aunt Daisy' (Daisy Basham).[36] By August 1939 a further six staff had been appointed. A men's and a women's officer were employed for each of three districts which presented contrasting settings for developing physical welfare and recreation programmes: Waikato, with a densely settled farming population and several town centres; Wellington, as a major urban area; and rural Southland. A Recreation Week was run in September–October to emphasise the culture-oriented recreational as well as the physical side of activities that were more prominent in the earlier Fitness Week. There was a lot on the go.[37] Brochures to accompany early morning exercise radio broadcasts, and music suitable for exercises were published in 1939;[38] two mountain tracks and sets of huts were under construction to meet rising demand from those keen to enjoy 'the great outdoors' and the popularity of what was known in New Zealand as 'tramping';[39] a Group Travel scheme was set up offering groups of twenty or more holidays costing no more than £1 a day;[40] an information section was collecting and distributing handbooks, guides and curricula – including a thick set of materials Helen Black brought back from a visit to Sydney in early 1940;[41] schemes for running holiday and playground activities were in the wings; and events were organised as part of the Centennial Exhibition that opened in Wellington in November 1939 and attracted over two million visitors in its five months to May 1940, marking the nation's founding in 1840. On Easter Saturday, 23 March 1940, physical welfare officer Noeline Thomson co-ordinated a major Girls Centennial Inter-House Display in the central Exhibition Court. Teams of young women from Masterton, Hawke's Bay, Palmerston North, Wellington and Wanganui took part in a series of spectacular gymnastic and exercise routines.[42] In the event Parry was not able to be in Wellington on the day, but his speech notes prepared for the occasion applauded what was on show: 'I very much admire the simplicity and gracefulness of your outfits. They exemplify the modern outlook of women of this country which is noble, matter of fact, clean and practical, necessary, no doubt, in peacetime, but more so when we are at war'.[43]

While the early stages of the physical welfare programme were set in action by the energetic Ruxton Bach and Helen Black, their recently arrived and more senior colleague in the Department of Education, Philip Smithells, also played a highly influential role. Smithells, at age 29, was appointed to head the newly formed Physical Education Branch within the Department of Education. He was responsible for physical education amongst school-aged children (5–15 year-olds). Overhauling and extending the existing curriculum and giving greater priority to physical education within primary and secondary schooling were part of the wider expansion of education driven by Clarence Beeby and his Minister, the powerful Fraser (who became Prime Minister following Savage's death in March 1940). Cambridge-educated, baritone-voiced and in demeanour the epitome of the public school Englishman, Smithells was anything but an orthodox product of that system. A background at the alternative Bedales School, the influence of R. E. Roper, a recent three-month touring scholarship in the United States, and a strong interest in drama and the humanities gave Smithells more of an interest in the cultures of body movement than in conventional sports and physique. At the Department of Education, and then as the founding director of the School of Physical Education established at the University of Otago in 1947, Smithells was highly influential in shaping physical education in New Zealand for more than forty years.[44]

Smithells, together with Rona Stephenson (later Bailey), one of the six physical welfare officers employed in August 1939, brought to the New Zealand programme a powerful commitment to physical activity that went further than Labour's notion

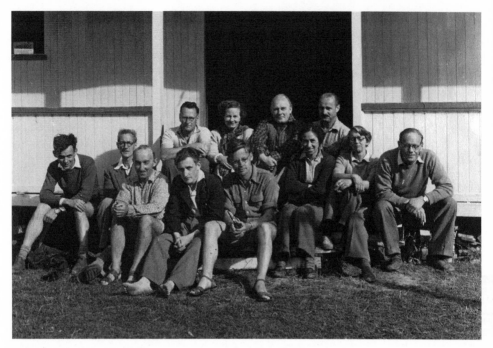

Philip Smithells (third from left in back row) at NZUSA Student Congress, Curious Cove, Queen Charlotte Sound, 1952. Smithells sought the company of literary and intellectual figures rather than 'sporty' types. Others present include W. B. Sutch, J. K. and Jacqui Baxter, Bob Chapman, and the Hulmes (Canterbury University). POO-045, Hocken Library

of constructive leisure. Both were drawn to the work by a radical vision of how the active body could be a basis for social as well as individual transformation. Rona Stephenson had been in the United States at the same time as Smithells in 1937–38, as a New Zealand student at the University of California, Berkeley, and then at Columbia in New York. She had been tremendously excited and inspired by contemporary dance and movement exponents such as Martha Graham and Josephine Rathbone. Originally from Gisborne, where she excelled in both sport and academic work, Stephenson attended teachers' training college but had been denied the third year 'phys ed' speciality because of the Depression. At the same time she had been selected in the first national basketball team to play against Australia. Returning to New Zealand from the United States, she worked briefly as a physical education teacher at Woodford House before joining the Physical Welfare Branch. To the Branch she was a rare and valuable find, having university training as well as possessing practical and physical abilities.[45]

Aged 24, Stephenson began work as the women's officer in the Waikato district office, based in Hamilton but travelling as far south as Taumaranui. In Hamilton she was keenly involved in the People's Theatre.[46] Moving to Wellington in 1943 to take up the position of Senior Women's Officer following Helen Black's return to

Australia, Rona also moved away from her first, brief marriage (to Ron Meek) and into a long-standing political commitment to the Communist Party. Smithells may not have fully shared Rona's political views, but they shared a great deal in their approach to physical education and physical welfare generally, and became close friends and colleagues. In July 1943 Rona spoke on sport and culture in the Soviet Union to a meeting of the New Zealand Society for Closer Relations with Russia, chaired by Philip Smithells. Smithells too found his first marriage did not endure, but his second wife, Olive Whitta, was a life-long exponent of fitness.[47]

Working through the Departments of Education and Internal Affairs respectively, Philip Smithells and Rona Stephenson were responsible for developing physical education programmes, training junior instructors and leaders, and encouraging various forms of exercise and movement. Both were keen to expand the scope of activities encompassed by their programmes. They were part of a political and cultural avant garde, interested in jazz, in coffee rather than tea, alive to American as well as British alternative ideas, and convinced of the politics of culture as well as the culture of politics. To those engaged in theatre, publishing and the arts in what Rachel Barrowman has described as 'a popular vision', Smithells and Stephenson sought to add the body in dance and movement as a site of radical expression.[48] With several others they formed the New Dance Group, 1945–47, exploring contemporary themes in the vocabulary of the modern dance ideas they admired.[49] It is a testament both to the critical role that could be played by individuals, and especially strong-minded individuals, and to the range of meanings that 'physical welfare' was open to at this time, that Philip Smithells and Rona Stephenson were able to bring a modernist, emancipist, strong vision of 'body work' to government-sponsored programmes of physical education and welfare. But the approach jarred with the more conventional notions of some of their colleagues, and of the majority of New Zealanders.

Working and Playing in Wartime

Rona Stephenson was still working in the Waikato district when war was declared. Prime Minister Savage's broadcast speech set out the basis on which New Zealand was going to war. Although Recreation Week (26 September–2 October) and the Centennial Exhibition (November 1939–May 1940) went ahead, the resources of government were quickly turned to supporting New Zealand's fighting troops and wartime production. Enlistment of men began immediately, the first echelon of soldiers leaving Wellington for the Middle East in early January 1940.[50] Recruitment of physical welfare officers stepped up and, while a number of them were called up for active service abroad, others were employed in a narrower range of work, providing physical training to the armed services, the Home Guard, the Air Training Corps and the women's auxiliaries.

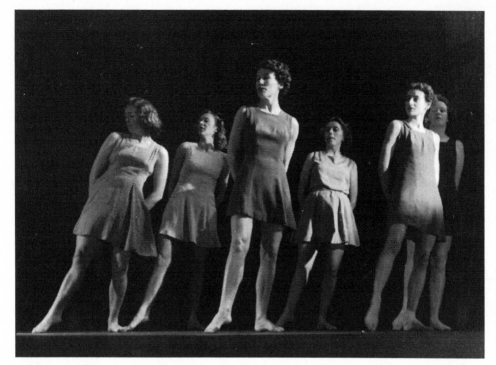

Rona Bailey (Stephenson), far right, performing with the New Dance Group, Wellington, 1947. Their style of movement, music and dance themes were highly contemporary. Items included those on the bombing of Hiroshima and labour relations in factories. Photograph by Neville Lewers. PAColl-6180-10-25, Alexander Turnbull Library

Work amongst the adult civilian population continued, but with a different focus. Women officers led keep-fit classes for the voluntary Women's War Service Auxiliary (WWSA), and stepped up work with women industrial workers and those under the sometimes tedious restriction of the 'manpower' control exercised by the Department of Labour (industrial conscription was introduced in March 1942).[51] It was in its contact with women and its organising work that some of the most innovative and enduring work of the Branch was achieved.[52]

While being active and fit were now regarded as necessities for women and girls, the style and practice of fitness were clearly distinguished from what was regarded as appropriate for men. Descriptions of the culminating display of the January 1942 Physical Welfare Branch officers' refresher course held in Lower Hutt illustrate the difference. The display was attended by the Minister of Health and Prime Minister Peter Fraser, the leader of the Opposition and various other Cabinet members. Reporting made it clear that the women's exercises, directed by Helen Black, 'differ from men's training, and are planned with due regard to the physiological and physical development of women. They feature rhythm, natural movement, grace, litheness, and general freedom.' On the other hand, the men's display was marked by a range of exercises that included boxing, wrestling and unarmed combat, with the programme 'top dressed' with 'clever acrobatic feats'.[53]

The provision of recreation for women at home as well as those in work was promoted by women's officers in various parts of the country. In Auckland, Gladys Gebbie started a highly successful recreation club for those later described as 'climbing the ladder of life': 40–60 year olds. Indoor bowls and swimming were particularly popular, with those participating in the latter adopting the name the Splash Club.[54] With 350 members at its height, the Auckland club drew out those reticent to use swimming baths during general opening hours, and to whom existing sports clubs and public facilities did not necessarily appeal. The Splash Club's success was noted as having brought 'considerable happiness to many homes, as the mother now has her recreational activities and is able to interest the family in the Club, instead of as before, having to listen to what the family have been doing [and] not being able to contribute anything of what she has been doing in the recreational line'.[55] In a series of radio talks broadcast on Christchurch station 3YA on Fridays at 11 a.m., Noeline Thomson, the local physical welfare women's officer, provided information and encouragement to women to get out and about, to play games and stay fit. She spoke as someone prepared to take up the challenge. In January 1938, Thomson cycled from her home in Oamaru to Auckland, and back. [56]

While women's physical recreation and sport were not invented during the war years or promoted exclusively by the Physical Welfare Branch, they had been significantly expanded and put on a stronger organisational footing. The YWCA had been by far the most important force and, by the 1930s, was employing the first full-time directors of physical activity programmes. In Wellington Helen Macdonald took up a post at the YWCA in 1938; she was followed by the highly qualified and inspirational Gisa Taglicht.[57] In the world of employment, interhouse sports associations, formed by workplace teams, were in existence in Wellington in the early 1930s, in Hawke's Bay and in Christchurch, and appeared sporadically elsewhere. Running annual sports days was their major activity. As in England, the Women's League of Health and Beauty drew a keen crowd when Millicent and Caroline Ward arrived fresh from London with their Bagot Stack training, setting up groups in Auckland (1937) and Wellington (1938). Within months of arriving in Auckland, Millicent was conducting a mass demonstration in the Auckland Town Hall, the evening presided over by the Mayor; while in Wellington, Caroline Ward attracted the endorsement of prominent orthopaedic surgeon and public figure Alexander Gillies for her Town Hall demonstration on 1 August 1938.

The Wards brought with them a dash of fame and glamour, and the kind of success that echoed that of the movement's central figure, Prunella Stack. The promise of health, beauty and fun, tied to the wider purposes of the age, had a winning appeal. Millicent Ward was widely admired as a public speaker, and appeared on the platform alongside Dorothy Graham, Ruth Niblock and Elsie Freeman (later Locke) in a debate organised by the progressive magazine *Woman To-day*. The topic was 'What I think of the outlook for world peace'.[58] But the League branches, like other popular dance and exercise classes offered by women teachers, were hard to keep going financially. Although branches of the League continued, in Hamilton and Wanganui as well as in Auckland and Wellington, they were never to recover their early prominence after Millicent's departure to Australia in 1941 and her marriage to neurosurgeon Anthony James. In the main cities the League's constituency was drawn more from single working women than from other groups.

Because of the time, organising skills, access to typing, duplicating and postage services the physical welfare officers had, they were able to extend the existing provision for women's sport. Although bowls was a popular sport throughout the country, the women's game was much less developed than the men's. There were local clubs and regional competitions in some parts of the country, but no national organisation or competition. Impeding the growth of the sport was women's limited access to bowling clubs and greens. Most greens were owned by men's clubs which showed a general reluctance to admit women for more than a few hours' play per week. Noeline Thomson, as physical welfare officer, was able to use the resources of her position to co-ordinate existing office-holders in the sport into forming a national organisation and competition, and cajoling the men's organisation to provide better access to the sport. Similar initiatives were taken by physical welfare officers in forming national organisations for volleyball, indoor basketball and softball. All of these national bodies have had a continuing life.[59]

While there were organisations and employers that promoted fitness for workers, especially their women workforces, in a piecemeal fashion, this commitment was a major focus of attention for the women physical welfare officers during and after the war years. Women employed in routine jobs on assembly lines, in biscuit factories, as clothing machinists, in meat and vegetable processing and packing, at the W. D. and H. O. Wills tobacco factory, and in bakeries; as shop assistants in specialist and department stores; and in service work in laundries and cafeterias, were among those at the forefront of the Physical Welfare Branch scheme. Recreation was seen not only as lifting morale during wartime, but, above all, as providing relief from the dull monotony of days spent on the assembly line and in routine tasks indoors.

These women were mostly the young, low-paid and junior ranks of the workforce. Before the school leaving age was raised to 15 in 1944, a larger section of the workforce was made up of 14–18 year-olds. They occupied an in-between status, not quite grown up but no longer wholly under the authority of home and school. Past school age, and perceived as having either too much or too little time for constructive leisure, the young women workers attracted the attention of the government scheme. It was this group Helen Black had in mind when she talked about the 'Miss

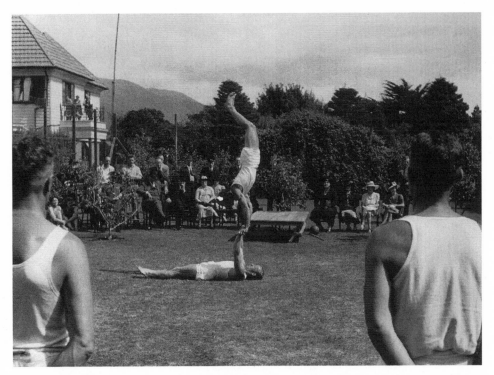

Men from the Physical Welfare Branch demonstrating feats of skill, strength and balance before Bill Parry, Minister of Internal Affairs (seated on left in central group), Prime Minister Peter Fraser and other dignitaries, c.1941. W. E. Parry Album, Ciochetto Family Collection

Fourteens' in her address to the Women's Social Progress League in September 1941. The 'girls' at Mercer whose plight was drawn to Bill Parry's attention on a visit in 1943 are others who belonged to this section of the workforce.[60] Employed in the Refreshment Rooms at the local railway station, the young women had very little opportunity for recreation of any kind. Apart from 'pictures very occasionally and ... a dance, again very occasionally', Parry wrote to Heenan, there 'is no tennis court, no basketball area, no facilities for indoor tennis, etc., and no club for cultural recreation. In consequence the girls are not contented and lack interest.' This was bad enough, but it was made worse by the social confines in which they lived and worked. 'The refreshment room girls are under the control of the head waitress both at work and at the hostel where they sleep. From what was represented, in some cases that control appeared to be irksome to the girls.' This was the situation that Parry saw as exactly one where 'great work for the welfare of the girls might be undertaken by one of the Department's physical welfare officers, or by a leader working under her guidance'.[61]

From these seeds – the YWCA, interhouse sports associations, and the provision of sports and fitness training by the Physical Welfare Branch, as well as the

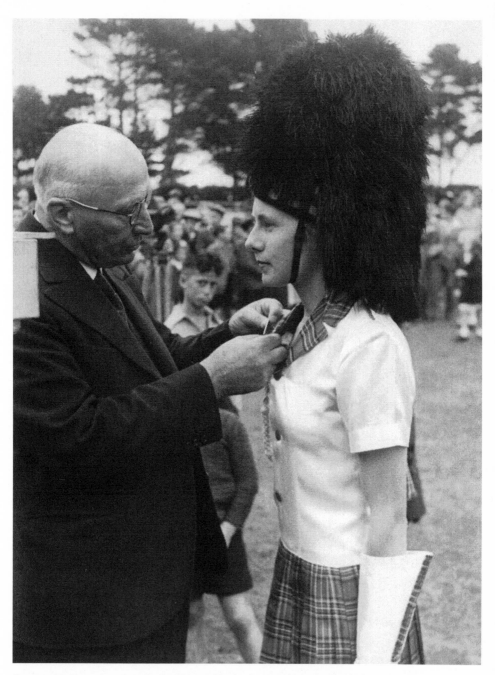

Encouraging the summer sport of 'girls marching' was something the Physical Welfare Branch regarded with pride. Bill Parry, Minister of Internal Affairs, awarding a medal to a member of a winning marching team, probably at the New Zealand Marching Association National Championships c.1947–48. W. E. Parry Album, Ciochetto Family Collection

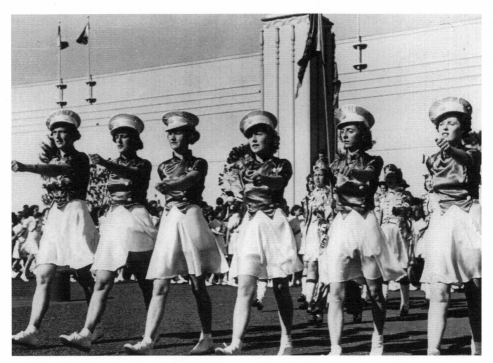

One of the marching teams taking part in the massed display of Girls' Interhouse sports teams on Easter Saturday, March 1940. The event was staged in the main concourse at the Centennial Exhibition in Wellington. The modernist style of Edmund Anscombe's buildings can be seen in the background. IA 62 4/38, Archives New Zealand

wartime pervasiveness of march routines and drill – came the inspiration for 'girls' marching' and its emergence as a major competitive sport. Teams of seven, and then nine, young women, dressed in identical uniforms performing military-style drill routines to the accompaniment of brass or highland pipe bands, were the core of the marching phenomenon. Under the encouragement of some of the physical welfare officers, this activity was fostered and developed into a competitive sport. Teams practised a set routine programme and then performed it before a judging panel in competition for points.[62]

Marching teams, as they became known, quickly became popular in various parts of the country. Leadership was provided by physical welfare officers, Miriel Woods being a guiding light in Timaru and around the Canterbury district. Coaches were found among retired sergeant majors and men from the forces familiar with military drill, now adapted to the competitive sports ground rather than the military parade ground, and performed by young women rather than military cadets. Members of the team generally designed and made their own uniforms, drawing on an ensemble of military dress and ceremonial uniforms, highland band accoutrements, including spats, Glengarry hats, busbys, epaulettes and lanyards, with chevrons, bell-hop caps and colours drawn from Hollywood glitz. It allowed for an inventive adaptation of a uniformed aesthetic, one that highlighted display and uniformity and drew attention to the legs and rigid torso – with white laced boots, short skirts, tight tunics and elaborate hats.

Marching became one of the jewels in the crown of the Physical Welfare Branch. Strongly supported by senior staff, especially Assistant Secretary Arthur Harper, marching was fostered by its officers throughout the country. The resources of the Branch and the Department of Internal Affairs as a whole were put behind the formation of a national marching association, and the codification of the activity as a competitive sport. In the late 1940s, national championships were attended by an impressive array of public figures – the governor-general, prime minister, leader of the Opposition, and other important political and public figures.

Marching was a local creation – a sport that was invented in New Zealand. It is distinguished from American cheerleading, with which it is sometimes compared, by being an independent competitive sport rather than an auxiliary activity to another game. It drew on some features of contemporary popular entertainment such as chorus girl routines, and especially the kind of highly synchronised performances made famous by New York's 'Rockettes', but it was always conceived as an outdoor sport and never as indoor entertainment. From the 1940s through to the late twentieth century, marching constituted a major summer sport for women and girls. While still in existence, it has faded from its earlier pre-eminent position. In 1952 the champion senior team, Dunedin's Blair Athol, travelled to Britain and Australia. The trip was partly proselytising and was intended to showcase the new sport. Audrey Paine, a member of the team, later recalled the lengthy preparations and fundraising undertaken by the thirteen members of the touring team, aged sixteen to twenty-three years, on what turned out to be the 'tour of a lifetime'. Britain's Central Council for Physical Recreation was involved in devising the itinerary and arrangements. While teams were for a time in operation in England and Australia, marching has not thrived outside New Zealand.[63]

Marching's success resounded with the predominant conservative and conventional strands in New Zealand's society and culture in the mid-twentieth century, rather than the modernist avant garde represented by Smithells and Stephenson. Drawing strongly on royalist sentiments, pageantry, a diasporic enthusiasm for tartans, pipe bands and the trappings of royal Scotland,[64] and the controlled exposure of young female bodies (legs in particular), marching offered a performance of order and highly orchestrated synchronicity. It could hardly have been more at odds with the spontaneity, fluidity and simplicity of the free and natural movement that appealed to the New Dance Group, or that which was being taught at the Wellington YWCA and elsewhere by Gisa Taglicht. Taglicht, a European refugee, brought formal training in modern movement to her classes. But it was the loose tunic-clad, barefoot, free-moving members of Gisa Taglicht's troupe that drew a hostile response when featured in a National Film Unit documentary, *Rhythm and Movement*, in 1948 rather than the populist marching teams. While there were those who expressed distaste for the spectacle of young women performing highly rigid military steps to whistled commands, either because of its shades of totalitarianism, or because of the sight of middle-aged men coaching slightly clad young women, they were in a small minority. Marching's exuberant anti-modernism was appealing and popular in 1940s and 1950s New Zealand.

The most expansive phase of Parry's physical welfare and recreation scheme came in the years 1945–48. With the war's end in sight, Parry had gone back to Parliament with a case for greater funding for his scheme. Now more than ever, he argued, New Zealanders deserved a holiday from the stresses of the war years; now was the time for the forty-hour, five-day week to be fully realised; and now was the time for sports and leisure organisations and facilities to catch up after their wartime neglect. By 1944 Parry could also note that New Zealand's scheme, in legislation since 1937, was part of a wider initiative taken not only in Britain but also in Australia and Canada. In all these 'British countries', he noted, the schemes were similar in principles and practice, and regimentation just as absent across all four. Any differences were ones of procedure rather than substance.[65]

With a steep increase in funding, the staff of the Branch expanded to just over sixty at its height in 1948. Technical and clerical personnel at Head Office supported physical welfare officers in twenty-one district offices. Supporting recreation clubs, organising sports events of various kinds from specialist athletic coaching to teaching new games such as softball and indoor basketball, assisting in planning for community centres, running learn-to-swim classes, providing leadership training for church and other service groups, and distributing information about physical education and facilities were among the many activities undertaken by physical welfare officers. They participated in the design, commissioning and filming of a 'community playground' in the Hutt Valley suburb of Naenae, a model of planned, ideal living, and a project that was characteristic of the expansive mood of the era.[66]

The goal of the 1937 initiative, to support sport and recreation with public funds, finally became possible. In 1947, £36,440 was distributed to 'beneficiaries includ[ing] tennis, cricket, bowling, basketball, yachting, and rowing clubs'; to community centres and recreation grounds; to local authorities; to Boy Scouts and other youth organisations; and to church groups and branches of the YMCA and YWCA. Grants were made 'on the self-help principle', the Department providing £1 for every £1 raised for approved projects. That year it 'estimated that the result of the pooling of the departmental and local funds has been an increase of more than £100,000 in the value of recreational facilities'. Nearly half went to recreation grounds such as playing fields, tennis courts and bowling greens.[67] The detailed annual reporting

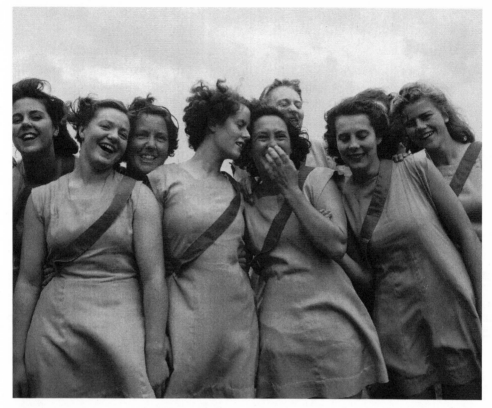

Physical Welfare Branch women officers photographed in a break in a training course, Hutt Valley, March 1944. The photographer was their fellow Department of Internal Affairs staff member, writer and keen mountaineer John Pascoe. John Pascoe Collection, F-977-1/4, Alexander Turnbull Library

of grants, by organisation and by region, was a response to tensions created by applications considerably outrunning the funds available, and the irritation caused by what was perceived as overly intrusive inspections by physical welfare officers on how monies had been spent. While funds were welcome, the associated scrutiny, and disappointed applicants, raised tensions.

Amongst the many activities undertaken in this highwater period of the Physical Welfare Branch's life were attempts to extend its work to the Māori section of New Zealand's population, both the majority still living in largely remote rural areas in the North Island, and the increasing numbers of mostly young adult working-age men and women now residing in provincial towns and the main cities. The work of the Physical Welfare Branch was seen as a useful part of a wider policy designed to modernise and 'develop' those whose standard of living, health and lifespan were markedly poorer than those of the Pākehā majority. Māori service in World War II, both in the armed services and in the war effort at home, propelled greater state action in what Māori statesman Sir Apirana Ngata termed 'the price of citizenship'.[68]

While there had been some interest in promoting physical welfare amongst Māori from the early days of the Branch, including an offer by Hirone Wikiriwhi in 1939 to set up keep-fit classes in Hawke's Bay, these efforts remained scattered and piecemeal.[69] By 1948 the renamed Department of Maori (previously 'Native') Affairs, under its first Māori head, Tipi Ropiha, was actively charging Māori welfare officers in districts throughout the country with a range of housing, employment, education and social welfare responsibilities flowing from the 1945 Maori Social and Economic Advancement Act. Many of the Welfare Division officers employed by the Department were returned servicemen with distinguished war records, who brought to their work an outlook different from that of their predecessors. In July 1948 physical welfare officers were instructed to seek out opportunities to co-operate with these colleagues in district offices throughout the country, seeing what they could do to make sport and recreation part of the general 'welfare' work under way.[70] Sport and recreation were seen as valuable in promoting health and work efficiency; in forestalling 'problems' in the 'adjustment' of young Māori newly arrived in provincial towns and main cities, particularly in the evenings and weekends; and in instilling habits that would fit with the modernist demands of a waged workforce (as opposed to 'traditional' life in the pā).

Volleyball, badminton, softball, square-dancing, marching, tennis, athletics and indoor recreation clubs were among the activities supported by physical welfare officers in districts, variously working with their Maori Welfare Division colleagues. In Taranaki, Vilma Macdonald got a volleyball club playing once a week and formed a Māori marching team in New Plymouth; a softball team had started in Waitara and two Māori leaders had learned the basics of square-dance calling to teach others in their communities. From Whangarei, Norman Helleur reported that all his work was with Māori as they made up the majority of those living in Northland. From Hamilton, Thomas Heard detailed a range of activities including assisting with the construction of two asphalt tennis courts at the Maniapoto Lawn Tennis Club, organising a Māori athletic championship, and running a series of square-dancing instruction sessions that included a finale at the Hangatiki Hall in which the local Māori community provided the orchestra.[71]

Roy Sheffield, based in Gisborne on the East Coast, where the majority population was Māori, reported a similar range of activities.[72] In June 1949 Sheffield concluded his account of recent initiatives by especially noting that at

... Te Araroa – a difficult district in the East Cape – a special magistrate's report was submitted last year in which it was stated that never before had the figures for juvenile delinquency been so low. This was a direct result of the indoor sports club I established there in April of last year, and is an obvious commentary on its social value.[73]

Sport and recreation as a form of social control, as well as a source of enjoyment, was apparent. Sheffield may also have been anxious to provide a rationale for ongoing support of the work of the Branch when it was coming under greater scrutiny. Earlier in the year he had submitted a detailed report on the dearth of recreational facilities in the adjoining large and sparsely populated Urewera district, which had drawn a sharp and angry defence from the State Forest Service. The Forest Service was upset at Sheffield's criticism of the lack of sporting and recreational amenities in the new timber towns, citing a shortage of labour as the main reason.[74] The family and social tensions within new, remote and poorly serviced communities, and the large gulf that existed between the material and amenity life in towns and cities (and even better-off rural areas) and poorer, often Māori-dominated rural areas were starkly evident in Sheffield's survey of the district.[75]

How long any of these initiatives lasted, and their enduring impact – if any – are difficult to gauge. They did not arrive into a vacuum. Sporting activities were well developed in many Māori communities at this time and, in places where Māori and Pākehā lived side by side, sport was a site where intermixing was common.[76] On the East Coast, tennis and hockey tournaments had flourished in the 1920s and 1930s, as they had in some other places. Major hui such as those held to celebrate the founding of the Ratana movement were often accompanied by major sports tournaments. Several major Māori sports organisations including the Maori Golf Association (1931) and Maori Rugby League Board (1934) were formed during the 1930s. But many communities struggled to build and maintain good-quality sports grounds and courts, and indoor spaces suitable for evening and winter use. Halls with low ceilings were a particular impediment. Aroha Harris' recent powerful discussion of Māori–state interactions in this period invites an understanding that reaches beyond a story of government policy (right or wrong), or 'Māori adaptation' (successful or not). Instead, she depicts a careful, varying and skilful set of steps through which an 'intelligent, critical, vibrant Māori leadership [was] involved in highly nuanced and complex interactions with the state'.[77] At the 'complicated and congested nexus' at which tribal committees, branches of the Maori Women's Welfare League and the Welfare Division of the Department of Maori Affairs met, a number of moves were possible. Harris uses the metaphor of the dance to convey the multi-sided dynamic of the story; the square-dancing promoted by the physical welfare officers was one of the actual dances being performed around marae in the late 1940s and 1950s.

Māori games and physical recreation also travelled in the other direction. Indigenous pursuits were looked to by innovators such as Philip Smithells and Rona Bailey to give a local content to the physical education curriculum in general use. Applying for his inaugural position at the University of Otago at the end of 1946, Smithells made particular mention of 'the physical education activities of the Maori'

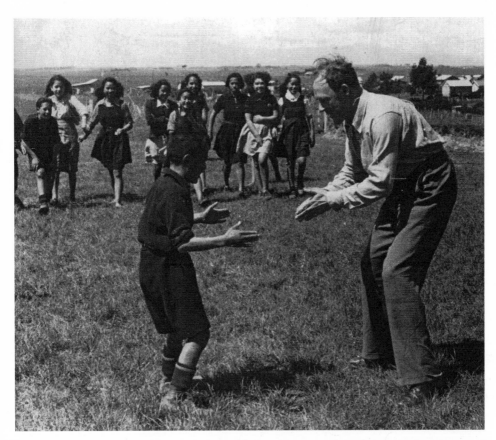

Philip Smithells playing the game 'Homai' with Māori children at Ratana, 1943. The game was played between pairs smacking hands on the thighs in response to calls. Smithells was keen to incorporate Māori games into the wider New Zealand curriculum for physical education. Games should reflect local culture was his argument. It was a progressive idea, but the terms on which such cultural exchanges took place would later be challenged. MS-1001/455, Smithells Papers, Hocken Library

that had been incorporated into the school physical education curriculum. 'That this portion of our cultural heritage has been spread so far, and is now recognised as a form of physical education, (as it was by the old Maoris), is the achievement of which I am most proud.'[78] Stick and poi games were among the activities to which Smithells was pointing. They had been incorporated into the physical education curriculum he developed first for primary and secondary schools at the Department of Education, and then as part of training teachers at the School of Physical Education at the University of Otago.[79] Smithells argued strongly that 'each country must evolve its own programme and method, and not just adopt those suited to other climates and traditions'. Such an approach meshed well with the nation- and culture-building impetus strongly driven at both the political and administrative levels in the Savage–Fraser government and more broadly amongst the 'cultural nationalist' generation. Wellington-born Brian Sutton-Smith, author of *The Ambiguity of Play* (1997), wrote his first study of the meeting of Māori and European cultures in the play of Māori children in the early 1950s; he went on to become the foremost theorist of play. In the eyes of a later generation, such activities could be seen less favourably as instances of cultural appropriation.[80]

A Welfare State but Not a Leisure State

Ironically, perhaps, the very flourishing of sport and recreation in the postwar years spelt the death knell for the Physical Welfare Branch and Parry's experiment in state-funded fun. After a brief spurt of activity from 1945–48, political, administrative and public support for the work of the Branch fell away, receding with the outgoing tide that washed away the urgency that the Depression and war had brought to government intervention. The 1949 general election marked the end of Labour's fourteen years in power; National was to govern for all but six of the next thirty-five years (1949–57, 1960–72, 1975–84).[81] While the differences between the two parties in New Zealand politics through this time were not large, being more matters of emphasis rather than ideology, they were evident at the margins of state activity such as those that had flourished under Parry and Heenan in the Department of Internal Affairs.[82] What New Zealanders did in their leisure time – cultural, sporting or recreational activities – were now seen less as things in which government might be involved. If public funds were to be used they were to be at minimal levels, or, preferably, through the transfer of funds from those raised in the leisure pursuit of betting (the government-run 'art union', TAB and Golden Kiwi lottery) and distributed by a grants board to sporting, community and cultural organisations. In the machinery of the 1950s and 1960s, lottery funds produced from state-run gaming continued as vital sustenance to meet the costs associated with sport and recreation. It was an era when amateurism was extolled, and when gaming proceeds, tobacco sponsorship and municipal funding paid many of the bills. Alongside all of this there was the considerable input of parental and other adults' voluntary labour and time, serving as fund-raisers, coaches, umpires and referees, uniform makers and maintainers, billeters of visiting players, transport providers and the like. As funding became a matter of competitive application to a single board, rivalry between sectors grew. Culture and sport, complementary under the Parry and Heenan regime, became increasingly positioned as rival groupings.[83]

Parry's precious scheme was not killed off under the new regime but was largely deprived of vital resources – both funds and people – and left to shrivel. Heenan's retirement in January 1949, after a lengthy and notable career of public service, marked the end of an era. Philip Smithells had left Wellington to start the School of Physical Education in Dunedin in 1947, the capital and the public service thereby losing a powerful and articulate champion of physical education.

Rona Bailey (formerly Stephenson), the influential senior women's officer, also became less involved in the late 1940s through absence overseas and then a period combating tuberculosis. She resigned from the Branch finally in 1952.[84] Even before the change of government, disquiet over the effectiveness of the Physical Welfare Branch had prompted a highly critical Public Service Commission enquiry. Its major recommendation, that the Branch be transferred to and amalgamated with the Physical Education Branch of the Department of Education, was stillborn.[85] As the Head Office of the Branch shrank to a staff of merely two by 1957, its focus became similarly defensive: providing support for Nevile Lodge's film *How to Drown,* which was part of a Prevent Drowning campaign, and similar work in mountain safety.[86]

As well as this general lean towards a greater role for private life and property as opposed to government ownership and control, the National government perceived little need for additional encouragement of sport and recreation in the postwar world. Up and down the country people were keenly playing every kind of sport, and enjoying their 'free' weekends and regular summer holidays. Even better, New Zealanders were winning on the world stage. The golden era of athletic triumph spanned from Yvette Williams winning gold in the long jump at the Helsinki Olympics in 1952 through to Halberg, Snell and Lydiard in the early 1960s. The main problem was not one of urging people to play but finding sufficient grounds and courts to enable all who wanted to play space in which to do so. Greymouth's basketball problem was typical of the time. The town had so many girls and young women's teams keen to play in the Saturday competition and so few courts that they closed off the main street for several hours on Saturday afternoons, converting the street to a playing space to make the winter competition possible.[87] In Dunedin, the demand for tennis courts was apparently insatiable. Even with the shortage of materials and labour, and the still rather straitened financial circumstances of many households, the combined tennis clubs of Dunedin raised £7,000 to build new courts to support demand for weekend and midweek play.[88] Throughout the country there was a major expansion of new housing on city fringes, driven by the unprecedented popularity of marriage and the consequent baby boom. Suburbs, rather than the city centres, which were largely deserted during evenings and weekends, became the place to find fun and company. Halls, courts and schools were all places for games and sport and recreation, as well as for meetings, films, church services, Boy Scouts and Girl Guides, and bible classes.

The characterisation of the 1950s as a decade dominated by 'rugby, racing and beer' may have been something of an exaggeration, but it captured the centrality of male sociability as the cultural keystone. Playing, and leisure in general, was people's private business, done – or not – in their own time and in their own way, not a matter of government interest. Voluntary efforts and amateur sport played by free citizens in free time as a matter of free will came to be reasserted as a cornerstone of civic culture, providing popular understandings of what it was to live in a capitalist democracy at a time when the Cold War gave 'the big state' a threatening rather than reassuring aspect.[89] Even the small flurry of disquiet that flared across the national stage after the highly respected wartime commander, Major-General Howard Kippenberger spoke out against the injustice of Māori players being ineligible for selection for the 1949 All Black tour to South Africa subsided quickly. If it was a concern, and it wasn't very much of one, it was a matter for the New Zealand Rugby Football Union rather than for the government.[90] Rumours that the Physical Welfare Branch was organising a national square-dancing competition only fanned smouldering suspicion about the Branch's work. Hilda Ross, National MP for Hamilton and Minister Responsible for the Welfare of Women and Children, was withering in her attack on this waste of public funds at a time when other demands were patently more pressing.[91]

Labour did not breathe new life into the Physical Welfare Branch when re-elected in 1957, but reactivated the issue of physical fitness and leisure in the very different circumstances of the early 1970s. A Ministry of Recreation and Sport and the New Zealand Council for Recreation and Sport were established by statute in 1973 to provide policy and distribute funding rather than to direct the activities themselves.[92] These new initiatives were also prompted by Christchurch's anticipated hosting of the Commonwealth Games in 1974 and the major public resources such events by then demanded. They also drew some momentum from recent concern at the over-abundance of sedentary leisure perceived as the product of the television age, and a fear that volunteer-supported community organisations were entering a period of crisis.[93] The widely promoted Come Alive campaign in 1975 urged New Zealanders to get up from their overly comfortable armchairs arrayed before the blue-lit TV sets in their homes and to do something active in the open air. A sense that outdoor activity held greater virtue persisted.[94]

A different kind of controversy about government involvement in sport came to occupy a central place in New Zealand political life from the late 1960s. It involved the same issue of rugby contact with South Africa as had been raised in 1949. The Norman Kirk-led government of 1972–74 was also confronted, as were its National predecessors and successors, with an increasingly vocal lobby group demanding a stop to sporting contacts with the apartheid regime in South Africa. Rugby tours between arch rivals the New Zealand All Blacks and South African Springboks were the most anticipated of sporting clashes, the pinnacle of the national sport, and thus fuel for a rapidly escalating controversy. Alongside those calling for support for New Zealand to join the international boycott isolating the apartheid regime came equally vociferous calls to 'keep politics out of sport'. The Kirk government was the only one to support the boycott, refusing to issue visas to the Springbok team scheduled to tour in 1973. The Muldoon-led National government in power from

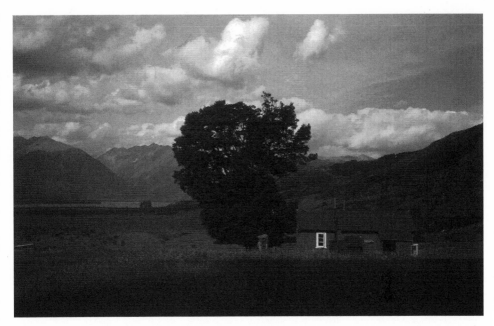

Hut Number 2 in the Hurunui Valley at the head of Lake Sumner, Canterbury, one of five built as part of the Harper Pass tramping track by the Physical Welfare Branch. Imagination seems to have paused when it came to the naming of huts on the track, never advancing beyond Numbers 1 – Number 5. The hut (modified since first construction) was destroyed by fire in 1996. Mark Pickering

late 1975 to mid-1984 reversed the policy, leaving the matter to the NZRFU. The Springbok team's tour to New Zealand during the winter of 1981 was accompanied by widespread and violent protests. The Third Test, at Auckland's Eden Park, was the final game of the tour. It was played under siege. The Springboks spent the night before the game locked inside the ground, and during the game a small aeroplane dropped flour bombs onto the field. Sport had indelibly become political in what is often described as New Zealand's twentieth-century civil war.[95]

While National governments supported the existing machinery of sport and recreation administration (largely dependent on lottery funds), it was the Labour administrations which reconfigured it, first by turning the Ministry and Council into the Hillary Commission in 1987. The Commission, in turn, was superseded by SPARC (Sport and Recreation New Zealand, in operation from 1 January 2003),[96] which brought together support for high-performance and grass-roots participation sport in the early twenty-first-century pattern of a largely contract-based relationship between government and voluntary (increasingly termed NGO) associations. Despite a rising quotient of taxpayer-funded central government funding, both the Hillary Commission and SPARC retained the status of Crown entities – organisations at arm's length from government, the taint of direct government involvement lingering.

New Zealand's experiment with government involvement in supporting greater sport and recreation through the 1937 physical welfare and recreation scheme can be regarded as only a limited success. Most existing studies, looking at it within a national framework, have been harsher in judgement than this account. Within the broader ambit of the wider British world in which it was one of four connected, if separate, initiatives, it might be viewed differently. It is certainly easy to identify its flaws and limits. Ambitious, idealistic and broad in scope, the messy reality of running practical programmes with scarce resources, a lack of trained staff and on a national scale was fated to disappoint. Although it was only operative from 1939 to 1949, and had disappeared in all but a residual form by the mid-1950s, some of its achievements in providing organisational impetus in several sports – including marching, basketball, volleyball and women's bowls – endured. Enthusiasm for games, particular skills and the experiences of those who participated in camps, holidays, fitness groups, leadership courses and organised sports remains an unmeasurable quotient in the realm of collective as well as personal memory. Within the broader historical memory of the building of the welfare state and the consequent turning point in New Zealand's twentieth-century history from 1935, the physical welfare and recreation scheme has lain outside what has been lauded of that achievement.

In the work of the physical welfare and recreation scheme, attempts were made to expand and shift the terms of New Zealand's leisure culture and, in particular, to invest leisure with constructive possibility and to democratise the enjoyment of and opportunity for leisure more evenly through the population. In its work with women, this is most conspicuous. Even so, it did not satisfy all, and was but one step in a period noted for its sexual division of leisure as well as labour.[97] When New Zealand-born, British-based journalist Hector Bolitho visited in 1946, he was reported to have found his home country 'dreary'. Bolitho was especially scathing of the country's men. They were 'silent, prone to melancholia and short of wit; the women neurotic and active, shouldering the many burdens forced on them by the legislation of the Government, which carefully assures the men of a five-day week while the women still work seven'. 'Nothing shocked me more on my arrival in New Zealand than to find the uneven distribution of labour between men and women.'[98]

Bolitho was not the only commentator to make such an observation. The stark divisions between women's and men's social worlds were also a feature of life in 1930s Australia. For all their political progressiveness, as places where women had won the vote in 1893 (New Zealand) and 1902 (Australia), the social fabric in the 1930s was much more conventional. The strong sporting culture in both societies was renowned for its male character. Yet when New South Wales and then the federal government of Australia introduced national fitness schemes in the late 1930s, they too sought to make this a provision for women and men. It is to that story we now turn.

3 Education or Health?

National Fitness in New South Wales and Across Australia

Gordon Young's arrival in Sydney, from Toronto, a week before Christmas 1938 was noted by the *Sydney Morning Herald* under the headline 'Education for Physique'. Young told the paper that he 'came with an open mind. He was not a faddist ... he believed that physical education should be adapted to the country.' Nonetheless, Young was eager to prove that he was a follower of the 'new conception of education – the training of the man or woman mentally, physically, and socially'.[1] As the first Director of Physical Education and executive head of the National Fitness Council in New South Wales, Young's appointment was a major achievement for those who had been pressing to make modern physical fitness a priority on the public agenda. With his landing in Sydney there was the first tangible realisation that better bodies and a better future lay ahead.[2]

With plenty of sun, fresh air and beaches, not everyone was convinced that Australians needed to be trained to enjoy themselves. Wasn't there ample evidence that people were already healthy and fit? Cricket had never been more popular, Manly and Bondi beaches were crowded, the surf lifesaver was a national hero and local athletes had won a sweep of medals at the Empire Games held in Sydney in February. Newly arrived from the Canadian winter, Gordon Young put himself in the position of the sceptic: 'the visitor to Sydney beaches must ask himself was physical education necessary?' But he quickly gave the answer consistent with the new scientific thinking: 'while sun-bathing and swimming were splendid, they did not constitute the end of a healthy life'.[3] The national fitness campaign in Australia was born out of a civic movement of progressive reform, one that was more alive to the threats modernity posed to the body than to the freedoms it promised.

Civic agitation rather than government initiative lay behind the national fitness scheme in Australia, with the first steps being taken at state level in New South

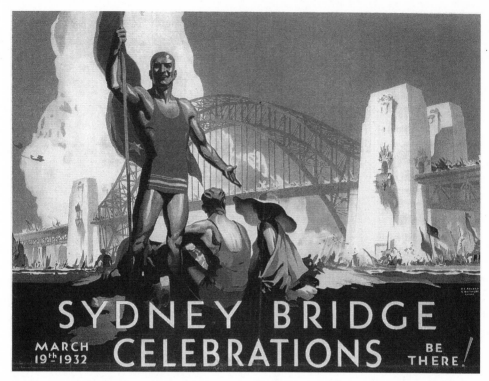

Douglas Annan celebrated much more than the completion of an engineering marvel in his poster for the opening of the Sydney Harbour Bridge. A heroic confidence in man and machine, nature and city, human and material spoke strongly of an optimistic modernity. Douglas Annan, Mitchell Library, State Library of New South Wales

Wales and Victoria. Although the scheme was inaugurated nationally in 1939, only in mid-1941 did it gain legislative endorsement in the National Fitness Act.[4] 'National fitness', the colloquial title by which the British campaign was known, became the pervasive term in Australia – applied both to the formalities of legislation and to the activities it sponsored. National fitness programmes lasted longer in Australia than in Britain, New Zealand or Canada. When they finally disappeared in the late 1960s and early 1970s, they did so as part of a wider reorganisation of government support for sport and recreation rather than through neglect or abolition.[5]

Modern Australians: A Movement for Civic Progress

The body had never been as central to Australian life as it was in the 1930s. Everywhere, enjoyment in the body was evident. Images of healthy and attractive bodies adorned objects and places as never before. The single greatest step in Sydney's transformation into a modern city, the opening of the Harbour Bridge in March 1932, was depicted on posters in which a bronzed and muscular lifesaver stood taller than the Bridge's highest arc, with lightly clad beachgoers occupying the foreground. The following summer it was Don Bradman's body that was under fire from English bowlers in the Ashes cricket test matches, drawing accusations that Douglas Jardine's team was playing outside the rules of the game. Bowling at the man rather than at the stumps was not the game of cricket as Australians understood or wanted to play it. The 'bodyline' tour, as it became known, raised a national furore, causing many Australians to question whether their country should continue as a loyal Dominion in the wider British firmament. The celebration of Australia's 150th anniversary in 1938 placed the story of successful development from convict and settler origins to modern nation within a theme of natural abundance and social progress, an achievement of past endeavour and a promise of future success. Still a young country in the eyes of the predominantly British descendant white population, the nation's vigour was depicted in the bodies of sunlit, muscular citizens.

With less idealism but greater fervour, sport attracted larger and larger crowds to events such as the Melbourne Cup, cricket matches and football finals (league, union or Victorian Rules).[6] In the dark days of the Depression, the feats of the great racehorse Phar Lap thrilled Australian crowds, as they did New Zealanders. Playing sport had never been more popular.[7] Sporting and other forms of active bodies were in the public eye as never before. Radio made 'live' commentary possible for listeners far from the race course or sports ground.

Sports results were a staple of radio news broadcasts from the beginning of transmission. It is estimated that by 1938 two in three Australian homes had a wireless set, while most families without one could listen at a neighbour's house.[8] Advances in telegraph and printing technology meant readers of the metropolitan dailies – Melbourne's *Age*, the *Sydney Morning Herald*, Adelaide's *Advertiser*, Brisbane's *Courier-Mail*, Perth's *West Australian*– now received their news through more and better photographs as well as columns of text. Advertisers in these papers, and the new pictorial weeklies such as *Pix Magazine*, took advantage of the technology in the new photo-journalism.[9] Sport, body culture and the new media fed each other, offering readers an expanded visual diet. An early issue of *Pix Magazine* featured Jack Davey, the popular presenter on Sydney's commercial radio station, 2GB. Pictured in dressing gown with tea trolley and microphone, Davey was shown conducting his early morning exercise show, 'The tummy club'.[10]

In day-to-day life, Australians were also embracing what it was to be modern in a mood that has been called the 'romance of modernity'.[11] Department stores, dance halls and movie theatres, never more prominent in the cityscape, offered accessible places and affordable moments of escape and consumption. Sports clothes – Speedo swimsuits, sundresses, shorts or casual jackets – made up a greater portion of the goods on sale. Sports styles were the fashion look of the decade.[12] Getting fashionably fit and participating in mass displays was popular amongst

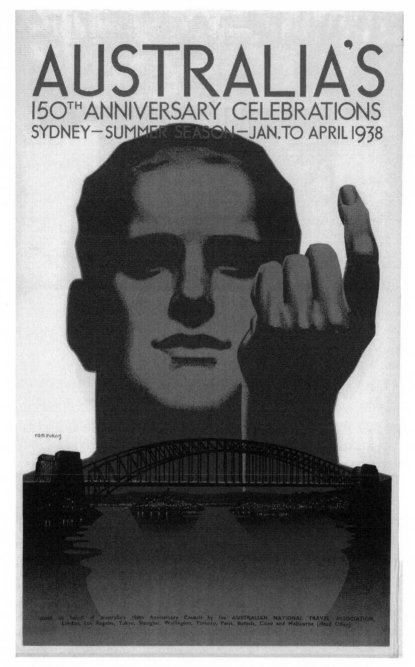

150 years of national development was celebrated in Australia in 1938 by the majority white population, an event that would be echoed in New Zealand's Centennial celebration in 1940. The colonial past was not yet a source of embarrassment or controversy. Sydney hosted the third Empire Games in early 1938 as an anniversary event. Tom Purvis, National Library of Australia

department store and other city workers. Encouraging workers to take up recreation and physical activity was part of a wider industrial welfare movement in Australia, and worldwide, at this time.[13] At Grace Brothers in Sydney, for example, the shop assistants had the opportunity of using the store gymnasium.[14] In the spring of 1939, a thousand young women performed in Melbourne's Olympia Park on a Saturday night. From business houses, the YWCA, sporting associations, Girl Guides, gym clubs and riding schools, they marched to music, performed rhythmic exercises and staged a fencing display. The horsewomen executed musical quadrilles. In the grand finale, all thousand participants marched through a blacked-out stadium creating an illuminated spectacle with each carrying a coloured lantern.[15]

Exercising for attractiveness as well as for fun and fitness was a thread in the contemporary appeal to women. While physical culture classes were still popular, new approaches caught the changing mood and the desire for novelty. When prominent activist and politician Ivy Weber was widowed for a second time in 1930, she returned to the profession she had learned twelve years earlier at the Weber and Rice Health and Strength College, but instead of giving classes in physical culture she took a job with the Berlei Corset Company, delivering lectures on figure control.[16] University-educated Thea Hughes found an eager response when she returned to Sydney from London in May 1935 bringing her Bagot Stack training.[17] Hundreds were soon flocking to a local branch of the Women's League of Health and Beauty. By October 1936 she led a large group of League members in a mass demonstration at Mrs Macquarie's Chair in the central city Domain.[18] The annual outdoor spectacle was a signature event for the League, marking its social and public prominence, its distinction from exercise classes that remained confined to halls and providing evidence that across the empire members belonged to a movement rather than an organisation. The Governor-General's wife, Lady Gowrie, 'a member of the League', and Lady David presided over the Sydney event of 1936.[19]

The appeal of the League, combining health and beauty, was part of the wider democratisation of beauty in the interwar decades. The promise of beauty for all, captured in Helena Rubinstein's famous declaration, 'there are no ugly women, only lazy ones', was not only a commercial slogan but part of a new ethos that made good appearance, as well as good health, a mark of self-respect and social duty. Beauty contests, popularised in the late 1920s, made physical fitness a criterion of judging. Judith Smart and Liz Conor's histories indicate the ways in which feminine beauty was argued about at this time as an expression of or distraction from national ideals.[20]

In the advent of beauty products as central to consumer culture, Australia had played a vital role. It was in her early years in rural Victoria as a Polish migrant, and then working in Melbourne around the turn of the century, that Helena Rubinstein first developed her line of beauty treatments and a highly successful method of

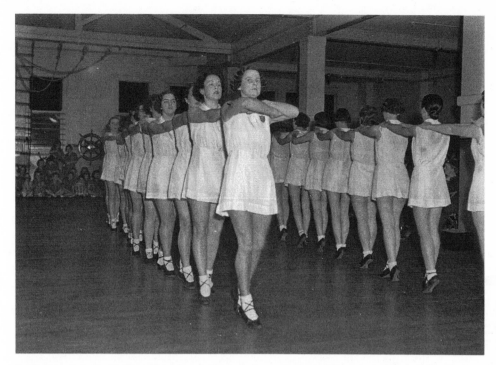

Employees at Grace Brothers Department Store photographed using the gymnasium built by the store for its workers. Industrial welfare facilities such as these were common in the interwar period, though some argued that they were tools for making workers efficient rather than opportunities workers might use for their own enjoyment. Hood Collection, State Library New South Wales

selling them. Combining 'medical treatment' with beauty care in her own range of products sold initially at her Valaze Institute at 274 Collins Street, Rubinstein parlayed her Australian experience and earnings to expansion in London (1908), New York (1916) and then across North America. With her great rivals Florence Graham ('Elizabeth Arden') and Charles Revson (founder of Revlon), Rubinstein was a leader in the creation of a mass market for affordable, branded cosmetics. The business thrived on mass production and mass advertising techniques developed in the early twentieth century, and on the growth of a market of women with small but regular disposable incomes. The promise of beauty for all was not just 'hope in a jar', a ruse sold to unwitting and passive customers, but part of the promise and possibility of self-invention – modern selves made, and re-made, daily as faces were put on to go out into the world.[21]

Looking good was one way of being modern; competing well in sport was another. When Decima Norman trounced all her opponents to win five gold medals on the athletic track at the Sydney Cricket Ground in February 1938, she was cheered wildly. Competing for Australia in the British Empire Games, Norman represented the 'athletic prowess of modern woman', according to the *Sydney Morning Herald*.[22]

The British Empire Games, just the third such event to be held, were staged as part of the 150th anniversary celebrations. The hosts did well. Australia proved to be the most successful of the fifteen empire countries participating in the Games' seven sports: boxing, athletics, cycling, lawn bowls, swimming, rowing and wrestling, winning twenty-four of seventy-seven events, far ahead of its nearest rival, Canada, with thirteen gold medals.

But for all these signs of vigour, health and success, not everyone thought the Australian body was as good as it should – or might – be. Or that modern times were all sun and no shadow. What was popular was not always what was good.

Modern living 'means to most of us an indoor, sedentary occupation, which allows us a bare minimum of sunlight and fresh air, and provides little of recreative or re-creative activity, which is an essential for true fitness'.[23] A sense that health and good living were threatened by urban life, by too much – or too commercial – leisure, by a lack of knowledge about how to exercise properly, by watching rather than doing, by a false conviction that physical exercise was the monopoly of youth, or by a limited notion of what it was to be truly healthy, prompted wide-ranging civic agitation in the 1930s. Among those leading it were C. E. W. Bean, official historian of Australia's Great War and founder of the Parks and Playground Movement; Edith Swain, Ellen Bingham and Zoe Benjamin of the Recreation and Leadership Movement; Dr J. H. L. Cumpston, Director-General of Health; Professor Harvey Sutton, professor of public health at Sydney University; Dr Grace Cuthbert, another prominent figure in public health and women's organisations; progressive educationist Professor George Browne at the University of Melbourne; Ivy Weber at the National Council of Women with its many affiliate organisations; and socially minded clergymen in the churches. Well-organised leisure, and physically fit bodies as the basis for a healthy and successful life and modern citizenship, were at the heart of their campaign. Through the 1930s these progressives joined forces to push for state and federal endorsement and funding for physical recreation and education.

Edith Swain founded the Recreation and Leadership Movement several years earlier, having become increasingly convinced that physical recreation held the key to contemporary problems, especially those faced by young people. When more and more people enjoyed 'free time', it was important that they be guided to use it constructively. 'Education for Leisured Citizenship' was the movement's goal through training leaders who could 'combat the increasing passivity of life'. As Zoe Benjamin told those attending a Movement Camp, 'Picture-shows, car-driving, wireless, bridge-playing and the necessities of mechanised industry, are causes for far too much passive sitting on the part of children and adults, to the detriment of bodily and mental health. People need much more creative activity.'[24] A leading figure in the National Council of Women, as well as a senior public servant in the Department of Labour and Industry, Swain was involved in the YWCA, convened the City Girls' Amateur Sports Association and represented several Australian organisations at the World Leisure Congress held in Los Angeles in conjunction with the Olympic Games in 1932.[25]

For C. E. W. Bean it was the 'ill-effects' of 'half of all civilized men' being driven 'from open country to crowded city' that cast a shadow over individual and national health. Also involved in the Town Planning Association, Bean argued loudly to protect and expand parks and open spaces across the Sydney metropolitan area. Leisure, sport and recreation were part of a modern citizenship, and space in which to pursue them was a necessary corollary. To the author of *The Anzac Tradition*, the influential statement of Australian nationhood for the interwar generation, it was in the country and open air rather than in the city and indoors that Australians were made. Preserving that possibility while becoming an ever more urban people meant active promotion of physical exercise on grass, sand and dirt under the open sky.[26] In its 1932 report, the Parks and Playground Movement found a mere 8,599 acres of park and playground across the 155,378-acre expanse of Sydney's city and suburbs, about half the old town planning standard allowance of one acre of recreation space for every ten acres of town land. The largest user of playing fields, the NSW Junior Cricket Union, reported a shortfall of ninety-one cricket grounds for teams seeking to play in the coming season.[27] For Bean, promoting open space, physical education and modern leisure was 'not so as to make champions, but so as to make citizens'.[28] Fitness and active bodies were thus also a response to geographical modernity. The pipe-smoking, shorts-wearing hiker had an urban equivalent – the walker in parks, children in sports grounds, all ages in swimming baths, and children in playgrounds that preferably had grass and trees rather than concrete or asphalt.

Although Gordon Young at one time described national fitness in Australia as 'a people's movement',[29] it drew more from the language and tradition of democratic liberalism and political vitalism than from the labour tradition that inspired Bill Parry in New Zealand. It was a progressive conservatism that saw physical fitness as a necessary counter to the deleterious effects of modernity (passivity, consumption, spectating and urbanism) and a bulwark against threats of social malaise to the nation. To the expanded domain of soldier, worker and maternal citizenship that had emerged from World War I was added the possibility, and duty, of active and healthy citizenship. Responsible and constructive use of time in leisure had become part of being a modern member of a local, national and empire-wide community. Progressive in its goals, what emerged as the campaign for Physical Fitness and Citizenship carried a streak of anti-modernism in its suspicion of the decadence of cities versus the virtue of the country, of technologies that removed face-to-face contact and of entertainments that were populist, especially those that were bought rather than created. The World Leisure Congress and the increasingly professional

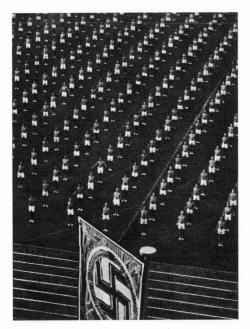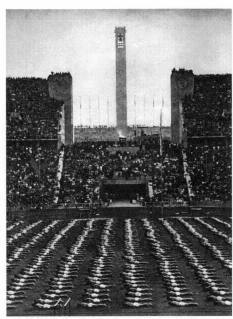

Spectacles such as this massed demonstration of 4,000 men and women from the Turner gymnastic movement held on the eve of the Olympic Games were what impressed visitors to Germany in the 1930s. NSW Premier Bertram Stevens and Minister of Education David Drummond were among the visitors, attending the Games in Berlin in 1936. *Berliner Illustrite Zeitung*, 1936, Ullstein A.G. Berlin, pp.70-71

welfare services run by churches and community organisations were more the origins of the movement and source of its recruits than the labour movement.

Eugenicist undertones flow through the progressive concern with preserving and enhancing Australians' physical fitness. In its seeking to secure adequate facilities for physical exercise and open space for outdoor leisure and games, the national fitness movement can be seen as part of a lingering environmentalism in Australian eugenicism. As Bashford and Levine indicate, eugenic discourses were broad responses to modernity. In Australia and New Zealand, Stephen Garton suggests eugenics in this period was 'everywhere and nowhere'. Proponents of government-supported physical education and physical exercise sought to better the standards of personal and national health universally, rather than by distinguishing 'fit' from 'unfit'.[30] 'Health to-day', as one of their pamphlets explained, 'means more than mere freedom from disease; it is something positive. It gives a sense of vitality and strength – of real joy in living. The National Fitness Council seeks to awaken in people a true "health consciousness".'[31]

At a conference held in Sydney on 2 July 1937 entitled 'Recreation – the Life Blood of Democracy', the various interest groups came together in an effort to push the federal government into action.[32] That the British government had, by then, published its White Paper and was seeing its Physical Training and Recreation

Bill through its final stages in the House of Commons only added urgency to the call that Australia should act. The main organisers of the conference were Edith Swain and others from the Recreation and Leadership Movement, Edgar Herbert (Principal of the Leadership Training College, operating in nucleus only at this time), and C. E. W. Bean.

The people attending the meeting in Sydney were also aware of developments in Victoria.[33] A similar civic campaign had been underway in Melbourne, with the dearth of adequate facilities and proper instruction in physical education particular concerns. Speaking to the National Council of Women in 1936, Professor George Browne of the University of Melbourne condemned Victoria as 'a backward State as far as Physical Education is concerned', lacking both trained teachers or any means of providing qualified staff.[34] The idea that physical fitness was something that needed to be learned rather than simply 'done', and where those teaching needed specialist training, was new in the 1930s, a progressive argument made by reform-minded educationists. That Australia lagged behind other places was also evident in the observation that not one of Australia's universities had a gymnasium.[35] Support for specialist physical education teachers also came from the New Education Fellowship that met in Melbourne in 1937.[36]

The combined efforts of the National Council of Women (Victoria), led by Ivy Weber and Browne,[37] resulted in the appointment of Dr Fritz Duras to the University of Melbourne to teach the first courses in physical education at an Australian university. Duras arrived in Melbourne from London, in March 1937, his appointment supported by the Carnegie Corporation's Academic Assistance Council. The Council gave help to German exiles. Because his father was Jewish, Duras had been forced to resign from his position as director and senior physician at the Institute for Sports Medicine at the University of Freiburg-im-Breisgau and to find refuge in England. With a medical degree and four years' experience, he brought an impeccable set of credentials to the new venture. Within a few months, what had been gingerly embarked on as a one-year course became a two-year qualification, and Duras' temporary appointment was renewed and upgraded.[38] Students from his courses were to play an important role in the unfolding national fitness story.

While the University of Melbourne was assured of its venture into the risky terrain of physical education by Duras' qualifications, the populist world of physical fitness continued to grab the limelight. In agreeing to judge the 'perfect girl' contest at the Pearce Bjelke-Petersen Institute of Physical Culture, one of the city's commercial gymnasia, in December 1938, Duras was alert to the accusations of elitism (that it took a university qualification to do 'phys ed', and that rubbing shoulders with the local gym compromised Duras' status). He may not have endorsed their methods but it was an opportunity to support the message of health and fitness.[39] Reaching across class was also in the mind of Harvey Sutton, public health exponent. He voiced special concern for 'the youth and maidens who leave school at the age of fourteen',[40] only a small number of whom were picked up by the YMCA and TocH.[41] Sutton was worried that such people 'form a lost legion...of onlookers and barrackers'. 'As a nation we need sportsmen, not barrackers: players, not spectators.'[42]

By the end of 1937 the impetus given to what was now known as the Physical Fitness and Citizenship campaign prompted New South Wales Premier Bertram Stevens to set up a Physical Education Advisory Committee.[43] Stevens, along with David Drummond, New South Wales Minister of Education, had attended the 1936 Olympics in Berlin where they had been hugely impressed by the levels of physical fitness in the population at large, as well as the sporting prowess in the stadium.[44] The Committee's first task was to draw up an advertisement for a Director of Physical Education for the state. Gordon Young's appointment was the result of an international search and the position carried a starting salary of £950.

The advertisement specified that applicants were to be 'natural-born British subjects',[45] who were also to provide certificates testifying to their physical fitness. They were to be graduates of an English, European or American university of recognised standing 'following a course of at least four years' training in Physical Education and/or Recreation'. They should also have '[p]ost-graduate administrative experience in England and/or elsewhere in relation to Physical Education and Recreation and should furnish evidence of good executive ability, personality, and driving force'.[46] The Toronto interview panel, comprising the University of Toronto professor of education Peter Sandiford; Dr Arthur Lamb, director of physical education at McGill (an Australian who had risen to a senior position in the Canadian physical education and sporting world);[47] and L. C. Robson, headmaster of the Church of England Grammar School, North Sydney, found Young at first 'a little too voluble and aggressive'. But the committee was assured by Lamb that he was 'tactful and that he has done sound work in other positions in association with men of various types'.[48] Young was selected from a field of over one hundred applicants. He was 34 years old, at the time the physical director of the Montreal YMCA, the largest and oldest in North America.

The different starting points in Victoria and New South Wales were to mark the longer term contrasts in physical education and national fitness in the two largest states. Where Victoria concentrated more on establishing an academic base for training physical education teachers, New South Wales' programme was more practically and community-oriented.[49]

Gordon Young's arrival in Sydney in December 1938 coincided with the federal government finally succumbing to pressure from physical fitness lobbying. Prime Minister Joe Lyons' government had been making noises of support throughout the year, but commitment had been elusive, testing the patience of the many coaxing voices.[50] Melbourne's *Age* published a cartoon of all the interest groups, including

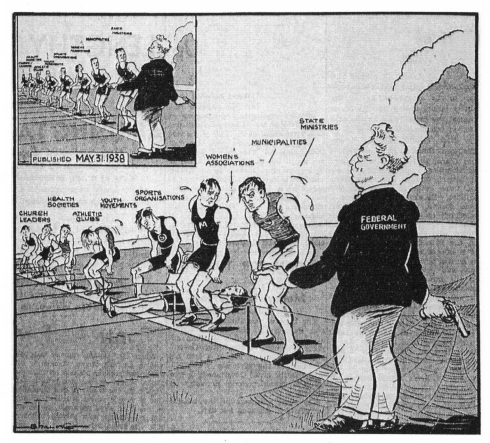

Impatience at the slow pace of government action on the national fitness scheme was captured in this cartoon printed in Melbourne's *The Age* in August 1938, months after politicians had made public promises that they would act. *The Age*, August 1938, from *Australians 1938*, 1987

state governments, as runners in athletic garb lined up under the starter's gun in May 1938 but now slumped with fatigue three months later, still waiting for the gun to go off. In the end, it was the insistent urging of public health champions that pushed Canberra into action. The announcement of a National Fitness Council and government support for a national fitness scheme in December 1938 came in the wake of strong resolutions passed by the National Health and Medical Research Council chaired by the Director-General of Health, Dr J. H. L. Cumpston.

Arguments made by the Council that promotion of physical activity and adoption of modern approaches to physical education were urgent matters of national interest were ones that had been aired by public health advocates for several years. They were also in keeping with Cumpston's leadership of the Federal Department of Health that he had shaped since being appointed as its founding director in 1921. Cumpston was driven by a strong commitment to public health in what has been described as an administration of 'progressive nationalism'. He is one of Michael Roe's *Nine Australian Progressives* (1984).[51] Cumpston worked hard to promote effective measures that extended understandings and practices of health achievable through public action. Initially in charge of quarantine, Cumpston led Australia's response to the 1918 influenza pandemic, which resulted in a much lower death toll than elsewhere in the Pacific region. With colleagues such as Professor Harvey Sutton, Cumpston was at the forefront of making health a central matter for civic attention in the interwar years. His promotion of a national fitness scheme was consistent with the priority he gave to preventive health. Cumpston was later to formulate the goals of the national fitness campaign in a way that linked personal duty with national action. As chairman of the Commonwealth National Fitness Council, he wrote: 'When we speak of national fitness we immediately evoke two concepts. The first is the concept of a state of personal fitness and the second is that this fitness shall be a condition universally enjoyed throughout the nation.' It applied to 'every age-period' and to both sexes.[52]

By 1938–39 many people held the view that Australia was 'lagging behind the rest of the world' in its failure to endorse a public campaign of physical fitness.[53] But by that time the various lobbyists had succeeded in getting some things going at state level. National fitness schemes in Australia did attract political support but they were not instigated by elected politicians. And it was to take a little longer to see results in people taking up greater physical activity.

Putting Fitness into Action

The first meeting of the Commonwealth National Fitness Council was held on 5–6 January 1939. Made up of the heads of health and education and representatives from the states, and chaired by Cumpston, the Council was more a loosely configured group of officials than of civic organisation leaders. Its work was placed firmly in the domain of health, with an emphasis on the 'scientific medical principles' underlying the federal government's early commitment.[54] By its third meeting, in July 1939, the federal government had made a commitment of £100,000 over five years to fund the programme of work the Council had devised. States beyond New South Wales – which already had a council – were invited to form state-level fitness councils and to contribute to advancing the work that had been given official endorsement. Victoria appointed Norman Brookes, the great tennis champion, as chairman of its National Fitness Council in 1939, the same year in which he was knighted.[55]

The sum of £100,000 voted was modest. It was derided in parliamentary debate two years later as a 'bagatelle' – but it was a start. When Sir Frederick Stewart, Minister of Health, took the initial recommendations of the National Fitness Council (initially named the Commonwealth or National Coordinating Council for Physical Fitness) to Cabinet in May 1939, he was acutely aware of the criticism the

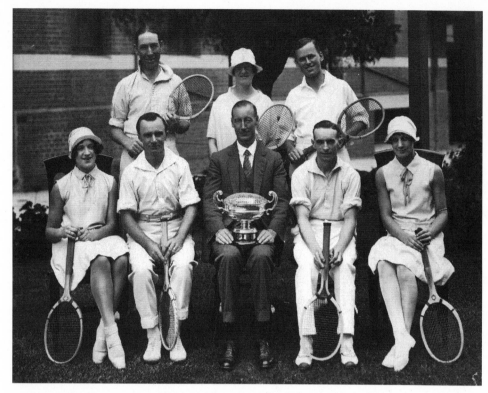

Match manufacturing company Bryant & May ran a series of sports teams, including this tennis team, 1928. Workplace sports were a big part of the sporting and recreation scene in the interwar period. Accession no. H92.401/155, Image no b31840, State Library of Victoria

Australian measure could draw, and the rather feeble support his government was putting behind the measure compared to commitments already made in Britain and New Zealand. He upbraided his colleagues:

> As sponsors, we must be prepared to assume an appropriate measure of financial responsibility. We can hardly claim that an aggregate of £18,000 spread over three years and distributed between six states fulfils that obligation in this respect. I recommend therefore that the Coordinating Council's recommendations be approved.... In the United Kingdom the government has made provision for a scheme of physical training and recreation involving an expenditure of two million pounds spread over a period of three years and in addition a continued annual charge of £150,000 ... the government of South Africa has approved an allocation of £50,000 toward a nationalist scheme of PE. In New Zealand, under the New Zealand Physical Welfare and Recreation Act, 1937 the Minister of Internal Affairs [is] authorized from time to time, to make grants to local authorities and voluntary organizations towards the expenses incurred in PT and Recreation.[56]

From this point on, the national fitness campaign in Australia was a complicated and overlapping mixture of federal, state and local provision, incorporating co-operation with voluntary organisations and co-operative arrangements with universities and teachers' colleges over training of specialists.[57]

The federal initiative meant that Gordon Young soon acquired a second responsibility as executive officer of the New South Wales National Fitness Council, in addition to his position as Director of Physical Education. He lost no time in getting into action in his new home. At the opening day of Edith Swain and Zoe Benjamin's Recreation and Leadership Movement Camp at Newport in January 1939 just weeks after his arrival in Australia, Young found himself fighting a bushfire alongside the Bishop of Armidale and the Minister of Health David Drummond. The camp was saved but the Minister's speech was sacrificed. Young's relationship with Minister Drummond remained close. As he later noted, with dual positions he served two masters: his civil service boss in the State Education Department and the Minister of Education, who was responsible for the state national fitness initiative. The wide and somewhat blurred brief suited Young's energies and his unbureaucratic habits.[58]

The lack of funds with which to undertake the ambitious programme of overhauling and upgrading physical education in schools, and launching a major community-wide fitness scheme, was something of a surprise. Before taking up the post Young had been promised a budget of £500,000. What materialised was something very much more modest, and he faced the task of putting physical education and community fitness on a professional basis without a means of training specialist teachers and leaders. Within a few months, however, he had a Flying Squad of teachers who had undergone several weeks' intensive training ready to take new programmes of physical education into schools around the state. Esther McRae's visit to Broken Hill in October 1939 as a member of the Flying Squad was typical of the work of the group. She visited seven schools, giving a variety of demonstrations including the new game of softball, met with the press, and gave encouragement to locals interested in forming a Community Fitness Centre for adult and evening recreation.[59] Both Gordon Young and his wife Pat were keen softballers and introduced at every opportunity a sport that was a highly popular summer game in Canada.[60]

Vacation Play Centres and supervised city playgrounds were organised as national fitness initiatives. The playgrounds were popular but struggled with poor equipment and served to underline the paucity of recreational facilities. When Helen Black made a short visit to Sydney from New Zealand to survey what colleagues in New South Wales were doing in February 1940, she commented on the dire need for more recreational space for children in the city.[61] The new 'Play Centres' for children run by physical education staff in the Education Department were a fresh venture and well subscribed, but the 'heat was so intense on the asphalt playgrounds that the children were hosed at 11 a.m. each day'.[62]

By September Young had also launched a well-produced monthly magazine, *Physical Fitness*, designed to promote fitness, sport and physical activity, and to provide a professional vehicle for what he envisaged as a growing number of physical educators. 'Physical fitness', the first issue explained, 'is no longer recognised as a matter of bulging biceps and outsized chests, but as a state in which man, to put it simply, feels well, eats well, thinks well and sleeps well. If he can do these things he may rightfully claim: "I am fit."'[63]

Public education was a major part of Young's task, as it was for his colleagues appointed to the more usual positions as organisers for National Fitness Councils in other states. Bert Apps, a graduate of Fritz Duras' Melbourne course and organiser for the South Australia Fitness Council, produced the *Keep Fit Book* in 1941. Readers were given a clear idea of the six simple elements needed for fit and healthy living:

> 1. A well-balanced diet – milk, butter, cheese, eggs, fruit, vegetables, meat, and plenty of water. 2. Enjoyable activity in the sunlight and fresh air. Health requires good muscle tone, which is built up through activity. Activity is the law of growth and development. 3. Sufficient sleep and rest. 4. Attention to personal hygiene, e.g. – Care of the teeth, Bodily cleanliness, Suitable clothing, Well-fitting footwear. 5. Regular medical and dental examinations. Many people spend more on the upkeep of their motorcar than on themselves. 6. Knowledge of the health rules. We are all suspicious of the extremist or faddist. A practical health education should be a recognised part of general education.[64]

The rules of health are simple, the author noted, 'but city life tends to complicate them'. The 'daily dozen' was recommended as being the best way to maintain regular fitness. Advice as to when and how to do these exercises was followed by detailed diagrams and instructions, from warming up to 'quietening' down to finish, with further points on posture, a 'word about the feet' and 'hints on personal hygiene'. Having a 'gramophone or wireless going' was recommended as music 'helps to make the exercises more rhythmical. March tunes and waltzes are ideal.'[65]

Posture featured prominently in national fitness public education. Standing, sitting and moving properly were important to proper physiology and efficient body functioning. Posture was also of greater significance at a time when tuberculosis and respiratory disease were still common, as good carriage was considered a guard against bronchial and lung infection. Posture also affected mood: improving one could enhance the other. Alongside silhouetted figures, one in bad posture, the other showing good posture, explanations such as these were common:

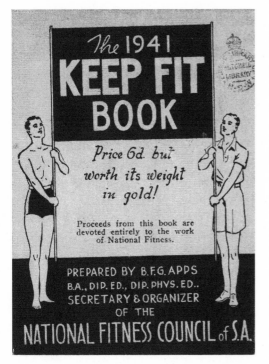 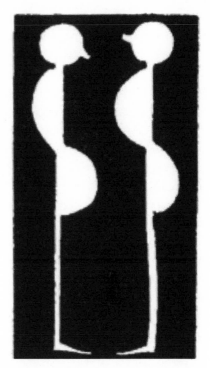

Compact, practical and cheap, Bernard Apps' booklet was designed for everyday use by all. Posture was considered central to health and good posture a key to feeling bright and happy. Posture was emphasised as essential to the balance that was essential to health and feeling good. A body out of balance, wrongly carried, was a body out of health and happiness. Later definitions of health in terms of well-being had less to say about posture. B. Apps, *The 1941 Keep-Fit Book*, 1941, Mitchell Collection, State Library New South Wales

Bad posture drains away our vigour. Observe the stance of the average, middle-aged man – shoulders humped, chest collapsed, stomach protruding. He tires easily, feels like an over-loaded ashtray. His lungs get barely a third of oxygen he needs; his slumping spine is throwing apparatus out of place, hampering digestion and elimination.

If this was all too recognisable to readers, a remedy was also at hand:

(1) Throw your shoulders back by rotating the palms of your hands as they hang by the sides. (2) Inhale deeply as though smelling a pleasant aroma. (3) Keep the midriff in position by imagining a pair of strong hands is supporting your diaphragm. (4) Plant your feet parallel, distribute weight evenly on both. Two weeks of this posture have cleared up many stubborn conditions defying diagnosis and drugs.[66]

Australians' casual and unsystematic approach to physical education and to care of the body in general were reflected in a tendency to slouch, in the eyes of

Fritz Duras. Duras was dismayed by Australians' neglect of posture given their fine physique. 'Your men and women slouch .... They are tired at the end of the day, but they do not lessen that fatigue by walking with their heads forward, their backs bent, and their feet shuffling.' To get over such a 'slovenly' approach, Duras recommended that they stand tall and walk 'with a loose-limbed action, taking long, purposeful strides', and urged everybody to perform daily exercise – 'even grandma'.[67] Professor Sutton's message that physical exercise should be a life-long pursuit was similar: physical education should be 'free, continuous, complete and universal...from the time the child begins to crawl until he becomes a doddering old man with a stick'.[68]

Recognising Australians' great love of games, especially the big sporting fixtures 'that draw enormous crowds to Australian arenas – Test matches, League football finals, and the like', Duras tried to coax people into thinking beyond these interests into a more 'systematic development of the body'. The big matches, he worried, filled an unwanted purpose, 'by providing the spectacle for an ever-increasing spectator class of playing age and physique'. These events could contribute more positively if the correct attitude towards them was adopted:

> Physical education could foster this attitude by producing children so keen on their own physical activity that they would be all eagerness to try to bat like a Bradman, drive like a Budge – not merely develop into round-shouldered and short-winded grandstand critics.[69]

The advice provided reflected the standard thinking of the time: people should aim to create their own healthy lifestyle rather than relying on patent remedies and self medication;[70] exercising and consciousness about health should become life-long habits; and efforts to maintain the health of the body would foster health of mind. Fitness, a state of good health that went beyond the absence of disease, opened up a realm of vital living that felt good and enhanced everyday enjoyment and happiness. Other forms of publicity produced by National Fitness Councils in Australia echoed those used in Britain, in iconography and message. 'Citrus for Fitness – in work and play', a poster produced by the Victorian Railways is a variation on the British 'In work and play – fitness wins' slogan.

The Minister of Health Sir Frederick Stewart urged Australians to think of physical fitness as their 'birthright'. But by the time Stewart's article appeared in the third issue of Gordon Young's *Physical Fitness*, the country was at war.[71]

With the war effort dominating attention, the importance of physical training sharpened around defence requirements. Conscription of men into the armed services (though not for overseas service) and of women into war work became the priority. The work of National Fitness Councils and organisers continued through the war, however, as the need for soundly based physical education and the value of physical exercise for civilian and service life were recognised. The national fitness scheme received statutory endorsement, a measure signalling its 'continuity and permanence', when the National Fitness Bill was passed in the Federal Parliament in June 1941. Debated in the dying stages of the Menzies United Australia government, it was not a partisan issue, but was voted in with a 54–3 majority. The vote also reflected the serious position Australia was facing in the war, with the Axis forces in the ascendant in the early months of 1941 in both Greece and North Africa. The government was under pressure. On this measure they were accused of both lacking urgency and creating a diversion. The Labor opposition's key dissatisfaction, however, was with the meagre provisions rather than with the principles of the scheme. A simpler measure than either the British or New Zealand versions, the Act gave statutory power to the National Fitness Council and established a National Fitness Fund. At federal level, national fitness was confirmed as a measure within the health administration even as it was more closely aligned with education at state level.[72] The Act was accompanied by a significant boost in funding, with a further annual grant of £50,000 being made available for distribution to the states.[73]

Money was granted within three institutional areas and for three purposes: to universities for the training of physical education specialists and for physical education activities for undergraduate students; to state councils for national fitness activities and facilities including camps, hostels, playgrounds, sporting events, keep-fit classes and leader training; and to state education departments for expansion of physical education in schools and teachers' colleges, including the provision of equipment.[74]

Bert Apps (South Australia) and Jean Thompson (Western Australia) were appointed to the newly created Canberra positions to direct the work of the National Fitness Council across the country. The central secretariat never thrived, however,[75] and the bulk of the drive for and provision of funding, resources, initiative and activity remained at the state level. In the parliamentary debate of 1941, Stewart claimed that New South Wales had put £27,000 into its national fitness programme, which was a much larger portion than that coming from the federal coffers. Stewart was drawing attention to the responsibility and commitment being made by states while the federal government dragged its feet.

Even at the height of federal engagement, the idea that national fitness was a movement reliant on popular support as much as on government policy was underlined. So, too, was the fine balance needed between federal funding and control, state autonomy, initiative and co-operation. The fact that national fitness sat between departments of health, education and defence further complicated the picture. In the booklet prepared for wide distribution in what had become Health, Milk and National Fitness Week, Cumpston admitted that the 'actual administrative

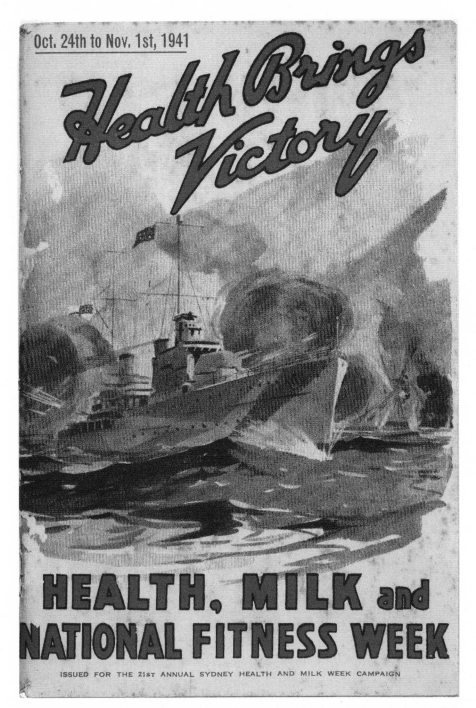

The long running New South Wales Health Week promotion gained two further priorities by 1941: milk and national fitness. The week long promotion in 1941 came at a critical time in the war, between the disasters in Greece and Crete and the entrance of Japan. *Health Brings Victory*, 1941, Mitchell Collection, State Library New South Wales expression of an organic unity of the efforts in the several States or of the work of the six State Councils [of National Fitness] has yet to be worked out'. He did not think it useful to 'attempt at a close organic unity under one central direction'. Treading a fine line between his central political masters, and state governments and administrations on which he was dependent for co-operation in getting anything done, he acknowledged that, while it 'is a natural impulse to look to the Commonwealth for at least a central inspiration on a national basis', it was not the place to look for 'actual direction and control'.[76]

The reorientation of national fitness around the demands of war was particularly apparent in promotions such as that made for NSW's Health Week in September–October 1941. Falling between the passing of the federal legislation and Japan's entry into the war, the slogan for the week was 'Health Brings Victory'. In the widely distributed brochure, the words were blazoned prominently in the skies above a warship. The message was that fitness was, for the moment, a matter of survival, while in the longer term it was a matter of enjoyment.[77]

In wartime the value of fitness needed little explanation. In a speech to the Travel League of New South Wales, Gordon Young pointed to the longer-term consequences of neglecting proper physical education and fitness at all levels: 'While our enemies had extensive youth-training schemes we were allowing children to grow like weeds on the macadam streets of congested suburbs.' Modernity in the approach to the body was as important as it was in buildings. In the same speech Young referred to Australia's children being stuck in outmoded buildings for their schooling, 'while the rest of the world is thinking in terms of chromium steel and modern high-speed engines'.[78]

Due to wartime restrictions there were no meetings of the federal National Fitness Council for the two years between October 1941 and September 1943. When the Council was finally able to meet again in Canberra on 29 September 1943, the session was opened by Minister of Health Senator Fraser.[79] With an eye to the common enterprise across the 'British world' and new friends in the United States, the Council's report was circulated to its sister bodies in London, Wellington, Ottawa and Washington DC.[80]

With qualified staff and ongoing funding for the national fitness scheme, physical education and recreation generally became less a matter of voluntary initiative and more a domain of professional control.[81] Physical education gradually gained a foothold in the universities – later in Sydney than in Melbourne, Queensland and Adelaide (and usually beginning with certificates and diplomas before subsequently moving to degrees). Federal funding made available to universities encouraged the beginnings of a university-qualified profession. Emphases varied: while Victoria had established a strong foundation for university training of physical education teachers – offering a two-year Diploma in Education course specialising in physical education – New South Wales had done more to devise community programmes. When Gordon Young failed in an attempt to persuade the University of Sydney to offer a qualification in physical education in 1943, training was offered instead through the Teachers' Training College. Nevertheless, while Young and Fritz Duras brought contrasting North American physical education and European medical backgrounds to their work, their protégés were able to gain their qualifications locally.

International networks continued to be important. Hector Kay, an Australian, replaced Young at the Montreal YMCA before returning to take up a similar post at the Sydney 'Y' in 1941.[82] Harry Le Maistre, originally from Melbourne, was one of twenty-three foreign students at Springfield College, Massachussetts, in 1939. He returned to teach physical education at the University of Sydney. While studying at Springfield, Le Maistre featured as one of the 'muscle men' in a photo essay published in *Life* magazine. Standing bare-chested in a physiology class, the lecturer painted ribs and organs on Le Maistre's torso in a striking manner. *Life* magazine was reaching an estimated 2.86 million readers with a high 'pass along' rate.[83] A new vocational and academic discipline reflected not only an emphasis on properly taught physical fitness in Australia but also a commitment widespread throughout Britain and the Dominions.

A Postwar New Order

That Australia's national fitness initiative was much more than a banging of drums for military training is evident in the character and longevity of its post-1945 life. Unlike Britain, where enthusiasm for national fitness evaporated with the war and the scheme was thankfully buried, or New Zealand, where the Physical Welfare and Recreation Branch had a brief 1945–48 flourish before fading out of existence, in Australia the national fitness scheme launched in early 1939 survived and endured well into the early 1970s. Becoming enmeshed in education, and focusing its efforts largely on young people, national fitness in postwar Australia avoided the distaste of government-directed adult sport and leisure that tainted it elsewhere.[84] With relatively little function as a grant-distributing institution to sporting organisations, the National Fitness Council largely avoided being a source of tension or of objection from a voluntarist society. Although representatives of cricket associations and rugby union (such as Herlihy) sat on the initial Sydney Advisory Committee, they did not continue to play a major part.

The widely perceived benefits of the relatively modest outlay on fitness projects gave pragmatic grounds for the scheme's continuance. But more important was the skilful association of national fitness with the goals of reconstruction. Recognising that the war was reshaping relations between state and citizen in profound ways, an article by Gordon Young in 1942, 'National Fitness and the New Order', marked a shift in discourse from what had previously framed arguments for government funding of physical education and exercise. Young emphasised that it was not just the immediate war and the enemy that were being fought against, but that sacrifices were being made *for* a new order, one in which human values and equality mattered more than property and old rankings. 'The interest of our Government in the happiness of its citizenship', he wrote, 'can be heralded as a great advance already in motion.' 'The most profound effects of this social revolution will be found in education.' Spelling out the detailed plans that national fitness officers were instituting, Young characterised the ultimate goals for which they were working as 'providing social unification and bringing a positive and dynamic approach to a new order'.[85] A more specific focus on young people (who represented the promise of the future), and on a goal of collective cohesion rather than the health of individual bodies, was more in keeping with the expansive vision of postwar reconstruction. That project, charted by the highly popular Labor Prime Minister Ben Chifley (1945–51), carried through into what has been described as Australia's 'golden age', the years from about 1946 to 1974 that were supported by the long economic boom.[86]

While activity at the state level remained lively, federal interest was flagging and the Commonwealth National Fitness Council met for the last time in 1954. Reviewing progress in the first five years of the national fitness scheme in 1944, Bert Apps, the national men's officer, reported that while there were 'encouraging signs' of the campaign's achievements, 'much, very much, remains to be done'.[87] The initiative rested with states rather than at the federal centre. Work across states varied. In South Australia and Victoria, youth associations and community centres were strong parts of the work undertaken; in Queensland and Western Australia, residential summer schools for leaders became part of a well-supported programme of activities.[88]

There were varying ways of imagining the path to reconstruction. A damaging row between Gordon Young and the Director of Maternal and Infant Welfare, Dr Grace Cuthbert, exposed sharp points of difference. Young sought to give national fitness an expansive definition, going public with a vision that encompassed family relations and the health of children. To Cuthbert this was unacceptable. Young was crossing professional turf and exploiting the blurry ground between his role as a public servant and, in the wider ambit, as executive officer to the statutory National Fitness Council. Cuthbert was also a member of the National Fitness Council.

In late 1944 Young published the first issue of a *National Fitness Newsletter*, a more modest version of the *Physical Fitness* magazine he began in 1939. Alongside articles introducing the newsletter's purpose ('We intend to get to know each other better, and let each of the team know what the others are doing. Our teamship, confidence and trust in each other are vital in building National Fitness and making our dreams come true'),[89] and reports of recent events such as the National Youth Association Conference, was a prominently placed feature entitled 'Diary of the

Community, No.1'. A photograph of 18-month-old 'Lois', face smeared with jam, accompanied a story telling how Lois 'had never seen her father until last week'. Her mother struggled to bring her up in an upstairs room in a 'residential' (a boarding house), where Lois had to negotiate a linoleum-covered floor and then find her way outdoors by precariously 'clinging hard to the dusty posts of the balustrade'. Turning to Lois' mother, the story continued: 'It was hard bringing up a baby in a residential, but this was the best she could find. "When would Jack be home? What would they plan together? Would he be changed after the war? Their marriage ... it must be a success, somehow. They hardly knew each other, really."' And then Jack returned, and saw Lois at the top of the stairs: 'Through the door, Jack looked up. His heart in his mouth. "Yes, that was HIS daughter!" The feeling of dry hate in his mind, the cynicism from seeing death too often, from living contrary to the beliefs you were taught as a kid – all were brushed aside in a moment.' The article ended happily with Jack bounding up the stairs to rescue Lois: 'She was warm, soft and alive. There was a strong feeling inside him – the desire to live, to work, to build again.'[90]

To Cuthbert, the newsletter, and in particular, the 'Lois' story, were highly objectionable. Depicting the young child Lois as slum urchin and her parents as the victims of a callous or non-existent public health system spoke of everything Cuthbert's Department of Maternal and Infant Welfare was striving to eliminate. The story reverberated with the bitter betrayal of returning soldiers from World War I. Current plans for reconstruction following World War II were striving to avoid a repeat of that experience. Young had misrepresented the work of Cuthbert's Department, had failed to consult members of the Council and had misrepresented his position by signing himself 'Director, National Fitness and Physical Education' (only the first part was true). Besides, what had such a story to do with 'national fitness'? Cuthbert was incensed. Hers was one of several resignations from the Council. Young's attempt to expand the borders of national fitness to the broader social and health universe did not prosper. The determination to make a better world from the sacrifices of the war years stirred up powerful debate. Gordon Young turned his considerable energies to making recreation and sport, in the broadest sense, part of the postwar programme.

Public support for national fitness and greater physical activity appeared undimmed. A characteristic sign was the enthusiastic offer by Mr Burwell of La Perouse in New South Wales's Botany Bay, an area frequented by tourists as a landing site of Captain James Cook, and the site of a major Aboriginal community. Writing to the Minister of Health in 1946, Burwell suggested that boomerang throwing be added to the physical training activities for school children. He offered instruction to teachers and pupils in what was required, without charge. After consideration, the Minister turned him down 'because of the element of danger associated with boomerang throwing in public school grounds or where young children are congregated'.[91]

The big success story of national fitness in the post-1945 years, particularly in New South Wales, were the national outdoor camps. Providing young people with a chance to spend one or two weeks away from home, in 'the bush', swimming, hiking, exploring and learning to work together while enjoying sports and recreation, the camps were well supported. They built on the interwar enthusiasm for fresh air, sun, camping, bushwalking and youth hostelling, all activities encouraged by National Fitness Councils across Australia.[92] Bringing the model of organised recreational camping for young people from North America, and in particular the Ontario–Great Lakes region, Gordon Young developed a series of sites with permanent accommodation and facilities.[93] Designed more around achieving education through recreation than the largely canvas camps of churches, Boy Scouts and Girl Guides, the national fitness camps were non-sectarian and 'fun'-oriented.

The first camp opened at Broken Bay at the mouth of the Hawkesbury River north of Sydney in 1941. Young recruited volunteer labour and funds as well as drawing on public resources in preparing the site and building accommodation. His membership of the Sydney Rotary Club proved valuable, and fund-raising efforts included a dance featuring actress Betty Bryant in a hall decorated with cartoons of vitamins and a competition for the person with 'the most attractive eyebrows'.[94] A camp for girls at Point Wolstonecraft (Lake Macquarie) was built soon after. Others followed, the most ambitious being Narrabeen Lakes, which Young hoped would serve not only as another camp site but also as a National Sports Centre. By 1969 there were ten camps in operation. Over three decades, from the 1940s to the 1970s, it is estimated some 700,000 young people 'had had an outdoor experience in the bush', around one in three of the young people in the state.[95] A Fresh Air Fund (on the Ontario model) raised money to enable young people from poorer families to attend camp.

'Camp' was both a place and a time. For twelve-to-eighteen-year-olds it became, for many, a common rite of passage, a time away from home, a place where you went to do some of your growing up. For parents, schools and the National Fitness Council, camps were regarded as playing a vital part in what, by the 1950s, was increasingly described as the 'proper adjustment' of teenagers in the transition from childhood to responsible adulthood. Becoming 'well adjusted' was most successfully managed through interaction with peers at camp. Opportunity and control were present both in the experience and the discourse around camp. National fitness camps were also attended by children from immigrant families and Aboriginal communities. Residents at the Cootamundra Girls' Home and the Kinchela Boys' Home, under the authority of the Aboriginal Welfare Board, were some-time users of the camps. National fitness facilities were, thus, part of the larger modernising

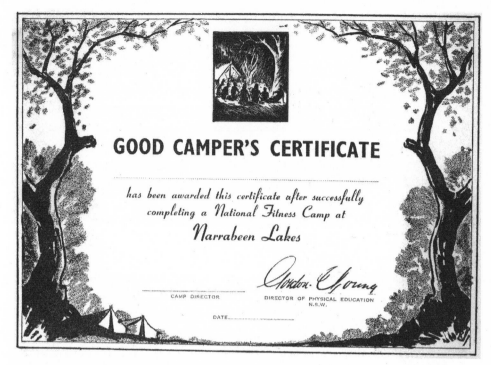

GOOD CAMPER'S CERTIFICATE

has been awarded this certificate after successfully completing a National Fitness Camp *at* Narrabeen Lakes

CAMP DIRECTOR

DIRECTOR OF PHYSICAL EDUCATION N.S.W.

DATE

Students attending the popular National Fitness camps established in New South Wales in 1941 received a Good Camper's Certificate at the conclusion of the camp. Around 1 in 3 young people in NSW attended a national fitness camp between the 1940s and 1970s. Precedent Book 11/19039, p.20, Agency 1728, State Records New South Wales

mechanisms directed to many Aboriginal young people at a time of transition from the older 'protection' to newer 'welfare' policies.[96]

In the postwar period, camps were also perceived as serving a crucial function in giving city children an experience of 'the bush'. A physical location, as the place beyond the city, the bush also carried a strong cultural meaning. While the sense of national culture conveyed in Russel Ward's *Australian Legend* (1958) was never universal, there was a residual notion that some authentic part of Australia lay in the bush rather than in the city. Learning to be an adult was also learning what it was to be an Australian. There was no better site to do that than in the bush. In 1950 a pledge to be used at the camps 'on such occasions as the Camp Director or Camp Principal considers desirable' was approved by the Secretary for Education. Campers would be encouraged to declare: 'In our hands lies the future of [this] great land, if we all work together doing our best for the common good, there is no limit to what our country can achieve. I salute my flag.'[97]

At the conclusion of their camps, which generally lasted fifteen days, young people went home with new experiences, sometimes new friends, ideally healthier, and, unless guilty of some misbehaviour, a 'Good Camper's Certificate' bearing the signature of Gordon Young, Director of Physical Education. They also took with them a sense of achievement as well as memories of good times.

While Fritz Duras retired in 1962, having reached the age of 65, Gordon Young enrolled as a student at the University of Sydney. Completing an MEd thesis, 'Physical Education in Australia: A Study of the History of Physical Education in Australia and a Forecast of Future Development', Young became the first substantial historian of the field he had spent a quarter of a century developing.[98] When he retired in 1969, the functions of the New South Wales state government were reorganised. His dual role was disentangled, the two parts becoming responsibilities of separate sections of government. Physical education was clearly demarcated as the responsibility of the Department of Education, while a separate National Fitness and Recreation Service was formed in 1970 to deal with what had previously come under the National Fitness Council's umbrella. The National Fitness and Recreation Service became part of a Ministry of Sport shortly thereafter (1972). The camps and other functions are now encompassed under the Sport and Recreation section within the NSW government agency Communities New South Wales. The work of National Fitness Councils in other states similarly became absorbed into departments of recreation, sport, culture and community. Their location within various government departments reflected differences in policy, between those emphasising participation and physical activity as part of community life and those emphasising public support for fostering competitive performance.

As Australian governments became more involved in sport, first with the emphasis on participation of Gough Whitlam's Labor administration, 1972–75, and then with a greater concern to ensure international competitive success from the late 1970s, the scale and nature of commitment has escalated substantially. The most prominent sign of this shift is the richly resourced Australian Institute of Sport (established in 1981). In Australia the 'national fitness' experiment exists much less as a distinct phase in the country's sporting and recreational history, than as part of a continuing story.

The Australian national fitness story is also one which follows some of the broad patterns of mid-twentieth-century Australian life: a complex struggle between federal, state and municipal authorities over powers, money, resources and responsibilities; a story of wartime adversity followed by expansive reconstruction and a blossoming in the golden years of the 1950s and 1960s; and the proliferation of areas of professional expertise. As a measure variously perceived as one of health, education, social service, recreation or defence, national fitness also interacted awkwardly across layers of government, and between government and voluntary associations. Driven by state education departments and universities providing physical education qualifications, it fell under the health portfolio in Canberra. As Imke Fischer argues, the years from the 1940s to 1970s were ones of 'silent control' by the federal government.[99] For David Kirk, the transition from the 1930s to the postwar period is one from 'disciplined' and regimented bodies to 'liberated' bodies.[100] While it is possible to see government extending its policy via voluntary organisations, as Melanie Oppenheimer suggests, in this case there is as much, if not more, evidence to suggest that voluntary organisations were pressing hard for government (at state and federal levels) to take up *their* agenda.[101]

National fitness in Australia was born from a period of intense interest in the body, when a civic language of citizenship promoted the healthy and fit body as a political aspiration. Democracy, leisure and physical fitness were wound into a language of citizenship in which the goal was individual physical fitness across the population. But the interwar era of progressive nationalism pursued within imperial loyalties gave way to a new order of social welfare; education for leisured citizenship to health was part of an era of prosperity. Recreation and physical activity remained important post-1945, but became encompassed within a more collective form of citizenship – within a sense of social cohesion. Sporting competition mattered, but remained in the domain of voluntary effort.

From the 1970s, national pride through sporting success was a populist thread in a more independently minded Australia. Being Australian remained closely connected with the outdoors, and with having an interest in and being successful at sport. Federal and state investment in sport became substantial in the late twentieth and early twenty-first centuries. Hosting the 1956 (Melbourne) and 2000 (Sydney) Olympic Games were occasions of massive national as well as civic pride. The success, and more occasional failure, of the nation's elite sporting teams (especially the men's cricket team) is often taken as a barometer of national mood. But in the later twentieth century the body was not a novel subject of attention, and making the case for investment in it no longer had to be done in the terms that civic campaigners urged in the 1930s.

4 Fitness for War and a Changed World

National Fitness in Canada

Canada's experiment with national fitness started late and finished early. The National Physical Fitness Act was passed only in 1943 and repealed in 1954.[1] But physical exercise and sporting success were central to the way in which Canadians became modern and imagined themselves as a nation from the 1920s through to the end of the twentieth century.[2] The decades that saw the opening of grand new stadia for ice hockey at the Montreal Forum (1926) and Toronto's Maple Leaf Gardens (1932) also saw the catastrophe of almost a quarter of Canada's workers out of jobs. From the misery came both a nationwide radio audience for the Canadian Radio Broadcasting Corporation's Saturday night show 'Hockey Night in Canada', and a publicly funded programme of sport and recreation that would serve as the model for the 1943 national initiative.[3]

Arguments for government funding for sport, recreation and physical fitness came from the remaking of relations between government and people, first through the crisis of Depression and then through the hopes of 'social citizenship' generated by wartime mobilisation. Fading idealism and Cold War scepticism led to the 1943 scheme being dropped by the early 1950s. But political interests, and especially national prestige, brought sport and physical fitness back onto the public agenda. Within two years of Prince Philip's widely reported Toronto speech in which he chided his audience with the comment that 'Canada's achievement in sports and games were hardly in keeping with a country which claimed almost the highest standard of living in the world', John Diefenbaker's Conservative government had passed the Fitness and Amateur Sport Act 1961.[4] The Act opened the door once more to government involvement in sport and physical fitness. Supporting sport and physical fitness became an enduring element of Canadian public life from that time forth.

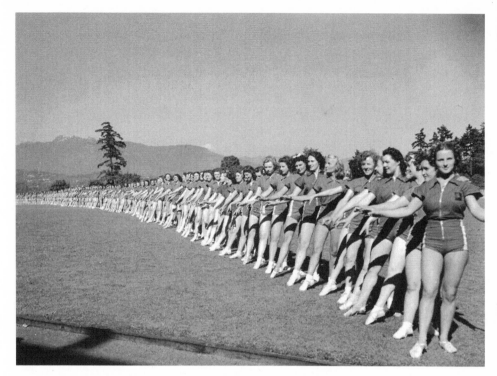

'Pro-Rec' – Provincial Recreation – programmes initially set up for unemployed people in 1934 proved so popular they were made available to all. Summer displays were part of a changing schedule of activities. CVA 586-226, Vancouver City Archives

The Canadian story is also the story of prominent 'un-Canadian' Jan Eisenhardt (1906–2004). Born in Denmark, Eisenhardt came to Vancouver in 1928 as a twenty-two-year-old, bringing with him a Scandinavian training and a dedicated commitment to physical health and activity as a means for securing social as well as personal freedom. In British Columbia he was responsible for what was arguably the most successful community sport and recreation programme of any national fitness initiative of this era: the 'Pro-Rec' (provincial recreation) movement. Appointed as director of the nationwide scheme following the passing of the 1943 legislation, Eisenhardt's career as a sport and fitness innovator came to an abrupt end when he was designated a security risk in the midst of the Cold War and was blacklisted as 'un-Canadian'. Eisenhardt always understood that the body was political, but this outcome was unimaginable.[5]

Canada played a key role in the dynamic world of globalising sport that Barbara Keys has described for the 1930s.[6] Eisenhardt's work adapted Danish models in developing public recreation programmes to a North American setting. The largest of the Dominions, Canada was at the forefront of fostering British ties of empire through sporting competition. John Astley Cooper's 1890s dream for a Pan-Britannic

Festival of cultural and athletic prowess had failed, but Bobby Robinson and the citizens of the lakeside city of Hamilton, Ontario, succeeded in hosting the first British Empire Games in August 1930. Robinson was a journalist and the prime instigator behind the event, and the city of Hamilton backed the Games with significant funding input. As opposed to the fractious tone of the 1920s Olympics, the Games were presented as an occasion to reinforce both the sentiment and 'blood ties' of empire and to re-assert British dominance in international sport. David Burghley led the English team and competed in the first event, a heat for the 400-metres hurdles. Percy Williams, the Canadian 100- and 200-metre national champion, took the oath on behalf of the athletes.[7] Canadian athletes were prominent competitors in the succeeding 1934 (London) and 1938 (Sydney) Empire Games, and hosted the second postwar event in Vancouver in 1954.

Radio listeners across the competing countries could follow the performance of athletes through the BBC Empire Service, and through 'special events' programmes such as those run by the Canadian Radio Broadcasting Corporation. Governors-general and games organisers described the value of these events in terms of the ties of 'blood' and 'family' that linked those inhabiting a common British world (such views said little to the substantial Francophone community within Canada). The values of family in the Anglo world were not just ones of sentiment but also spilled into the commercial world. Imperial Tobacco was just one company to take up the powerful exposure that sports broadcasting made possible. Their advertisements featured between CRBC reports at the 1934 London Games.[8]

At the same time, however, it was the fate of ice hockey teams that increasingly attracted popular national following amongst Canadians. In this realm, there was less of a common sporting culture shared between Canada, Britain, Australia and New Zealand. While the classic 'games of empire', cricket and varieties of football, were played, they had come to occupy narrow regional and class enclaves. The increasingly popular following commanded by hockey drew Canada much more into a North American sporting world. The US-controlled National Hockey League (NHL) formed in 1917 provided a competition in which teams such as Conn Smythe's Maple Leafs, and Saturday night broadcasts of the big games across the growing CBC network from the early 1930s, thrived. But the NHL was also the most prominent example of an ongoing tension in Canadian sports and games – between attraction to the larger and more professionally organised sports culture (and associated commercial broadcasting and press coverage) and determination to define and protect local amateur sports and athletic talent from the larger US enterprise. Observing the dual influences at work in Canada, although in relation to social policy at this time, Harry Cassidy noted: 'Like so many things Canadian, it is something of a cross between the British and the American versions, with some native ingredients added.'[9]

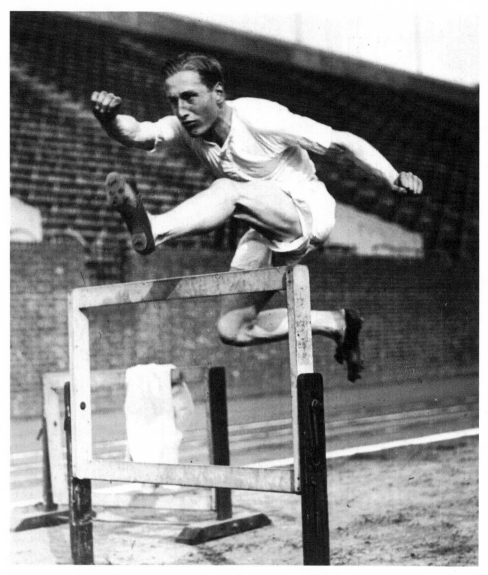

Champion hurdler, Lord David Burghley (1905–81), competed at the 1924, 1928 and 1932 Olympics, and at the first Empire Games held in Hamilton, Ontario, in 1930. He was a leading member of England's National Fitness Council, 1937–39, chairing its Publicity sub-committee, by which time he was Conservative MP for Peterborough. Burghley featured in *Chariots of Fire* (1981), one scene showing him training with glasses of champagne poised on either side of the hurdle. The Burghley House Collection, England

Sporting competition drew Canada into a variety of international arenas that consolidated imaginings of a common nation while also drawing on different strands within that imagining – British and American, historical and contemporary, amateur and professional. Those interweaving forces were still at work in shaping public debate and aspirations for sporting and physical fitness in the 1950s. Sporting and leisure culture provided part of the context for what emerged as the more focused national fitness scheme under the 1943 legislation. Physical fitness and the lobbyists for better physical education as part of a more widely conceived citizenship proved to be those most involved in shaping the Canadian scheme as it evolved in the early 1940s.

Playing Through the Depression

As early as 1918 members of the leading sporting association, the Amateur Athletic Union of Canada (AAU), took a delegation to Ottawa proposing a national sports and recreation programme to the government. Well-organised sport and recreation, they argued, could serve both as rehabilitation for returning soldiers and as a memorial to those who had fallen. The programme included an extension of existing municipal playground and related facilities, and an investment in physical education at all levels. The AAU would provide policy and technical direction to a government administration.[10] The delegation went away empty-handed, but it was characteristic of Canada's sporting associations that they made such an approach, and continued to do so through the interwar years. Unlike sporting associations elsewhere, Canada's amateur sports leaders, typically drawn from the same social and political elite that was represented in provincial and central government, regarded public support via funding and endorsement not as a threat to their autonomy but as necessary in upholding the practices of amateurism against incipient professionalism, and to protect Canada's best talent from being recruited to better-endowed college programmes and professional leagues in the United States.

By the time Dr Arthur Lamb led the Canadian team to the Olympic Games in Los Angeles in 1932, the fears of the AAU had been realised. Most of the medal-winning members of the team were athletes who competed and/or were coached in the United States. As manager of the Olympic team and member of the Canadian Olympic Association Executive, as well as Director of Physical Education at Montreal's McGill University, Lamb occupied a powerful and unique position in the Canadian sporting world.[11] He had already had to fend off a campaign to boycott the Games by the Workers' Sport Association, who condemned the event as 'boss' sport, another form of class oppression designed as 'an inducement to breed ... patriotism and militarism'.[12] He had also incurred the wrath of Alexandrine Gibb, head of the women's track athletes in the 1928 team, and others from the Women's Amateur Athletic Federation of Canada, for voting for the removal of women's events from the Olympic programme following the 1928 Games. Not only had Lamb voted to reduce women's already limited competitive opportunity at international level, but he had done so without consulting the athletes or their association.[13]

By the 1930s, it had become clear that competition in sport was not confined to what went on between athletes and players in the sporting arena. It was also about who could play, the terms on which people played and what they played for. As Bruce Kidd has so convincingly demonstrated, the 1930s witnessed a struggle for Canadian sport – between amateur and professional, workers and bosses, and between advocates of women's right to compete against those who believed competition was antithetical to modern femininity (including the majority of women physical educators). In this contest for power, public resources – whether in the form of direct funding grants, broadcasting access, taxation levied from entrance fee income at the gates, municipal grounds, patronage by public office-holders or physical education curricula – all became part of the tussle.[14] The contest between competing interests was also a sign of how valuable sport had become, in cultural and commercial terms.

The Canadian government's contribution of $10,000 to the AAU toward getting the national team to Berlin for the 1936 Olympics recognised some of the costs involved and the prestige that accrued from successful performance. But it dismayed Lamb and other AAU leaders who had to find the remaining two-thirds of the budget, and appalled the Workers' Sport movement who were part of an international coalition of worker, leftwing, Jewish and anti-fascist groups urging athletes and teams to withdraw from the Games in protest at the Nazi regime's policy towards Jews. In Canada, as in the other Dominions and in Britain, the campaign failed and teams were sent to compete. The British Olympic Association's decision to attend was crucial in determining the Canadian stance. The impressive demonstration of athletic prowess and youthful fitness generally on display throughout Europe and specifically in Berlin made an impact on Canadians as it did on Britons, New Zealanders and Australians. Arguments that the country's sport and physical fitness should be put on a stronger administrative footing and more scientific basis under government direction were aired in late 1936.

Early in 1937 the former hockey star, and now lawyer and Liberal MP, Hugh Plaxton put a resolution to the House of Commons proposing the formation of a ministry of sport. Plaxton's proposal was debated by Canadian MPs as the British government's White Paper on physical training and recreation was published. One of the arguments Plaxton made was that national interests implicit in top sporting events were now too crucial to leave in amateur hands. National prestige, the importance of sports to national health, efficiency in administration and a proposed 'national scheme of physical training' to be run with the provinces were other parts of his bid. While there was some support for the idea, it did not proceed.[15] But interest in the work of the World Leisure Congress and what was being done in Britain and Europe did not subside. On his visit to Berlin in June 1937, Prime Minister Mackenzie King met Hitler, was hosted by von Ribbentrop, and lunched at the British Embassy with Sir Nevile Henderson and his local guests General Göring and Baron von Neurath. He spent much of the Sunday of his visit on a tour of the Reich Sport Field and Physical Culture Academy, a labour camp, new roads and the work of the Strength through Joy labour organisation in the company of the Reich sport leader, Herr von Tschammer.[16]

Canadian athletes attending the Empire Games in Sydney in February 1938 did not have the advantage of such lavish sports facilities. Amateur sports organisers had, once again, to scrimp and save to gather together sufficient funds to send even a small team of competitors. Team members had to find their own way by rail to Vancouver and to be in a position to be away for nearly three months. They included seventeen-year-old sprinter Barbara Howard, 'the first woman of colour' to represent Canada on an international team. But even the successes of the team amidst the vicissitudes of 'hot climate, inadequate living conditions, insect bites'[17] and the lengthy journey did not give any further impetus to the AAU's argument for government support.

Competitive sport played on an amateur basis (the AAU model) was only one kind of 'body culture' attracting the attention of Canadians in the mid-1930s.[18] The National Hockey League was now a major feature in the national as well as sporting landscape. Toronto's Maple Leafs team was quickly attracting a following through much of Anglo-Canada, thanks to its success on the ice and exposure on Saturday night broadcasts to the network of public stations by national radio. If professional hockey emphasised a spectacle of combative masculinity, a modern physicality for women was presented in a popular alternative. When Prunella Stack sailed to Toronto in 1935 bringing the message of the Women's League of Health and Beauty to the women of Canada, she was received by eager adherents. A group of over one hundred women gave a demonstration of rhythmic exercises clad in the League's distinctive black shorts and white tops following her address to a large audience at the Eaton's auditorium in Toronto in September. Within a year the membership had grown to a thousand, and within two years to over five thousand in Toronto alone. Other League branches were founded across Ontario, and in Montreal. Although the League continued after the war, and still maintains a small presence, its popularity never reached the heights of the late 1930s.[19] Workplace sports and exercise teams such as the basketball team made up of employees from Woodward's, a large department store in western Canada, were also popular through the 1930s.[20]

All these activities, and the extensive coverage of sport in the daily and magazine press, testify to the same popular enthusiasm for fitness and sport in Canada by the mid-1930s as was evident across Britain, Australia and New Zealand. Calls from physical educators, public health advocates and some sporting associations for more to be done to promote physical fitness along the lines of national campaigns under way in Britain, and prompted by the League of Nations in a report in 1936, failed to win a political constituency either among Conservatives, in office until 1935, or the Liberals who replaced them at the start of a long hold on power. But

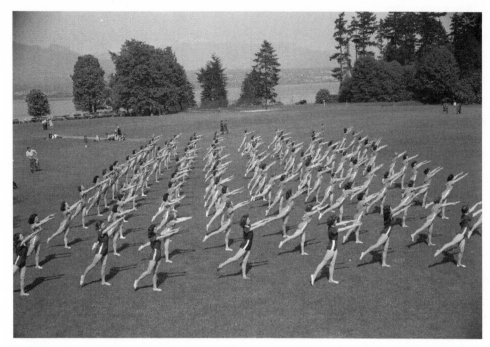

Calisthenics demonstration by 'Pro-Rec' group, Stanley Park, Vancouver, 1940s. CVA 1184-2357, Vancouver City Archives

political action was finally spurred in response to the dark rather than light side of modernity, by the prospect of idle rather than active bodies.

The great shadow of the Depression that cast thousands of people into misery and lassitude across Canada hit British Columbia and the city of Vancouver particularly hard. In the parks, streets and among the abandoned car wrecks around rubbish dumps, groups of men who had gone west in hope of work, a passage out or simply a milder climate congregated in what were described at the time as 'hobo jungles'.[21] City authorities were faced with providing what relief they could to thousands of people, and maintaining order in the midst of desperation and poverty. Under the Liberal premier Duff Pattullo's 'little new deal', a more constructive and less punitive regime towards those out of work was possible.[22] The hated labour camps were discredited and new directions were pursued. In late 1934 Jan Eisenhardt, with the backing of provincial Minister of Education George Weir (a professor of education at the University of British Columbia before entering politics), proposed a scheme of volunteer-run games and recreation classes for those unemployed aged 15 and over. Eisenhardt had started work in the city as a playground supervisor with the Vancouver Parks Board when he first arrived six years earlier aged twenty-two. By 1934 his energy and ambition had taken him to being supervisor of all the city playgrounds.[23] These public parks and recreation areas, developed through the work of women's organisations from around the turn of the century, were valuable amenities within the city, designed to offer safe and attractive public space, and constructive recreational areas especially but not solely for children and young people. They were first staffed by volunteers, but by the 1920s the city had taken over responsibility for their supervision.

Eisenhardt and Weir set up what came to be known as Pro-Rec: a publicly funded, free, genuinely popular community sport and recreation programme. Offering classes for free, initially to those unemployed and then, under popular demand, to all aged fifteen and over who were no longer in school, Pro-Rec membership grew rapidly. Members took part in a wide range of activities – exercise and fitness classes in local halls two or three times a week, bowling (the most popular participatory sport at the time), basketball, volleyball, boxing, wrestling and apparatus gymnastics for men; keep-fit, gymnastics, dancing and some games predominated in the women's classes. Hiking, picnics, youth hostelling, and various outings and social activities were also organised depending on season and facilities. The constructive and purposeful nature of recreation was evident when defined against 'mere loafing or off-side amusement'.[24] Eisenhardt's familiarity with the popular Danish adult education system known as the Folk High School, which promoted co-operative principles, and the rhythmic gymnastics of Niels Bukh were influential in shaping the recreation programme that developed in Vancouver and then across British Columbia.[25]

Registered participants grew very rapidly from an initial 2,700 in 1934–35 to nearly 27,000 in 1938–39. The number of centres from which the programme operated started at nineteen in 1934–35, the first year, expanding to 135 by 1938–39.[26] Pro-Rec members came from 'all walks of life ... and all ages', encompassing unemployed youth, housewives, young working women and businessmen seeking exercise.[27] In the second year, a membership crest was sold to participants for 15 cents. It featured the letters PRC over an embroidered British Columbia coat-of-arms. Members were encouraged to wear simple uniforms, if they could be afforded: dark shorts and gym shoes for men, shorts and a blouse for women (later supplemented by the light-blue one-piece gymnastic suit that became known as the women's Pro-Rec uniform). As a cost-saving measure, a special soft shoe was designed for women to make from canvas or heavy cotton and elastic, with felt from an old hat used for the sole.[28]

The spectacular demonstrations by young women's fitness classes staged at Stanley Park in the summer were highlights on the annual programme of events. Akin to the big demonstrations of the Women's League of Health and Beauty, Pro-Rec displays combined exercise, health, fitness, grace and a splash of glamour. Quite unlike old-style physical jerks, or the controversial involvement of women in competitive, exertion-demanding sports, fitness demonstrations had a highly contemporary feel. They proved very attractive to a wide range of young women in the city.[29]

Unusually for sports and physical recreation programmes, Pro-Rec drew in more women than men. The success of the keep-fit classes and especially the mass displays was partly responsible. The slogan 'Health, Beauty, Diet and Sports' encapsulated the same sort of winning combination as the Women's League of Health and Beauty's 'Movement is Life', emphasising the glamour, goodness and modernity of physical health and fitness. Eisenhardt encouraged women leaders as well as women members, doing much to foster professional advancement.[30] The strength of women's civic culture in Vancouver also provided something by way of leadership and impetus to the Pro-Rec phenomenon. In 1928 a Women's Building had opened in Thurlow Street in central Vancouver, providing a meeting place for the city's women's organisations.[31] Political mobilisation, which had had franchise as its focus – won in 1917 – did not subside but turned to a range of local and national issues.

The success of British Columbia's Pro-Rec scheme proved an inspiration to a series of limited-term initiatives taken by Mackenzie King's Liberal government when it was returned to office in 1935 by an electorate desperate for relief from continued recession. Ian Mackenzie, the new Minister of Health and National Pensions, represented a Vancouver seat in the Ottawa Parliament and was familiar with Eisenhardt and the Pro-Rec programme. From briefings given to the National Employment Commission came recreation schemes for unemployed people aged eighteen to thirty under the Unemployment Agricultural Assistance Act (1937), Youth Training Act (1939) and Vocational Training programmes (1942). Funding from the Dominion (Ottawa) government was provided to provincial authorities on a 50:50 basis to run recreational programmes designed 'to sustain morale in times of idleness', 'maintain employability' and find 'releases for inner life through recreation'.[32] Around $1.5 million dollars per year was committed to support the schemes.[33]

They fell well short of what the small but vocal lobby pressing for a national physical fitness programme on a scale similar to that under way in Britain was aiming at. Prominent figures in the physical education and public health professions, including Arthur Lamb at McGill and A. A. Burridge at McMaster, ran a public education campaign through the National Physical Fitness League formed in 1938.[34] Unlike their colleagues in Britain or Australasia, they failed to make national fitness a political priority in the years c.1937–39. Saving rather than spending money remained a government priority, as the numbers of unemployed and the effect of the Depression lingered. The federal government took the view that recreation and preventive health were the responsibility of local and provincial governments – and not necessarily a public priority.

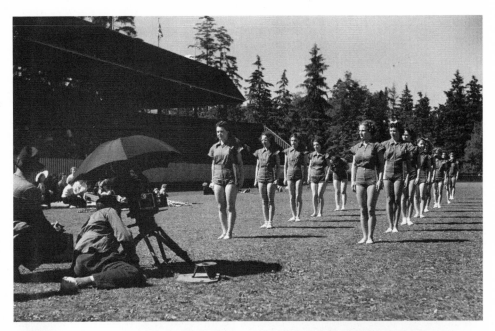

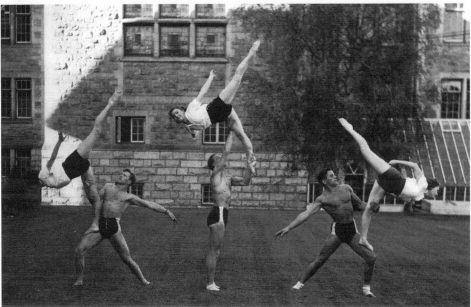

Top: The summertime mass demonstrations by 'Pro-Rec' groups proved popular with spectators and with the press. This group was being filmed by movie and still photographers. CVA 586-235, Vancouver City Archives

Below: Spectacular gymnastic displays showing strength, skill and balance such as this one performed by 'Pro-Rec' participants took much practice to perfect. They were popular among groups keen to present a daring demonstration and to convey abilities of the collective rather than the individual. Sp P46.4, Vancouver City Archives

Wartime Promises and Peacetime Ambitions

Only in 1943 was a National Physical Fitness Bill put before the parliament in Ottawa. Concern over the level of fitness of men called up for service was the immediate rationale, but the wartime measure owed at least as much to the political consequences of the country's mobilisation for war as it did to a sudden awakening to levels of health and fitness in the population. Providing for the establishment of a national council led by an executive director, whose purpose was to promote 'the physical fitness of the people of Canada',[35] the Bill signalled the government's commitment to an ongoing and universal programme supporting adult physical health. The proposed legislation followed the Australian model in establishing a national organisation to distribute federal funds to regional governments responsible for running programmes, and to provide technical oversight. Funding of an initial $250,000 per year was to be allocated to provinces on the same 50:50 basis as applied in the preceding unemployed youth recreation schemes. The scale of financial support hardly denoted the measure's urgency in the context of the government's wartime administration. As Lamb commented the following year, against the $11 million being spent daily 'for death and destruction', the total annual sum spent on national fitness 'would only last our fighting forces approximately thirty minutes'.[36]

Canada's national fitness scheme came into existence as the political expectations of Canadians moved to the left. The Bill was one product of a series of debates beginning in late 1942–early 1943 in which the Mackenzie King government rehearsed possible shapes for a peacetime welfare state in efforts to fend off the challenge by the socialist Co-operative Commonwealth Federation's (CCF) rapid rise in popularity, and strong support for the Communist Party. Offering an alternative to the two main parties, the CCF's promise of guaranteed jobs and social security held strong appeal. A draft National Physical Fitness Bill (first named the National War Fitness Bill) emerged from the overlapping mesh of politicians' and officials' deliberations instigated by the parliamentary Special Committee on Social Security. Leonard Marsh's *Social Security for Canada* (often described as Canada's 'Beveridge report') and a report on health provision from a group of officials headed by Dr J. J. Heagerty, a sympathiser with the cause of national fitness, were presented in March 1943 along with the draft Bill. A national physical fitness scheme had been in Minister of Health Ian Mackenzie's sights for some months. The measure's uncontroversial ideal and ready wartime focus on the need for fit servicemen, along with its very modest budget, made it a useful measure for the Liberals to signal a response to immediate circumstances, as well as a forward-looking attention to matters of health for all Canadians. The more difficult commitment to national health insurance was put on the table but not resolved.[37]

Introducing the Bill to his colleagues, Mackenzie raised expectations that the work of the National Council would do much to address 'the standard of physical fitness among our people', which had 'not been as high as we should have liked it to be'. Acknowledging that the resources provided were small relative to the task, he was reassuringly hopeful: 'at least it is a beginning; perhaps tall oaks may from little acorns grow'.[38] The Minister's description of the legislation as 'non-contentious and non-controversial'[39] was largely borne out. Opposition members questioned matters of detail rather than the underlying principles at stake. Tommy Church, Conservative MP for the Toronto seat of Broadview, argued that the funds should be available to municipalities rather than provincial governments as this would get it to places where the money could be used more directly and effectively. Strongly supporting federal action on physical fitness, Church underlined the impact the war had had on exposing the need for greater action not only in Canada, but also as a result of the 'great change in thought of the people of the British empire':

> The war brought to light that a large number of our young people were not physically fit; it showed the need of a national movement to promote physical fitness among men, women and children, and our whole system of education from elementary schools to the universities seemed to have been lacking and deficient.[40]

Church also urged more action on promoting sports and games, decrying the government's lack of a sports policy. He told the House that 'Canada has excelled in this war, as it did in the last, largely through sportsmanship of all kinds and branches'. Now 'that we are in the fifth year of the war there should be a national statement from the government to clear the air as to what shall be done to finish the war and then what shall be done afterwards'.[41] Speaking for the Cooperative Commonwealth Federation, G. H. Castleden, Member for the Saskatchewan seat of Yorkton, gave his party's strong support for what he hoped would be the beginning of something larger. Like others, he considered it 'disgraceful that there had to be a war to bring out the records of the standards of Canada's health'.[42] In the Senate, Iva Fallis gave her support to the measure, noting that 'anyone interested in the future well-being of the citizens of Canada cannot do other than give support to the principle and ideas involved in this legislation'. She pointed to the associated importance of proper nutrition to physical fitness and also made a plea that women 'have a greater voice ... in the carrying out of post-war programmes'. The physical fitness provided for in the 1943 measure was a cause in which she believed women 'can be of great service'.[43]

The Act passed through all its stages on 21 July 1943, taking effect from 1 October.[44] Jan Eisenhardt was subsequently appointed National Director, and members of the National Council named on 15 February 1944.[45]

Pressure on the government to convince electors that there would be something worth fighting for intensified from 1943 to 1945. The political situation highlights the significance of the National Physical Fitness Act as a small flag raised to a brighter peacetime future. As Peter Elson notes, Canadians carried the legacy of deprivation from the Depression with them 'as they were being asked to fight for Canada in the Second World War': social as well as national security was the goal.[46] Sensitivity over the terms on which Canada had agreed to enter the war – notably, that conscription would be accepted but on the condition that none of those called up would be required to serve overseas – was under severe strain by 1944. The government finally broke the agreement, incurring strong opposition.[47] The continuing popularity of the CCF meant that the Liberals went to the polls in 1945 having provided a generous Family Allowance scheme, a Veterans Charter and a Green Book of promises for health insurance, unemployment assistance, social housing and universal old-age pensions. The newly constituted National Council for Physical Fitness embraced its task in this context of an expanding 'social citizenship', a significant remaking of the relations between government and people.

To Eisenhardt the goal was ambitious, a promise of health that meant much more than the absence of disease, and a sense of social duty. At the first meeting of the Council, he set down an understanding of the work ahead in a resolution that described physical fitness 'to mean the best state of health, to which has been added such qualities as strength, agility and endurance as are necessary for a life of maximum service of one's family and country'. Further elaboration was given in noting that 'although the purpose of the Act is to develop the physical fitness of the people of Canada, this Council stresses the fourfold nature of fitness which is spiritual, moral, mental and physical and that total fitness must originate in the home, the church, the school and the community'.[48] In a 1944 article, Arthur Lamb's warm endorsement of the initiative he had long lobbied for was similarly idealistic. Noting that the 'greatest asset of any nation is the health of its citizens', he urged his readers not only to think of the immediate needs of manpower, rehabilitation and reconstruction, 'important aspects of any plan for social security', but also to ask whether it was 'even more important that most aggressive steps be taken towards pre-habilitation to enable the forthcoming generation to live more wholesomely and happily?'[49]

British Columbia's Pro-Rec scheme got a considerable fillip in funding under the population formula of the National Physical Fitness Act.[50] Its activities expanded to include community centre projects and school sports championships. In Alberta and Saskatchewan, public recreation programmes developed under the preceding schemes of provision for unemployed youth were also consolidated. Physical education became the focus elsewhere. Quebec did not enter into the scheme, its funding allocation dropping from what it had previously received under the 1930s youth and unemployment initiatives.[51] (The impetus behind national fitness was largely drawn from Anglo-Canada, and the wartime circumstances in which it became a federal initiative were symptomatic of the distance between 'the two solitudes' of Francophone and Anglophone Canada.[52]) At the Ottawa national office a series of pamphlets outlining exercise and posture were published between 1946 and 1948. The Council's existence also provided a stimulus to the longer-lasting Canadian Sports Advisory Council.[53]

Although Ontario joined the federal scheme later, in 1947, it was already running publicly funded recreation under the Ontario Community Programmes Branch. Activities like those available in the city of Brantford were typical. John Pearson, the local recreation organiser, emphasised community action and citizen participation, and encouraged local residents to form groups themselves rather than at his instigation. To the comment, 'We need more tennis in this town', Pearson would reply, 'Well, what are you doing about it?' Mobilising neighbourhood energies was the best way to build community and was consistent with the underlying ideal that such programmes were ultimately about teaching and promoting 'democratic living'. The community committee rather than the paid official became the driving force. But there were many impediments to such an ideal, among them the time and effort for committee work as well as the recreation activity. Having 'to work to play' was not always what residents most wanted to do in their precious time 'off'.[54] But for a period, however, a thriving, largely volunteer local recreation scene buzzed with things to do – euchre games, playground activities, folk dancing, movie nights, craft classes, current-event discussions and garden parties.[55]

Government support for physical fitness and active recreation was not confined to the work of the National Council. It also appeared in other areas of federal responsibility. Sport and physical recreation as a tool for the 'advancement' of indigenous people – as an aspect of the wider project of 'remedying backwardness' – was also part of the immediate postwar story in Canada.[56] Eisenhardt left his position with the National Council for Physical Fitness to take up a job with the United Nations in New York at the end of 1946. When he returned to Canada he was employed by the Department of Indian Affairs in the newly established position of Supervisor of Physical Education and Recreation. Taking up the job in February 1950, Eisenhardt joined the Department at a critical time in its history. A wider re-direction in federal 'Indian' policy, away from explicit assimilation and more towards integration, was codified in the Indian Act 1951, a descendant of the original Indian Act 1876.[57] The 1951 Act removed prohibitions on indigenous people's access to alcohol, engagement of legal services and certain cultural practices such as the potlatch, while also giving incentives to various forms of 'advancement'. In Eisenhardt's parlance, as for many non-indigenous Canadians, potlatch ceremonies were still referred to as 'orgies'.[58] While the era of universal human rights, racial 'advance' and urbanisation brought new forms of interaction between indigenous

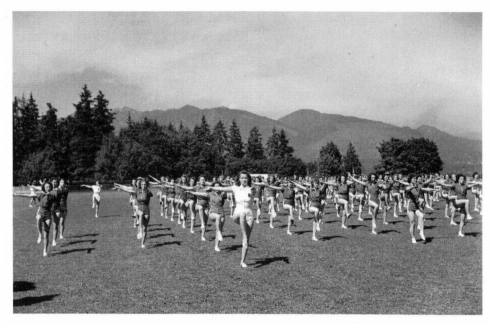

Exercise in the open air was a central part of the 'Pro-Rec' system. The healthy properties of sunlight, fresh air and open space were seen as life-giving along with the exercise routines. CVA 586-234, Vancouver City Archives

and non-indigenous peoples in Canada, as it had in New Zealand and Australia, it took some time for cultural understanding to develop.

Sports, recreation and physical education programmes were looked to as part of the remedy in tackling poor health conditions in mission schools and on reserves. Games were considered a good way to facilitate the integration of aboriginal young people into the public school system.[59] Not only were sport and games useful in teaching skills and teamsmanship, they were also looked to here, as elsewhere, to instil the virtues and rewards of individual achievement, healthy competition, and the disciplines of time and adherence to a common set of rules. Such attributes were regarded as inherently valuable, but were also usefully transferred to participation in schoolroom, workplace and modern social life. Sport, games and physical recreation programmes offered a means whereby 'Aboriginal peoples' resistant and residual cultural orientations might be contested and transformed',[60] where 'traditional' people could become modern Canadian citizens.

The position filled by Jan Eisenhardt required 'a man of considerable tact and diplomacy'. The Department of Indian Affairs only controlled day schools for indigenous children and relied on church organisations to run the more numerous residential schools. The Department had to persuade the churches to change their practice, but could not direct them to do so. Janice Forsyth and Michael Heine, writing in 2008 with the benefit of contemporary records and an interview with

Eisenhardt, emphasise Eisenhardt's long-standing desire 'to work with Aboriginal people', albeit from a rather romanticised view formed in part by James Fenimore Cooper's novels. Eisenhardt's duties in his new role –

> ... included developing and implementing a comprehensive program of physical education and recreation for students in day and residential schools and for the inhabitants of reserves, conducting physical education and recreation courses for field agents and teachers of Indian schools, and cooperating with provincial authorities in joint programs of physical education and recreation.[61]

Undertaking a survey of the recreational facilities that existed was Eisenhardt's first priority, a task he undertook from April to October 1950, visiting thirty-two residential schools, twenty-one day schools, and twenty reserves in Quebec, Ontario, Saskatchewan, Alberta and British Columbia.[62] Eisenhardt's suggestion that consulting with 'the Indian chiefs' would be useful as he surveyed what currently existed and devised recommendations was sternly rebuffed by his superiors. New, not old advice was what was required: the expertise of a professional, not timeworn 'tradition'. A modernising agenda could still be contained within departmental paternalism. Most reserves and schools had very limited sports equipment or grounds, even for simple games of volleyball and football. But alongside this material poverty, Eisenhardt also observed some very rich practice, most evident in the popular Sports Days. At Cowichan, British Columbia, he described one such event 'where nearly 800 people attended the field day competitions in 1950. The festivities included races for all ages, ranging from the seventy-five-yard dash to the mile, softball and soccer games, "comical" contests, and a bone game.'[63] Such occasions were as much about communality and socialising as competitive sports. In Eisenhardt's view, the Sports Days did not necessarily encourage the best physical performance and, thus, could have indifferent outcomes, but nonetheless he appreciated the inclusiveness they fostered. He also recognised that play and games might take a range of cultural forms, some emphasising participation while others might encourage high-level competitive performance that would draw on the skills of those regarded as 'natural' athletes.

As Forsyth and Heine suggest, Eisenhardt shared many of the views of his progressive contemporaries in appreciating the different aspirations of indigenous Canadians and, in particular, their desire for greater autonomy and self-determination, while also pressing a need for 'a higher degree of social organisation' in health and recreation.[64] His recommendations with regard to sport, games and physical recreation were designed to inculcate greater aspiration towards competitive achievement within a wider programme of 'cultural advancement'. The 'cultural skills' achieved by participation in such activities would, in turn, 'help the Indian to achieve the social and economic progress necessary to enable him to take his place in the modern world and will enlist his active participation in the shaping of the future of his people'.[65]

As well as putting these views forward in reports for his superiors, Eisenhardt also published them in an article in the professional journal of the American Association for Health, Physical Education and Recreation, under the title 'The Canadian Red Man of Today'.[66] The article put Eisenhardt in trouble with his bosses. He had not consulted them over the publication of the article, the contents of which, he was told, would be sure to inflame relations between the Department of Indian Affairs and the churches running the residential schools. Effectively thwarted thereafter in his role in the Department, he resigned, after less than two years, in December 1951. The low pay carried by the position was a further precipitating factor.[67] From Eisenhardt's brief tenure, however, came an achievement of enduring value: an award recognising the significant history of indigenous sporting success with which to inspire contemporary athletes. Named in honour of distance runner Tom Longboat (1887–1949), a member of the Onondaga Nation in the Six Nations of the Grand River, and winner of the 1907 Boston marathon in record time (2:24:24), the first award was made in 1951. It carried with it considerable prestige.[68]

The Cold War was to prove the death knell for Canada's early experiment with government-supported physical fitness and the career of its most effective exponent. From the Department of Indian Affairs, Eisenhardt took up a position in the staff training section of the large airplane manufacturing firm Canadair. Within months of being hired, he was dismissed with no reason being given. When he asked for one, the only reply he received was: 'You got more enemies in Ottawa than friends.' Unbeknownst to him, he had become the subject of a security investigation in the midst of Cold War panic and had been blacklisted from employment. Unlike the McCarthy era trials in the United States, Canadian investigations were conducted out of public view. Accusations could not be answered and any evidence behind them remained secret. Among thousands of citizens subject to such investigations, Eisenhardt was later one of those termed 'un-Canadians'. Interviewed on Len Scher's documentary film of 1996 *The Un-Canadians*, he likened the experience to being 'dirtied' but with a stain or mark that would never wash off.[69] Towards the end of his long and active life (he led fitness walks into his nineties), Eisenhardt's reputation was restored with public awards and honours, but 1952 marked the end of his career as Canada's leading physical exercise director.[70]

The Cold War and postwar prosperity also brought calls for less rather than more government. By the late 1940s and early 1950s, 'social citizenship' arguments that had been used to make sport and physical exercise a national and public responsibility were receding. They were eclipsed by new definitions of freedom that endorsed a restricted rather than expansive role for the state, and leisure time as one of private rather than state involvement. When a delegation of sports officials met the new

Minister of Health and Welfare, Paul Martin, in 1949, their request for support met with a rebuff: 'Government had urgent questions before it', and, moreover, 'there were many things in a free society that people should do for themselves'.[71] The response was a clear echo of Lord Beveridge's views in *Voluntary Action*.[72] Martin's response reflected the changed context of a retreat by government in the wake of the end of the war, a distaste for political interference in sport, and where prosperity meant there was no return to the 1930s conditions requiring schemes to occupy unemployed young people. People enjoying rising living standards for the first time in a long while did not want to hear the language of discipline.

When a new bout of anxiety raised questions about the physical fitness of Canadian men, the suggested remedy was in keeping with the notion that staying healthy and fit was a private rather than public matter. In a series of articles in Toronto's *Globe and Mail* in 1952 and 1953, Josephine Lowman drew readers' attention to the contemporary problem of 'the tubby hubby'. Far from being facetious, Lowman pointed to the crisis posed by the expanding waistlines of modern men. The newly discovered obesity was described as a 'top killer' and 'one of [Canada's] top national health problems'; it was depicted as part of a worrying decline in overall male physical fitness.[73] But the solution to the 'problem' of overweight husbands who posed a weakness to the nation at a time of possible threat lay principally with the fat men's wives. Rather than requiring a public response, the obesity needed responsible housewives to pay close attention to diet in the realm of marriage, home and family. As Deborah McPhail has argued, the way the Cold War raised uncertainty about the correctness and appropriateness of the social order reasserted the 'normal order' of work and family organised around gendered divisions. Social order was linked with national security.[74] One of the consequences of the obesity 'scare' was that it gave some fillip to sales of exercise advice books developed by government agencies and to popular fitness broadcasts such as those run by Lloyd Percival on CBC radio. The '5BX' programme for men and later the 'XBX' programme for women, first developed for use by the Royal Canadian Air Force, commanded huge sales across Canada, the United States, Australia, New Zealand and beyond.[75]

Cold War Demise and Royal Revival

In this climate it is not surprising that support for the National Council of Physical Fitness was not forthcoming.[76] Apart from an additional $7,000 granted in 1949 in recognition of Newfoundland joining the Canadian confederation, the National Council received no increase in funding. Eisenhardt was not replaced as director until 1948 and then his successor lasted only a short time. For most of the period from the end of 1946, the direction fell to the acting chair Joe Ross and the departmental executive secretary, Dr Doris Plewes. Postwar Minister Martin and his deputies were less personally tied to the measure than their predecessor Ian

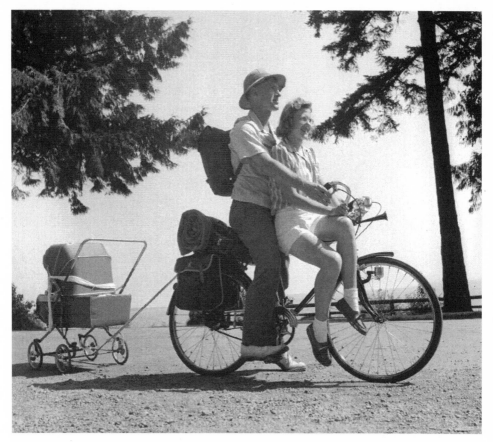

Summer activities organised by 'Pro-Rec' included bike hikes that this family is enjoying. Douglas Park, Vancouver, July 1943. CVA 586-1344, Vancouver City Archives

Mackenzie. In some frustration, the National Council took legal advice over its powers in a failing attempt to maintain some authority.[77] But the net result was to further reduce support in Ottawa where the Council was increasingly seen as a provincial institution seeking federal resources rather than as a central organisation directing a national scheme.

As had happened elsewhere, the problem of putting very ambitious and broadly conceived goals into practice, and establishing their 'effect' through a happier, healthier and fitter mass population was a very difficult administrative and political task. As Schrodt noted in 1973, 'the Act had not been sufficiently precise in its statement of purpose, or clear in its delineation of responsibilities'.[78] The Council met for the last time in 1952. When the Citizens Research Institute of Canada, a conservative small-government lobby group, published their 1951 challenge 'Abolish the National Physical Fitness Undertaking?', it took little extra push for the 1943 legislation to be repealed and the scheme rendered extinct. The Citizens group argued that a measure of this kind was unnecessary because recreation was a responsibility of local and provincial governments, and that it prompted unnecessary bureaucracy and unjustified expenditure.[79] The National Physical Fitness Act was repealed in 1954. Political journalist Blair Fraser's comment at the time, 'now that the National Physical Fitness Act is dead and buried, there's a fair chance that some of its objectives may at last begin to be achieved', pointed to the stalemate reached between the Council and its political masters.[80] 'Small p' politics in the form of disagreements between Council members had also played their part. The timing of the Canadian scheme's demise almost exactly coincided with that of New Zealand's Physical Welfare Branch.

A distinction between local recreation in peacetime and national fitness in wartime was an easy one to make in arguing *against* continued support for the National Physical Fitness Act and its National Council by government in Ottawa. But it turned out not to be quite so simple in practice. While the early 1950s saw the retreat from a social agenda and with it the rationale for federal involvement in recreation-oriented national fitness, the later years prompted government action to shore up sporting success in the international arena. As the Cold War shifted from the tense military standoff of the early 1950s into the larger contest between power blocs in the middle and later years of the decade, international sport became a potent site for ideological as well as athletic contest. Soviet athletes competed for the first time at the Helsinki Olympics in 1952, while other eastern bloc nations sent teams to subsequent games. National reputation on the sporting stage carried prestige, but also wider cultural and political significance. For all nations, the popularity of sport, and the increasingly televised spectacle of the victories and defeats of competitors wearing national colours, made the sporting arena one of considerable power.

When Prince Philip chided Canadians in his speech to the Canadian Medical Association in 1959 he jabbed at the nerve of national prestige. Remarking on Canadians' recent lack of achievement in sport, he mused as to whether the country's high standard of living 'was having the same effect upon the community as a plaster cast had on the muscles of the body'.[81] His audience was all too well aware of what he was referring to. The national ice hockey team had been defeated by Soviet opponents in 1954, and again at the Winter Olympics in 1956. The performance of Canadian athletes at the Olympic Games in 1952 and 1956 was considered disappointing. The one silver medal won at the Rome Games in 1960 would only confirm such perceptions. Promoting general health and fitness through increased priority to physical activity would yield better sporting results as well as other benefits. Urgent action was needed to combat what Prince Philip termed 'sub-health'. National interests were once again linked to the physical state of bodies en masse.

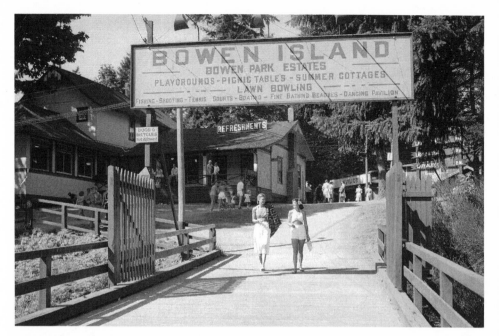

Picnic and camping grounds for summer recreation were also part of the 'Pro-Rec' initiatives. Bowen Island proved a popular destination for Vancouver residents looking for relaxing Sundays and summer holidays. Bowen Park Estates Recreation Area, August 1946. CVA 586-4605, Vancouver City Archives

By the late 1950s international sport had once again become a highly politicised arena. The tests of strength performed by weightlifters, discus throwers and gymnasts were not just about athletics but also competitions for ideological and political supremacy. For Canadians their 1954 defeat in ice hockey gave added charge to the sense of national sporting pride. Television, beaming into Canadian homes first from US stations, and then from Canadian broadcasts from 1952, brought the victories and losses ever more vividly to public attention.[82]

The case for government to take some role in advancing the incontrovertibly good ideals of better physical health and sporting success was not long resisted. Within two years of the Prince's speech, the Conservative government of John Diefenbaker had passed the Fitness and Amateur Sport Act 1961.[83] With a budget of $5 million, wider functions and clearer responsibilities, the Act provided a basis for an enduring if developing sports and fitness policy over the next four decades. Only in 2002 was it replaced by the Physical Activity and Sport Act ('part of a strategy to affirm the important role of sport in Canadian culture and society and to give effect to the Government of Canada's policies on physical activity and sport'). 'Fitness' was replaced with 'physical activity' in the 2002 legislation, in order to refer more 'to the action of being active than to a particular end result'.[84]

Generally speaking, Canadian historians have depicted the National Physical

Fitness initiative as a false start to the more substantial story of government support for sports and physical activity inaugurated by the 1961 Fitness and Amateur Sport Act. The earlier story is told as one of failed opportunity in winning a place for sport and/or recreation within the wider remaking of relations between government and people in the wake of economic depression and war. Such accounts place national fitness within a history that sees government support for sport and recreation as a progressive measure in upholding participation and values of competition against business values and interests, and in defending a local and national culture from subordination to powerful commercial and cultural influence from the United States.[85] Extending this story to one that connects the Canadian experience to the wider British movement for national fitness allows a broader view of the shared features and a sharper perception of specific national circumstances. What happened in Canada departed considerably from that which unfolded in the other Dominions, Australia and New Zealand, as well as from the British original.

The Canadian story, if confined to the life of the Act, 1943–54, and the scale of commitment, was of shorter duration and more modest than similar stories elsewhere. But in a longer view, taking cognisance of the beginning of British Columbia's Pro-Rec scheme, which provided the inspiration and leadership for the nationwide programme in 1934, and the re-engagement of central government with fitness and sport in 1961, it can be considered as more enduring. Government support for recreation and fitness was spurred first by the crisis of unemployment. The prospect of fit and healthy bodies, and of publicly sponsored sport and recreation, became part of the vision of the new order in a peacetime world imagined in the midst of the Second World War. The rationale expressed by sponsoring ministers in 1941 (Canberra) and 1943 (Ottawa) was one propelled by wartime immediacy, but based on an expansive notion of political responsibility: the prospect of fit and healthy bodies becomes a promise of the future. The Canadian experiment with national fitness, nonetheless, ran up against many of the same obstacles as were encountered elsewhere: a political initiative that was then not given space to develop; a great chasm between ambitious ideals and the parsimonious sums voted to achieve them; and a tension between central and provincial (and in turn local) authorities about distribution, and between the facilitating organisation established by legislation and its political sponsors.

Canada's story also presents us with the conundrum of ties with Britain that lingered well into the twentieth century. With less of a shared sporting and leisure culture linking them to Britain, tensions between the Anglo and Francophone communities, and the increasingly powerful pull of the United States towards a North American orbit, Canadians may well have shrugged off the imperial bonds earlier and more emphatically than Australasians. In retrospect, this was definitely the story told by the great majority of Canadian historians. In the early twenty-first century, the lingering British ties of the pre-1945 era proved unpalatable.[86] References to Canada as a 'Dominion' and to 'Dominion government' faded quickly in the post-1945 world. The adoption of a new national flag in 1965, the red-and-white paneled maple leaf, signalled a clear departure in perceptions of nationhood and a strong marker of independent nationhood (even though 'nationhood' remained difficult for a society whose history and geography encompassed strongly distinct regions, languages and dispositions). The post-1945 era also brought a simultaneous tug towards the new world power in the US and a continuing desire to define a distinctive Canadian-ness against what it was to be 'American' – especially in cultural terms. But British ties and membership of the Commonwealth continued to hold some sway, especially within Anglo-Canada. They took on increasingly symbolic and even nostalgic forms. Royal tours remained popular. Canadians continued to play a leading role as hosts and participants in Empire and in Commonwealth Games (in Vancouver in 1954). Prince Philip spoke about health and sport in Toronto in 1959 as president of the Canadian Medical Association. His power and position may have been more the relics of a passing era than expressions of the confident age of empire, but it was a platform and a voice that lobbyists within Canada used to their advantage. The subject he addressed was of wider interest than simply to the medical fraternity. Sporting prowess and physical fitness invoked a modern, popular and apparently apolitical common bond between people that spoke to a continuing cultural and sentimental linkage. There was also, in Prince Philip's speech, an echo of the sentiments of George VI's speech that had launched the national fitness campaign in Britain in February 1938.[87]

5   Healthy Bodies, States and Modernity

A Twentieth-Century Dilemma

The call for Britons to 'get fit – keep fit' in 1937 was one that echoed around the wider British world. In Melbourne, Auckland and Toronto, newspapers carried reports of the national fitness campaign underway across England, Wales and Scotland. The prime ministers of Australia, New Zealand and Canada were in London to attend the coronation of George VI and the Imperial Conference when the scheme was before the British House of Commons. It was a model many thought should be emulated. In New Zealand later the same year, in Australia a year later, and in Canada in 1943, national governments did follow, instituting their own schemes of physical welfare and recreation (New Zealand) and national fitness (Australia and Canada). Funding, public education and legislation flowed. All shared a common aim: to encourage people to continue with sport or some form of physical exercise once they left school. Political support and funding from central governments were made available for sports, for physical recreation and for physical education.

But as the preceding chapters have outlined, in all but Australia these initiatives were short-lived. They were regarded by contemporaries as having fallen short, or having failed outright. In 1948, Englishman Philip Smithells, writing from the newly established School of Physical Education at New Zealand's University of Otago, referred dismissively to 'the rise and fall of the abortive and futile National Fitness scheme' in Britain.[1] The few studies that have been made have leaned towards Smithells' judgement. *Strong, Beautiful and Modern* does not overturn that picture. But it does see in these histories something more instructive about how politics and play interacted in the twentieth century in the contest for what might be termed 'sporting citizenship'.

In histories of failure, or of limited achievement, lie clues to the meaning of the past. Antonia Maioni and Matthew Worley, addressing related aspects of this period, have both reminded us that the 'right kind of failure' was often the most productive catalyst for historical change. Worley quotes Michael Biddiss' observation that initiatives that do not work out may be more 'accurately representative of an age than ultimately more profitable ideas'.[2] Sporting citizenship refers to the way in which sport and physical exercise became part of the dynamics of power linking individuals to government and state. These dynamics operated in a variety of ways, at times drawing the lines between governments, sport and 'better bodies' closer together, at other times driving them apart. It is these paradoxical, attracting and repelling forces that pose the dilemma in relations between active, healthy bodies and states through the twentieth century. These dynamics can be seen at work in the powerful place that sporting teams came to occupy in the ways that societies imagined themselves as nations. The cultural significance attributed to Australian cricketers and New Zealand rugby players had parallels in other national cultures. Sporting success on the international stage proved difficult for politicians to resist. Photo opportunities alone proved valuable currency in efforts to link sporting victory with political popularity. Physical education in schools and places for leisure such as national parks, became part of what was expected to be provided as public services. But at the same time, sport and physical recreation were viewed firmly as activities that were the concern of autonomous associations and matters for individuals to choose, or not, as they felt inclined. In this way there was a strong line of separation drawn between governments and healthy bodies. The lines of sporting citizenship were not constant, but in flux, part of wider trends in the expansion and contraction of state power, economic conditions, cultural forces and social movements.

In Britain and the 'white Dominions', this 'sporting citizenship' took on a distinctive character due to the strong and resilient civil culture of games-playing. The commonly expressed 'natural' love of sport and British preference for games above all other pursuits carried a resonance beyond the sports field. Notions of 'fair play', 'abiding by the rules' and decency extended far beyond descriptions of what went on in the field of play. Together with this ethos of behaviour was an equally strong adherence to volition – the idea that play was an end in itself and taken up (or not) entirely at the will of those who wanted to play. In keeping with that notion, play was organised on an independent basis, typically in associations of those who shared an interest in the game, whatever it might be. Sporting and recreation organisations comprised a large section of the dense associational life in Britain and the Dominions in the early twentieth century. The civil culture of games-playing conveyed central ideas about freedom, and of its exercise within bounds of a sanctioned authority. In the civilised restraint of violent contest confined to the sports arena, within a society organised by rule of law and parliament, lay the essence of what it was to be 'British'.[3] The fate of the national fitness and physical

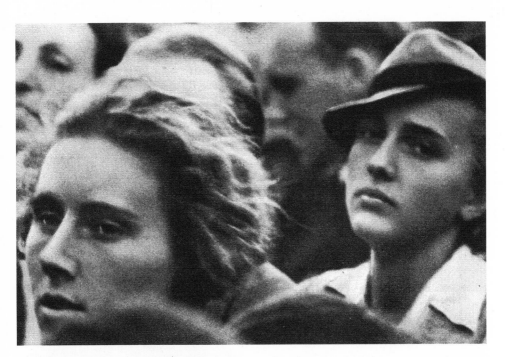

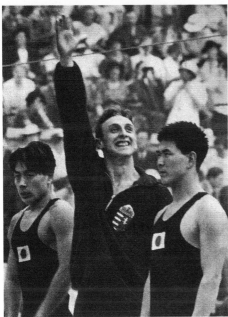

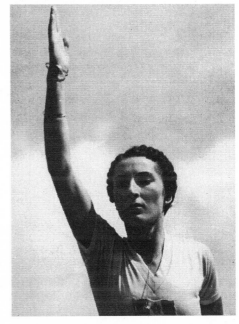

Photo journalism reached new heights at the 1936 Berlin Olympics capturing the beauty, strength, skill and competitive tension of athletes and those who gathered to watch. *Top*: among the crowd were champion winter sports athletes skier Chistl Cranz (left) and ice skater Maxi Herber (right). *Lower left*: Hungarian swimmer Ferenc Csik won the 100 metre freestyle gold medal, upsetting Masanori Yufa and Shigeo Arai, from Japan, silver and bronze medal winners. *Lower right*: Eighteen-year-old Italian Anna Avanzini on the balance beam. *Berliner Illustrite Zeitung*, 1936, Ullstein A.G. Berlin welfare schemes as they came into being and then passed out of sight can be placed within this larger framework of a distinctively British sporting citizenship. While the schemes themselves lasted only a few years everywhere except in Australia, the purposes and aspirations they encompassed did not disappear. The schemes inaugurated in 1937–43 proved to be the first major salvo in what has proved to be an enduring area of contest and negotiation.

The national fitness schemes were products of the highly charged context of the late 1930s. Hugely popular, sport and physical exercise were part of the polarising politics and cultural tumult of that decade. Energetic, active bodies spoke of modernity. But was it a modernity of individuality and freedom or of mass conformity and national duty? That problem was never far from the minds of contemporaries. It remains a problem that is not easily solved. As an historical episode, the fate of national fitness and physical welfare across the British world presents challenges for interpretation, connection and evaluation. As an ongoing theme, the questions of how far governments can or should go in urging healthy adult citizens to be physically active, or in guaranteeing security of leisure as well as livelihood, remain matters of contest.

Together with the question of the relationship between governments and healthy bodies, two other themes run through the national histories discussed in Chapters 1 to 4. One concerns the continuing close bonds between Britain and the Dominions well into the twentieth century, and their enigmatic demise. When did the empire come to an end for these former settler colonies? Alongside the unravelling of constitutional and trade links sits another story of sporting ties. *Strong, Beautiful and Modern* suggests a 'British' history that was strongly connected and more than the sum of its parts. While New Zealand, Australia and Canada inaugurated their own fitness schemes, they are unlikely to have done so had Britain not started its campaign and given it statutory power with the Physical Training and Recreation Act. Products of the era when the British Empire was still intact and links between Britain and the Dominions were close, the schemes enable a closer examination of the character of what was often lauded as a common 'British world'. But what remained strongly intact in the late 1930s and early 1940s had evaporated with the 'end of empire' twenty years later.

The other theme concerns the question of what it was to be modern, as seen from the vantage point of the 1930s. What does this history tell us of that pervasive yet elusive moment when to be modern was to embrace the fashion of an active life in the body, to be surrounded for the first time with radio, talking movies, passenger air travel, cheap cigarettes, branded lipstick – the commodities and habits of everyday consumerist modernity?

Flexing and Relaxing the Sinews of Empire

Looking across the national fitness schemes as they were introduced in Britain (1937), New Zealand (1937), Australia (1941) and Canada (1943) reinforces the familiar story of the close bonds between Britain and the 'white Dominions' persevering well into the mid-twentieth century. But it also reveals marked differences in how a common purpose, and similar legislation, was put into action. In Britain a Conservative government sought to boost local and voluntary effort through publicity, district committees and a grants scheme; in New Zealand legislation was presented as part of a wider provision for workers and for welfare generally, with physical welfare officers employed directly by central government. In Australia and Canada, federal ambitions were slow to catch up with state and provincial initiatives. Civic-minded groups in these places pressed their governments to act in the fear of falling behind the British lead. The most active programmes were instigated by community-minded directors of physical education supported by influential backers.

A strong degree of connection across the four countries was recognised by contemporaries. Arguments for supporting national fitness or physical welfare may have varied, along with detail in how the schemes worked, but there was common acknowledgement of their importance. In this respect alone, the history of the national fitness schemes across Britain, New Zealand, Australia and Canada constituted a wider movement. In the legislation itself, the resemblance is striking: Britain and New Zealand, Canada and Australia replicated each other's statutes. The White Paper produced in London in January 1937 was widely circulated, reported and discussed. So too was the British Medical Association's 1936 Report on Physical Education. Copies of the HMSO publications of early 1937, *Recreation and Physical Fitness for Girls and Women* and *Recreation and Physical Fitness for Youths and Men*, were found on shelves across the world as authoritative guides for contemporary instructors and leaders. Women and men occupying positions in the newly professionalising field of physical education were part of lively networks joining disparate points in the British world. The career and educational paths of a number of people who feature in the preceding chapters, including Gordon Young, A. S. Lamb, Helen Black and Philip Smithells, provide evidence of this.

While the wider British world formed the principal circuits along which people and professional exchanges ran, it did not form a hermetically sealed realm. Canada's leading figure in developing publicly funded physical fitness schemes was Jan Eisenhardt, born and educated in Denmark. The United States also provided important opportunities. Gordon Young and Harry Le Maistre both attended Springfield College in Massachusetts, originally established as the training institute for the YMCA, and had a huge impact on the uptake of national fitness in Australia. C. Ruxton Bach, the first men's physical welfare officer in New Zealand, was a graduate of the University of Southern California. The time that

Philip Smithells and Rona Stephenson (a New Zealander) spent in the United States in 1937–38 did much to shape the philosophy and practice they pursued subsequently. A less common path was that taken by Dr Fritz Duras, who arrived in Australia as a Jewish refugee and took up a position teaching physical education at the University of Melbourne. Drawing on expertise from beyond the British realm was necessary, given the lack of training and experience that had evolved in the empire, itself a characteristic of the tradition of 'games culture'. While Eisenhardt managed to innovate, Duras found it necessary to adjust more significantly to the local sports and leisure culture. Duras' qualifications in medicine, and his formal training in the science of healthy movement, were most unusual areas of expertise in the strongly sports-based leisure culture that predominated in Australia. Gisa Taglicht, the Laban-trained instructor at Wellington's YWCA, faced a similar gap between local improvisation and formal European approaches.

Whatever their origins, people employed in the promotion of sport and physical fitness found themselves in a world that was strongly marked by the common mesh of 'British' values, commodities and events. The Union Jack and 'God Save the King' were seen and heard in many places where people thought it unremarkable to describe themselves as British, when they had never stepped on British soil. Manufacturers saw the British Empire (and especially the prosperous Dominions) as a common market. From Aertex shirts to Slazenger tennis racquets and Gunn & Moore cricket bats, Bournville cocoa and Lane's emulsion – products that were already familiar to both British and Dominion markets could be given an added push by association with health and physical fitness. It was an opportunity that Dominion producers also exploited.[4] Cinema audiences across the world equally recognised the singing comedian George Formby and were able to buy sheet music for the songs he made popular through his many films, including the 1938 release *Keep-Fit*. Sound film was one of the new ways in which the long-standing ties of empire were made modern in the 1930s.[5]

As David Cannadine has noted, empire was 'an imaginative construct, existing as much (or more) inside the minds of men and women as it existed on the ground and on the map'.[6] In sport and the 'love of the game', there were fertile seeds for that imagination. Connections of empire were strengthened and popularised in the 1920s and 1930s through new technologies of communication. Newspapers could now print stories and photographs relayed across the world within hours to meet daily deadlines. Even more powerful were the invisible sinews of sound and voice through the wireless. The BBC's Empire Service gave immediacy and substance to links between people across the globe. While public utterances of shared interests and values across the empire might have been invoked ubiquitously, to the point of becoming platitudes, radio infused them with vitality, variety and currency. In the regular listening routine, those connections became part of everyday lives in disparate parts of the world. Sporting events and results were topics of recurrent and intense interest that drew in an audience, and kept it tuned. 'Live' radio broadcasts enabled every listener to take part in the excitement of play as it happened, for every home to be inside the grandstand. For cricket followers in England or Australia during an Ashes series, or rugby followers in Wales and New Zealand, this was irresistible. While the new modes of communication did not alone spur the realisation of an empire-wide sporting competition in the first Empire Games held in Hamilton, Ontario, in 1930, they did much to make it a success – as well as to support successive Games in London four years later and in Sydney in 1938. Cultural ties between Britain and the Dominions (the main participants at the Games) were amplified through such events.

Connections were also matters of practical co-operation. Events such as the Empire Games and international tours by sports teams relied on close contact, including tense negotiations at times, between national associations.[7] They were reinforced also in the pavilions created for the Sydney Exhibition (1938), the Glasgow Empire Exhibition (1938) and the New Zealand Centennial Exhibition (1939–40). Although falling within a tradition of international exhibitions stretching back to 1851, these were insistently modernist in design and content. Fitness and good health were introduced to visitors by robots in the government courts at Glasgow and Wellington ('Godfrey' and 'Dr Well-and-Strong').

The special bonds shared between Britain and the Dominions (and sometimes the wider empire) were also emphasised in this period by a range of independent organisations. Whether by patriotic bodies such as the Imperial Order Daughters of the Empire or Victoria League, the Home Reading Union, the Red Cross or new entities, the links were underscored as of special value.[8] The ballooning membership of Girl Guides and Boy Scouts through the interwar years represented what Kristine Alexander has identified as 'imperial internationalism'.[9] The cultural bonds comprising such an empire-based internationalism were significant both in the modernity of their form, and in the way they interacted with the new dynamics of international politics. They complemented the newly formed but weak League of Nations in its attempts to restrain the aggressive nationalism that once more came to the fore. And they were part of the explicit reaching across national boundaries that was such a large, if doomed, part of the post-1918 world.

When Prunella Stack and other leaders of the Women's League of Health and Beauty looked to spread their message, it was to Canada, Australia and New Zealand that they first turned. The effervescent League came alive in branches, halls and parks throughout the Dominions as it had in Britain. As readers and film viewers, women outside Britain already knew about its grand demonstrations and its charismatic founders. The pattern of connection supports the argument of Martin Daunton and Bernhard Reiger that Britain's modernity rested on its intermeshed

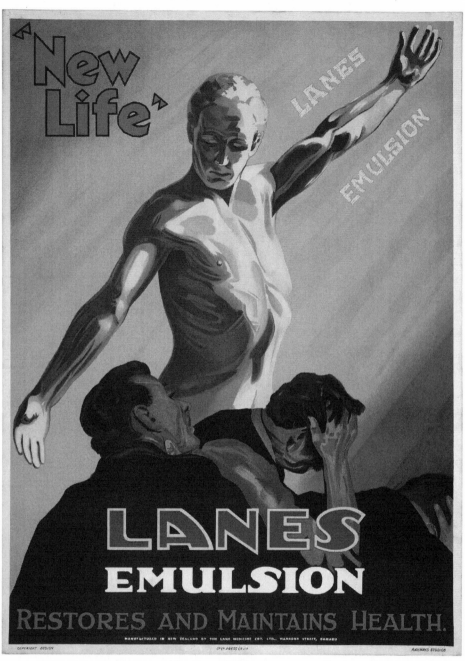

Lane's Emulsion promising a remedy for most common ailments was not new in the 1920s and 1930s, but its promotion in the visual and written language of vitality, strength and light was very much a product of the period. The body of the main figure was lit in warm yellow and pink while the cowed figures at the base were depicted in dark greys and brown. Eph-E-Pharmacy-1927-01, Ephemera Collection, Alexander Turnbull Library links with the Dominions and wider empire. In their exploration of the meanings of modernity in Britain from the late-Victorian era to World War II, they argue that 'imperial dimensions exerted a deep influence on contemporary understandings of Britain as a modern nation'.[10]

Politically, the interwar period was a time of important reconfiguration in relations between Britain and the Dominions. Initiatives such as the Empire Settlement scheme, the Empire Marketing Board (1926–34) and the Ottawa Agreement (1932) signalled some innovation in the continuing processes of emigration and trade. The most significant constitutional change came when the Statute of Westminster of 1931 formalised the agreement made in 1926 making the parliaments of Britain and the Dominions ones of equal stature.[11] In his opening address to the Imperial Conference of 1937, the first held under the new arrangements, British Prime Minister Stanley Baldwin described how those present had 'become an association of peoples, each with sovereign freedom of its own but accustomed to co-operate closely with each other in matters of common concern and all associated under the Crown'.[12] All delegates commented fulsomely on the oath that George VI had made at the Coronation immediately preceding the conference, which recognised the 'direct and immediate' relation between the King and the people of each Dominion.[13] Whereas George V had been 'King of Great Britain and Ireland and Ruler of the British Dominions beyond the Seas', George VI had promised 'to govern the peoples of Great Britain, Ireland, Canada, Australia, New Zealand, and the Union of South Africa', along with 'possessions, and the other territories to them belonging or pertaining' and the 'Empire of India, according to their respective laws and customs'.[14] Canada's Mackenzie King was widely applauded when he noted that the changes, far from disrupting the ties of loyalty, affection and co-operation, had done the opposite. What made British institutions strong, he said, was their combination of continuity and change.

Mackenzie King's statement might be interpreted differently. So, too, might the histories of national fitness as presented in *Strong, Beautiful and Modern*. Mackenzie King was speaking from London amidst the abdication, the highly volatile situation in Europe and the pressure being applied to British authority by the Indian independence movement. What is significant is the Canadian Prime Minister's need to make such a specific statement of the ongoing loyalty of 'British' citizens throughout the world. Similarly, Michael Savage (New Zealand), Joe Lyons (Australia) and Barry Herzog (South Africa) took positions at the Imperial Conference that were aimed at domestic constituencies. Within those, loyalty to Britain remained the predominant sentiment but it was less something that was assumed. Rather, it was something that coexisted with nascent national feeling, a growing sense of the irrelevance of British formalities of class and hierarchy, and which had become qualified by the price of loyalty exacted by World War 1.

Against the argument that has been made here, that the national fitness histories confirm a picture of a connected and common British world, can be placed an interpretation affirming the uniqueness of local histories in Britain, New Zealand, Australia and Canada. Such an argument would emphasise the differences in the schemes, in their timing and longevity, their political drivers and the contexts in which they took shape. The grounds for making such an argument are most strong in the Canadian case. There, a Liberal administration adopted programmes developed in pre-1939 circumstances, as part of wartime political compromise. The Canadian context diverged significantly from that in Britain, Australia or New Zealand in its sporting and leisure culture, in its proximity to the influences of the United States, and in the tensions British ties presented to a dual Francophone and Anglophone settler society. Australia and New Zealand might, similarly, seek to explain their histories in terms that look to a strong civic movement, and to a markedly progressive physical welfare tradition, respectively; and, more generally, to a political culture of active social democracy. But those arguments have not been considered sufficient, in this study, to overturn the overriding interpretation of the national fitness history as one of a connected movement across the 'British world'.

Another term that might have been used to describe the history set out in these chapters is transnational. Joan Tumblety, writing about the healthy body movements of this time across France, Germany, Australia, the US and UK, identifies them as 'genuinely trans-national'.[15] The scope of the connections can be broader yet. Chiang Kai-shek and Soong May-ling's New Life Movement, founded in China in February 1934, emphasised vitality, self-cultivation, and personal and public health as part of a wider political purpose. Its existence, and subsequent denunciation by the Communists in favour of a more collective notion of bodily fitness, expands the scale and raises the question of a non-Western modernity.

One might also look usefully to Ian Tyrrell's critique of transnationalism before 1900 and in imperial contexts from the perspective of someone for whom United States history is central; or to James Belich's ending point for what he charts as the uniquely successful Anglo world.[16] While links and overlaps with the United States and thus the broader Anglo world feature at points in this study, they are minor and largely fall outside the 'British world' more specifically imagined. The British world encompassed by a common games culture that is at the centre of this history was permeable. It did include United States and to a lesser extent some European links; but only within very important limits.[17] Empire and British links, and, specifically, a British games-playing culture, lay at the centre. In the Empire Games, in games-playing to participatory ends, in the educational and organisational links of physical education, in the Women's League of Health and Beauty, in the network of the medical profession, the 'British world' is supported as a specific case. The permeable limits are seen in the YMCA and YWCA, in the influence and inspiration of other body cultures and educational systems, in encounters with United States experience that had an impact on the thinking of people like Ruxton Bach, Philip Smithells and Rona Stephenson. The logic that the original British initiative, including legislation, provided a necessary but not sufficient basis for initiatives taken up in New Zealand, Australia and Canada might be assessed differently if this context is considered. While the term transnationalism is not rejected, the notion of the 'British world' in this instance comes closer to the kind of transnationalism that was at work. In the current quest to write history beyond national borders, 'transnational' has become widely invoked. That has its attractions, but also its dangers – the term can be so widely applied as to lose meaning.

Strong, Beautiful and Modern has sought to depict the way in which Britain and the former settler Dominions of Australia, Canada and New Zealand continued to comprise a British world linked by cultural bonds of sport, fitness and ideas about use of the body, as much as by trade and constitution. At a time when the international situation was highly volatile, poised between extreme ideologies and regimes, such bonds took on additional significance. Evident for the first time in the 1930s also was the immense potential for power offered by the international stage of sporting contests seen on movie screens and in the popular press. The contests for control over *international* events staged by *nation* states, such as the 1932 and 1936 Olympics, were to become long-running features of the twentieth century. Indeed, it could be argued that organisations such as FIFA and the IOC wielded greater influence than international bodies such as the United Nations. Here, too, the term 'transnational' does not quite capture the new form of modern power politics that encompasses the apparently ephemeral yet pervasive activity of sporting contest.

The argument emphasises British and imperial links in the themes and questions that have been pursued, and in the context of the historical literature (the 'new imperial history') within which the discussion is located. Written at a time when the 'ties of empire' have given fresh and pressing urgency to historical and contemporary debate in the former colonies as well as in Britain, the interpretation has leaned more towards the connections and common movement than the national or local story. Connections may also hold greater significance for residents in smaller and distant societies. Completing the study from a place often thought of as at 'the edge of empire' may also have contributed to the interpretation that is set out. To imagine being at an edge is also to presume a centre somewhere else.

A shared civil culture of physical fitness based on sport is another important thread uniting Britain and the Dominions. The instigation of national fitness and physical welfare schemes was a testament to anxieties that games-playing might not be sufficient in the world as it was in the late 1930s. Everywhere a common 'British' approach to sport and games was invoked, as too was a conviction of the shared priority of adult physical fitness. Contrasting contexts gave the schemes their local shape. New Zealand followed the British model quickly but with a political impetus that diverged sharply from that of Chamberlain's Conservative government. Minister Bill Parry's championing of physical welfare and recreation (greater opportunities for recreation and sport for working people) was tied to a wider manifesto of a workers' welfare state. In Australia, an active but more conservative civic progressivism was the driving force. In Canada, the political consequences of wartime finally prompted the Mackenzie King government to introduce the National Fitness Act in 1943 as part of a wider promise of peacetime reconstruction under pressure from the socialist Co-operative Commonwealth Federation.

Contrasting sports and leisure cultures in each place also contributed to the differences in histories. With the longest history of sports and sporting organisations, Britain's leisure culture was the most profuse and complex. By the 1930s, the world of mass commercialised sport was growing fast. But the British sporting world was still essentially divided between professional and amateur sports, and leisure patterns that mirrored class (and gender) divides.[18] In Australia and New Zealand, the dominant sporting culture was one in which the imperial legacy was strongly evident in the popular codes – cricket and rugby union being the dominant 'national' sports, respectively. But the style in which they had come to be played and the strongly associational nature of sports made the Australasian sporting world a more egalitarian and less variegated one. Professional sports did exist but in smaller pockets (horseracing, wrestling, rugby league). In Canada, the 1930s represented a time of particular contest between the established amateur associations (many of which had strong links to political and social elites) and new entrepreneurs keen to shape new followings and audiences for commercially organised contests. The associational model and the local activities were under pressure, and national interests were threatened by the greater commercial and cultural power exerted from the United States.

If the origins of the national fitness schemes reveal something about the degree of connection between Britain and the Dominions, their endings also tell us something about the fate of those bonds in the later era we know as 'the end of empire'. In England and Wales, and Scotland, what began with a zest came to an end with the beginning of World War II. Nonetheless, a major public education campaign had been undertaken, and a number of projects funded. And in Scotland the policies pursued under the Central Council for Physical Recreation mantle in the 1950s drew considerably from experience and people involved in the earlier national fitness episode. In New Zealand and Australia, fitness for wartime service kept the schemes going during 1939–45, with attention in New Zealand particularly being paid to the usefulness of recreation and physical health among women war workers. A brief postwar flourish, amid expectations for leisure from a peacetime population, was not sustained and the scheme soon collapsed. A similar pattern was witnessed in the shorter-lived Canadian story, the national fitness scheme moribund by 1951. Reoriented around the needs of 'youth', the Australian scheme lasted longest, providing a range of sport and recreational programmes at community level until overtaken by reorganisation of state departments in the late 1960s. There was no sustained common enterprise after 1945, and no broader outcry at the demise of the schemes started with considerable commitment just a few years earlier. No subsequent British initiative drew wider emulation.

Belief in the value of sport and games had not diminished, however, in the aftermath of the national fitness experiment. If anything it was stronger, with people like Philip Noel Baker arguing vehemently that sporting exchanges could make an enormous contribution in rebuilding shattered international relations. George Orwell remained sceptical, famously likening international sporting fixtures to war without the shooting.[19] The voluntary and independent basis for sport was strongly reasserted. There was no role for government in coaxing people to play. It was in this context that postwar sporting exchanges resumed. The London Olympic Games in the summer of 1948 were staged despite severe austerity. The first postwar Empire Games were held in Auckland in 1950. The schedules of international tours in major sports were also restored.

For Canada, Australia and New Zealand, all losing their Dominions status by the late 1940s and moving to stronger expression of nationhood, sport has proved paradoxical. In Australia and New Zealand the most popular games tend to be ones of British origin, while sporting contests offer some of the sharpest moments of national pride. Where in earlier decades Australian and New Zealand successes at the Olympic Games or in other international contests might have been viewed as triumphs for empire *and* nation, the two were now un-coupled. In the process of coming to 'the end of empire', as Curran and Ward note, Australia shifted towards seeing nation as something mutually exclusive to empire, a state beyond and antithetical to that former affiliation.[20] Yet sport continues to provide strong links in what might be described as the time of 'disconnected connection'. The Commonwealth Games have continued to be staged, with Britain, Canada and Australia most frequently providing the host cities for the Games. Sports with very strong followings in Britain and Australasia – cricket, rugby and netball – are still largely, and most competitively, played between nations that were former members of the empire.

The status of the former settler colonies is also exposed within the international ambit of 'sporting citizenship'. Within the Commonwealth, from the 1960s to 1980s struggles around sporting contacts with South Africa pitted white and non-white members of the Commonwealth against each other. Decolonising in sport could prove more difficult, and take longer, than in constitutional arrangements.

Relations between governments and the governing authorities in sport, such as the International Cricket Council and the New Zealand Rugby Union, reveal the limits of the ability of representative governments to control events. Decolonisation, it could be argued, continues in the field of sport. The status of member countries and players in some of the most popular sports remains highly unequal in the conditions of participation. Control has recently been wrested from old hands in cricket, with power passing to the Indian subcontinent. In rugby, however, the shape of the game as a whole, and the playing status of smaller nations (such as Samoa, Tonga and Scotland) is still determined by the International Rugby Board which remains in heavily British and 'old world' control.

As the political, defence and economic ties between members of the former empire have become attenuated, the discourses that continue to link the Commonwealth often focus on the shared love of games. Articulated by members of the royal family, such ideas serve to reinforce the popular and symbolic threads that still link together parts of the old imperial world. As recently as December 2010, Queen Elizabeth II invoked the value of sport in her Christmas Broadcast. One 'of the most powerful ways' of building communities and creating harmony, the Queen noted, was 'through sport and games':

> In the parks of towns and cities, and on village greens up and down the country, countless thousands of people every week give up their time to participate in sport and exercise of all sorts, or simply encourage others to do so. These kinds of activity are common throughout the world and play a part in providing a different perspective on life .... Sportsmen and women often speak of the enormous pride they have in representing their country, a sense of belonging to a wider family. We see this vividly at the Commonwealth Games, for example, which is known to many as the Friendly Games and where I am sure you have noticed that it is always the competitors from the smallest countries who receive the loudest cheers.[21]

The links between sporting events and the royal family are ones of mutual benefit. The presence of the Queen and other members of the royal family at major events continues the project of modernising and popularising the monarchy – a process that began early in the twentieth century when members of the royal family began attending places such as Wembley as well as Ascot. For sports, the presence of royalty adds prestige, media interest and distinction in the constant competition for profile.[22]

State Intervention or Individual Responsibility?

Providing money for sport and recreation, and launching public campaigns to encourage adult physical recreation and fitness, represented the first significant involvement by central government in these activities. In New Zealand and Canada,

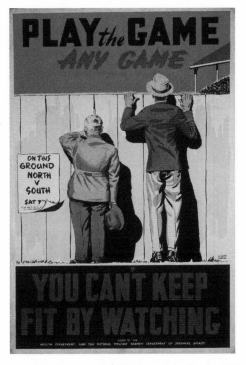
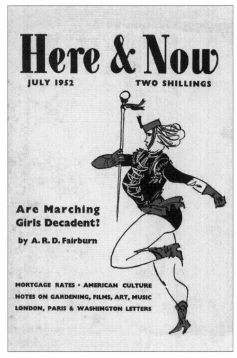

Sport continued to be highly popular in the 1950s but too much watching and not enough playing prompted campaigns to urge people out of the grandstands and on to the field. From the dissenting edge of the 1950s came digs at the kind of play appropriate for the age. A. R. D. Fairburn's article in the leftwing *Here & Now* questioned the conformist, even reactionary, tendencies in New Zealanders' enthusiasm for military-style marching as a summer sport amongst the country's young women. *Left*: New Zealand Railways Studio poster produced for the Health Department – Physical Welfare Branch. Eph-D-Health-1940/50s-01, Ephemera Collection, Alexander Turnbull Library; *Right*: Dennis Knight Turner cover sketch, S-L-732-cover, Alexander Turnbull Library

the arguments justifying public involvement were part of wider programmes of 'social citizenship'. New Zealand's Labour government supported a physical welfare and recreation scheme as a natural corollary to reductions in working and shop-trading hours and its major commitment to social security. In Canada, federal support for the national fitness programme extended to recreation schemes that had been running for several years and indicated a promise of more in the future. Bound up with discussions of a national health service, the 1943 National Fitness Act came at a time of political pressure on the government from the left. In Australia, the progressive civic campaign urging government action on a physical fitness scheme linked leisure and physical fitness in a notion of modern citizenship. 'Education for Leisured Citizenship' was the goal of one of the key lobby groups. In Britain the case was made more in terms of national duty. Posters proclaimed the message: 'England expects every man and woman to be healthy and fit.'

Longevity of the schemes is one measure of effectiveness. But it is not the only one. In general, as has been indicated, contemporary and historical judgements have pointed to the limits, if not outright failure, of the schemes – especially in Britain where they were short-lived, and in Canada where they never gained much momentum. Elsewhere there has been some tendency to point to the schemes as examples of 'social control' and to their advocates as more punitive than permissive. *Strong, Beautiful and Modern* suggests that this is not the full or perhaps even the principal story. In the area of recreation, the broader historical difficulty of bringing fairly into view those who *did* as well as those who *said* is compounded. Those who put on sandshoes, hiking boots, swimming togs, or picked up a volleyball, did so largely from an immediate desire for enjoyment. The satisfaction of *doing* is its own end. The great pointlessness of games is their defining paradox. But those who argued for the opportunity to play, and who set out rationales in order to establish the importance of these activities were engaged in a different task. Their efforts were directed to writing, arguing and setting out the case for devising and funding schemes, and (often) in making that case to governments. Inevitably, the historical record tells us more of the latter (the writers) than the former (the doers). But we need to be cautious in reading it.

Jobs, wages and holidays represented the labour agenda in the 1930s. Second to securing employment for all, parties of the left had as their priority the achievement of the forty-hour week and paid annual holidays. Even a Conservative British government passed the Holidays with Pay Act in 1938, which urged but did not make mandatory the requirement for employers to pay workers for a week's annual holiday. Regulating time for leisure was an important backdrop to the wider public discussion of the uses of leisure, and a factor in governments' readiness to take the next step into promoting activities within that new 'time off'.

Whatever the arguments, or political circumstances, in all four countries, contemporaries emphasised that improving fitness and access to active leisure were goals so evidently beneficial as to need little explanation. While there were debates over detail, in each place legislation establishing the schemes was supported by the major political parties and regarded as a matter largely beyond partisan divisions. Providing greater time for leisure was already a political issue, and the prospect of increasing leisure as a permanent feature of contemporary life dates from this era. The importance of leisure as a birthright and a state-supported goal appeared to be realised in the years of prosperity following World War II, before the end of the economic boom and deregulation brought what Juliet Schor describes as 'the unexpected decline of leisure'.[23] Regulating time for leisure was one thing. Going further to provide the means and activities through which people were to spend their leisure time was another.

With postwar welfare states and the era of prosperity came full employment and the shorter working week. Common time for leisure existed in the evenings and weekends. With the deregulation of the economy from the late 1970s, and diminution of the strength of organised labour, the lines between work and leisure also eroded. By the end of the twentieth century, a sign of the increasing disparities between sections of society was not just in monetary wealth but in those described as 'time poor' or 'time rich'. A common distinction began to be made between those with jobs where the demands extended far beyond a five-day, 40-hour limit leaving them time poor (but cash rich), and those either unemployed or under-employed with too much time and little cash. The widespread lament for the demise of volunteering and community associations needs to be set in this context.[24] Robert Owen's nineteenth-century notion of an eight-hour day and a socially shared rhythm to the working and non-working week once more became an aspiration rather than a reality. In the longer span, while the early twenty-first century has not yet come to replicate an eighteenth-century society divided between leisured and labouring classes, it has seen the rise of greater disparities in opportunities for leisure alongside the rising disparities in distribution of wealth and meaningful work.

In all four countries the conundrum was raised of reconciling government action to encourage sporting and recreation pursuits with the voluntary, independent and discretionary nature of such pursuits. Governments sought to resolve the tension between asserting that sports and physical recreation were something that people should do of their own volition, while simultaneously urging them to do more, by shying away from any hint of compulsion, and by making the fitness campaigns the responsibility of organisations at arm's length from core government administration. The National Fitness Councils of England and Scotland, and their parallels in New Zealand and Australia, were statutory bodies. That pattern has endured. Only in Canada has sport and physical activity found a place within direct government administration.

Strenuous efforts were made to reassure people that sports and physical recreation were, and would remain, matters of individual and voluntary choice. In Britain suspicions that the Physical Training and Recreation Act was nothing more than a first step towards conscription drew strong denunciations. But there was every reason to believe that the scheme's promoters were sincere – the projects were diffuse, women's activities were included along with men's, and physical recreation along with sport. Moreover, the national fitness schemes were abandoned at the outbreak of war. While the tense international situation contributed an urgency to action, the national fitness initiative was far from being militarism in disguise. Lord Aberdare, chairman of England's National Fitness Council, had at times to dampen those who were over-zealous in suggesting that compulsion was needed to make the measure effective. The independence of sporting and recreation organisations that received grant monies from national fitness councils was also guaranteed. Bill Parry's eager suggestion that New Zealand's sporting organisations might be usefully co-ordinated under one centrally run organisation was the only attempt to bring sporting institutions under any central direction in any of these countries (the idea was soon dropped). National sporting and recreational federations did not become branches of state. So, for all that the physical fitness initiatives drew from an admiration of European models of the mid-1930s, they did not emulate them. The raggle-taggle appearance of the British delegation to the Lingiad festival in Stockholm in July 1939 turned out to be a reassuringly untidy proof of the freedoms enjoyed in the games-playing world.

The goal for which people were urged to take up greater physical activity – whether in England's 'Fitter Britain' campaign, New Zealand's 'Fitness Week' or under the 'Health Brings Victory' national fitness programme (New South Wales, 1941) – was one that linked individual to national health. Advice on sleeping and eating well, exercising regularly, good posture and the benefits of maintaining a bright outlook were standard components of health education. But how far governments could, or should, go in making citizens have 'better bodies' was a more difficult line to draw. 'National fitness' became a much less palatable term after 1945, and largely dropped out of use. Loaded with discredited eugenic distinctions between 'fit' and 'unfit', and suggesting subservience of individual freedom to national authority, national fitness carried a very different meaning in the post-fascist and post-Nazi era. While the physical fitness schemes instigated in Britain and the Dominions were a long way from the regimented mass movements of Germany and Italy, (and did not reflect their more extreme population policies), the extension of government into the lives of healthy, adult citizens proved a discomfiting precedent. This disquiet contributed to the short life of the schemes.

In some places in these histories there is evidence of a contrasting orientation: where the promotion of sport, leisure and physical activity forms part of a social-democratic or progressive agenda. State action in sport and physical recreation becomes part of social innovation, using the powers of state action and public resource to redistribute opportunities for sporting competition and physical recreation. The most obvious examples are New Zealand c. 1939–48, Scotland in the 1950s under the Central Council for Physical Recreation, and British Columbia's Pro-Rec in the 1930s. In these instances public investment in sport and physical activity was advanced on a wider agenda of social equality and redistribution. The more predominant strand, however, is of sport and leisure being set outside the bounds of the state, something designated as 'private' and left to the vagaries and highly uneven discretion of independent associations. Discussing Britain through the mid-twentieth century, McKibbin identifies this pattern as evidence of the enduringly narrow notion of democracy even at the height of Labourist ascendancy in the immediate post-1945 years.[25]

Although the national fitness schemes took shape at a time when governments of varying political colour were expanding the scope of the state, they did not secure a place in those expanded boundaries. The difficulty of reconciling the voluntary principle at the heart of sport and recreation pursued within a games culture (on the one hand), and the taint of government involvement in the healthy bodies of adult citizens (on the other), made governments in Britain, New Zealand and Canada draw back from their earlier commitment. In doing so they reasserted the value of voluntarism, the independence of local and community organisations, and the centrality of individual initiative and drive. Sport and recreation were once more established as a realm at a distance from politics. There was to be no 'leisure state' to parallel the 'welfare state'. William Beveridge, whose 1942 Report was widely lauded as providing the blueprint for Britain's welfare state, produced a less well-known work *Voluntary Action* in 1948. In this, and on his 1948 tour of New Zealand and Australia undertaken in the same year, he emphasised that, while there was an ongoing role for voluntary effort in providing social services even in an era of expanded state responsibility, there were other activities in which the state had no place. Sport and recreation clearly lay in this domain – outside the boundaries of the state. Politics should have no part in how people played. Moreover, Beveridge emphasised the distinctive Britishness of voluntary activity, noting that the 'vigour and abundance of Voluntary Action outside one's home, individually and in association with other citizens, for bettering one's own life and that of one's fellows, are the distinguishing marks of a free society. They have been outstanding features of British life.'[26] The special place of volunteers, and the ethos of voluntarism in British life, have continued to be noted, most recently in Prime Minister David Cameron's championing of community responsibility and local action as part of the 'Big Society'.[27]

The Pursuit of Better Bodies

The national fitness story is also a history of a modernity lived in the body, a history shaped by an era in which strong, fit and beautiful bodies carried powerful currency in politics and culture. Sport had never been more popular – to play or to follow – than it became in the 1930s. The 1932 Los Angeles and 1936 Berlin Olympic Games, staged as mass spectacles, were the most elaborate of a series of international events, one the product of American capitalism, the other of the Nazi state. Both Games were theatrical in scale, reaching worldwide audiences for the first time through the work of press, radio and film reporters whose presence was central in the planning of both cities' organising committees. The 1930s was the first truly global sporting decade. But the meaning and purpose of sporting competition was, itself, a matter of contest. If the Olympic Games in the 1930s offered a newly powerful stage for rivalries in national supremacy in international competition, events such as the Maccabiah Games, the workers' sport and women's international festivals offered an

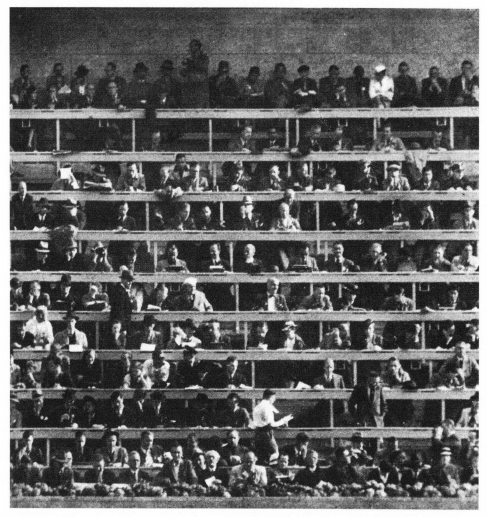

The press box built into the Olympic Stadium, Berlin. 800 representatives of the world's press covered the Games. As the *Berliner Illustrite* proudly told its readers, 'from here many hundreds of thousands of words found their way to uncounted million readers'. *Berliner Illustrite Zeitung*, 1936, Ullstein A.G. Berlin, p.49

internationalism based on common identities outside the nation state. The Empire Games were also, to an extent, a reaction to the escalating stakes of international contest. They drew some of their impetus from a desire to restore a 'games spirit' to competition within a distinctively British domain, against what was perceived as the overly ruthless pursuit of competition at all costs in the Olympic Games.

The powerful demonstration of sporting prowess on display at the 1936 Berlin Olympics, however, proved hard to resist. Representatives on the National Fitness Council for England and Wales included those who had been or still were top athletes: David Burghley, Philip Noel Baker, Dorothy Round, Wavell Wakefield,

Lord Aberdare (C. N. Bruce). They sat alongside those who were prominent in the many non-sporting 'healthy body cultures' that flourished in this period. Among them were Margaret Morris, founder of the Margaret Morris Movement; Phyllis Spafford of the Ling Association; Prunella Stack from the Women's League of Health and Beauty; and Major Gem, organiser of physical training for the London County Council. A similar span of sporting, fitness and outdoor recreation interests was present in New Zealand, Australia and Canada. It is a reminder of the diverse range of sporting, dance, movement, keep-fit and outdoor recreation activities that existed in the 1920s and 1930s. By the second half of the twentieth century, the dominance of competitive sport had not entirely eliminated all other forms of physical recreation, but it had very much come to overshadow them.

The idea that the healthy body was an active body gained a new intensity in the post-World War I world. Exercising for competition, to keep fit or slim, or simply for fun was now something many people were keen to do, and something voguish. It was an idea promoted commercially as well as by medical professionals. And it rested on a rejection of the old duality of mind and body conveyed in the 'mens sana in corpore sano' (a sound mind in a healthy body) motto. A modern person was an integrated whole. The physical fitness campaigns in Britain and the Dominions linked individual health, fitness and enjoyment with national interest. Public education campaigns aimed to raise awareness of the benefits of physical exercise and opportunities to participate in sport, games and physical recreation (hiking, camping and cycling especially). Fitness and physical activity were defined and justified as worthy of public expenditure because they had a national as well as individual purpose. People were urged to see their own fitness and health – through physical activity – as a duty of citizenship. Personal benefits from increased health and happiness would accrue along with benefits to the nation as a whole. In this way, the national fitness campaigns went further and were more ambitious than the post-World War I project of reconstruction that Carden-Coyne has described.[28]

Strong, fit and beautiful bodies were also central as ideals and symbols to modern life. In modernist aesthetics – painting, design and sculpture – and in commercial and popular culture – movies, magazines and advertising – the human body was highly conspicuous. Bodies in action – dancing, leaping, swimming, running – were highly evocative images of contemporary vitality. Jack Lovelock was just one athlete whose picture appeared on cigarette cards. Adonia Wallace, winner of many beauty competitions, was the face and body for Wright's Coal Tar Soap in 1938. An advertisement shows her clad in swimming attire under the heading carrying her advice: "'My rule for fitness and beauty," says Britain's Perfect Girl, "is simple exercises and the daily use of WRIGHT'S COAL TAR SOAP".[29] To be judged 'perfect' was part of promotional hyperbole, but also a hint of modernism's utopianism.

That utopianism points in a further direction: to modernism's quest to create the world anew. In that ambitious, sometimes authoritarian, dream lies its vigour, but also its danger, its dark and light shades. For both the progressive left and the authoritarian right, active and strong bodies were part of a reforming agenda. Within the national fitness schemes, the promotion of physical activity and recreation took on progressive contours (in the work of Rona Stephenson (Bailey) and Philip Smithells, for example); but could also present the complete antithesis in the promotion of strong and fit bodies as part of totalitarianism. Exalting the strong body as an instrument and metaphor of the strong nation, and physical strength and 'racial purity' as national virtues, were prominent elements of this period. Modernism's slippery nature presents a puzzle for interpretation. The contradictory character of modernity, a state defined by opposing forces, helps describe if not resolve such stark contrasts. One solution, and a useful one, is to recognise the active body as part of the defining contradictions of modernity: its wonder *and* terror, excitement *and* fear, light *and* shade. Taking a step beyond this Bermanesque point leads to the problem of fascism's relation to modernity, a question complicated by the divergent nature of fascist movements. In Mussolini's Italy, in the chrome belts and bare heads of the uniformed members of Mosley's British Union of Fascists, were clear signs of modernism – in contrast to the social and aesthetic conservatism of culture under Nazism. Going further, Roger Griffin argues for the inherently palingenetic (rebirth) project of fascism as a form of modernism. The 'healthy body culture' movements were part of that radical re-making. His explanation teases out a resolution to the problems of both fascism and modernity – both are entities that are easily recognisable but hard to account for beyond very specific historical contexts.[30] Susan Sontag's 1975 article 'Fascinating Fascism', an indignant response to the uncritical reception of Leni Riefenstahl's photographic work, offers another perspective on the difficulty of disentangling modernism from its political context. For Sontag, the failure both to distinguish sufficiently *and* to connect aesthetic and political assessment was objectionable. Riefenstahl and her extensive work output provide an ongoing subject for exploring the contradictions of modernity.[31]

Another way to understand the problem of fit, active and strong bodies in the cultures of left and right at this moment in the twentieth century is to consider them as a form of anti-modernism. Much less developed than modernity, and often conveying little more than a synonym for 'reaction' or 'tradition', the utility of the concept is amply demonstrated in Alison Light's work in explaining the popularity of non-literary fiction in interwar Britain. In *Forever England*, Light advances the argument of a 'conservative modernity' to explain the massive contemporary popularity of Agatha Christie's detective fiction, and to repudiate its dismissal by literary critics and labour historians alike.[32] Neither simply nostalgic nor modern in its form or style, such work 'went straight to the heart of new kinds of anxiety about English social life'. Christie was a popular modernist, Light suggests, offering an engagement with the new but in a conservative guise. It is the era of Hercule Poirot rather than Miss Marple. Similarly, Sharon Walls offers a useful analysis in *The Nurture of Nature*, her study of the hugely popular Ontario summer camps between the 1920s and the 1950s (in which a ten-year-old Pierre Trudeau participated). Wall explains in a fine-grained discussion the appeal 'wilderness' holidays had to city-dwelling Canadians searching for meaning in modernity. In the anti-modern pursuits of camping, lighting fires with sticks, fashioning wood, paddling canoes, and living in tents was an antidote to over-civilisation. In the 'wilderness' a child might grow into an adult. For Light and Wall, it is the combination of conservative setting and modernist pursuit that defines a 'conservative modernity' or 'anti-modernism'. Such combinations might also be seen in some of the national fitness and physical welfare activities discussed in the preceding chapters.

Sport and body cultures did not sit outside the polarising politics of the 1930s, but were part of it. Both liberal democracies and totalitarian states became involved in promoting some form of 'fitness' amongst their populations. A key argument of this study is that interest in fit, strong and beautiful bodies in the 1930s was not the monopoly of totalitarian and right wing regimes. At popular, commercial and government levels, the fit and healthy body was also a central figure in Britain and across the wider 'British world'. Against the background of increasing time for leisure, and the novelty of the principle that healthy bodies were active bodies, a wide range of body cultures proliferated. Out of this milieu came the government-initiated schemes for promoting greater physical fitness through encouraging more sport, building sports and recreation facilities, and supporting the professionalisation of physical education. The history of national fitness across the British world reminds us of the much wider, and more varied, body cultures that existed in these years, and of the intermixing between ideas and practices across places with very different political ideologies.

Gender, the meanings of urban vs 'outdoor' space, the issue of race and the presence of radio have also run through the national fitness story. They add further contours to the historically specific meanings of modernity depicted by Bingham's study of gender and the popular press in Britain, Matthews in her portrait of Sydney, Carden-Coyne's argument for the body in the Anglo world, and Daunton and Rieger's discussion of contemporary understandings of a specifically British modernity.[33]

The concern with bodies, state and modernity was centrally organised around gender. Women wearing short skirts, short hair, even seen smoking, playing sport or performing exercise constituted some of most striking signs of the difference of modern times. The debate over the degree to which the interwar decades remade relations of gender has attracted considerable attention in British historiography. While this has not been the prime question here, clearly national fitness schemes gave a fillip to women's sport and recreation. In each country programmes were aimed at both women and men, and women as well as men were employed as organisers and officers of state-funded fitness organisations. Physical education as a recognised speciality within higher education was advanced, a significant innovation for men who had lacked such an opportunity. Although the national college planned for England was not realised, elsewhere impetus towards providing training and qualifications for those who would become physical education professionals was facilitated by the schemes.

Geographies of modernity are evident in the significance attributed to the spaces in which people were encouraged to take exercise. The contradictory nature of modernity was also played out through exercise in the outdoors. In all four countries, recreation in 'nature' was valued highly. Camping, cycling, hiking and youth hostelling counted as top priorities in grants distributed by national fitness councils. The symbolic image of the free-striding hiker under the open skies was not just an ideal, but a product of the genuine popularity of these pursuits in the interwar years. The value of 'nature' was, it was argued, all the more important for people whose lives were constrained, as never before, by urban living and routines set by clock and machine. In a contradiction characteristic of modernity, 'nature' was both more accessible through advances in transport, regular weekends and holidays, and portable tents, but also more necessary. In supporters of physical fitness schemes such as Australia's C. E. W. Bean and the schemes' provision of these kinds of outdoor activities, there was an element of an anti-urban, even nostalgic hankering for a simpler past. Individual activities and collective meanings were brought together when Scottish hikers, English ramblers, Australian beachgoers, Canadian wilderness venturers and New Zealand trampers were depicted as representatives of a national culture.[34] In the context of the 1930s that outdoor space was imbued with the essence of what it was to be British, Australian, Canadian or a New Zealander. Urban and city space was less specific, less weighted with local features, more universal. If modernity and city space stood for the universal, sophisticated and metropolitan, then 'nature' and the 'outdoors' offering space for hiking, camping, youth hostelling, represented the local, particular and national.

In Canada, New Zealand and Australia, government-sponsored physical exercise and sport programmes formed part of modernising policies adopted by governments towards indigenous peoples. Jan Eisenhardt at the Canadian Department of Indian Affairs, physical welfare officers in New Zealand working with colleagues in the Department of Maori Affairs, and staff in Education and the Board of Aboriginal Affairs in Australia identified sport and recreation opportunities as useful in addressing disparities in health and education levels. Sport and organised recreation

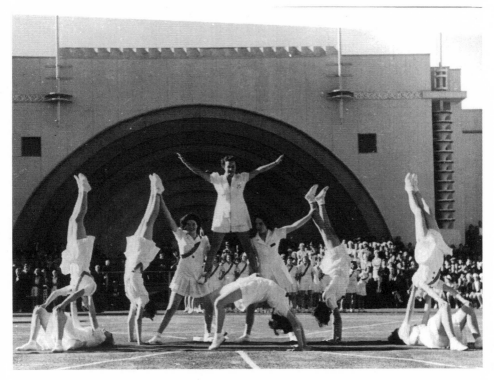

Months of practice culminated in an elaborate demonstration of symmetry and balance. One of the interhouse teams performing as part of the massed display at the Centennial Exhibition concourse in Wellington on Easter Saturday, March 1940. IA 62 4/38, Archives New Zealand

were seen as helpful as many indigenous communities were making the transition to urban settings and wage work, particularly in the post-1945 period. As had been the case throughout much of the twentieth century, for a very small but highly visible group of indigenous men and an even smaller number of indigenous women, it was professional sport that opened opportunities for social and material advancement. Amateur sport generally was organised in such a way as to maintain barriers.[35]

Technological advances were also an instrument in the convergent forces of modernity. Radio has been a running thread through the national fitness histories. Centrally important in revolutionising communication, and in creating new communities through such innovations as the BBC's Empire Service, radio occupied a particularly significant place in promoting physical fitness. In its intimacy and simultaneous anonymity, it was able to reach listeners while they were still in their pyjamas getting ready for the day – an ideal moment in which to perform ten minutes' exercise, 'the daily dozen'. The listening habit and the exercising habit, it was hoped, would reinforce each other. These were the aims of those responsible for physical fitness campaigns, hopes that were realised everywhere except in Britain. There, the BBC's implacable opposition had a number of roots, but ultimately baulked at programming that came too close to endangering the freedom of an Englishman not only in 'his castle' but also in his body.

In telling the story of national fitness campaigns across Britain, New Zealand, Australia and Canada, *Strong, Beautiful and Modern* sets out a fuller and more connected history than exists to date. The history emerges from the world of the late 1930s and the early 1940s, in which a particular convergence of the broad strands of state, body and modernity resulted in the first major involvement by central governments in sporting activities and physical recreation undertaken by adults. The world from which the campaigns emerged was, however, soon swept away, the scale of events of World War II obscuring and diminishing its existence. The moment of convergence has perhaps been lost sight of, the influencing forces separately evolving or dissipating. Those forces include the politics of fascist nationalism, the aesthetics of modernism, the unprecedented reach of mass communication, and the novelty of active adult bodies. Fitness movements are particular in time, as they are in place. *Strong, Beautiful and Modern* also connects to another important topic – health and medicine. At all levels – scientific knowledge, political debate and commitment, social experience and material things – the 1920s–40s was an immensely significant period in the development of modern health. As a response to the ailing rather than healthy body, health services have come to occupy a central place in all the societies under discussion here. In contrast, government schemes for adult sport and physical recreation did not.

While the demise of national fitness schemes saw governments withdraw from direct involvement in sport and physical recreation, by the 1960s changed circumstances brought a demand for government to engage once again. The imperative by then had become the pressure to perform competitively in an international sporting arena shaped by the Cold War. President-elect John F. Kennedy appeared on the cover of *Sports Illustrated*'s special Christmas issue of 26 December 1960, warning readers of the dangers of 'The Soft American' and, in particular, of 'our increasing lack of physical fitness' as 'a menace to our security'.[36] The contest for supremacy between the Soviet bloc and the west was one played out in Olympic medal tallies as well as in missiles. Canada's Fitness and Amateur Sport Act 1961 was followed soon after by Britain's first ministerial portfolio for sport and a national Advisory Sports Council (1964). A ministry of sport and recreation was established in New Zealand in 1973, while state governments in Australia made similar moves. A more substantial commitment was made when the Australian Institute of Sport was opened in 1981. With narrower goals and a trickle of funding, the focus was generally on supporting national sporting associations in an era when amateurism was still intact, and costs of competition relied on perpetual fund-raising (such as contributions from tobacco companies for coaching schemes). In all places discussed here except Canada, a sense that sport and recreation were properly kept at a distance from government was maintained by ensuring that responsibility rested with statutory bodies at arm's length from government.

From these new beginnings, there has been a continuous, if uneven, history. Substantial development has occurred in the first decade of the twenty-first century with a noticeable rise in public funding and profile for UK Sport, SPARC (New Zealand) and their equivalents. In arguments over the balance between attention to be paid to elite vs community-level sport and recreation – the gold medals or grassroots, and the shifting rationales for investing public monies in such activities – some of the same tensions evident in the national fitness era can be seen. Is sport part of national culture, or a national 'culture of excellence' – and if so, is it successful only if winning or coming first is the outcome? If encouraging people to be physically active is justified in terms of improving health – fighting obesity, reducing heart disease, improving mental health – how far can people be coaxed into such things? In framing the 'obesity epidemic' as a social and political crisis whose solution lies in better exercise of individual will, Christine Halse is among those who have suggested that a new discourse of power surrounds the virtuous 'bio-citizen'. 'Right body size' is judged on a measure resembling the older categories of deserving and undeserving poor.[37] Instead of analysing the worldwide production and proliferation of high-fat, high-sugar cheap 'foods' (a fast-fat economy), the 'obesity epidemic' defines the problem in terms of individuals as isolated consumers succeeding or failing to exercise willpower. Political debates over whether to tax high-fat foods or publicly fund 'stomach-stapling' operations pose the current problem between individual aspiration and collective responsibility. How do governments encourage adults to be healthy without endangering individual freedom?

The idea that 'doing exercise is good for you', a new message in the 1930s, is now a commonplace. The pursuit of a 'better body', that defining condition of modernity, endures. But what is understood as fitness, and the circumstances in which it is pursued, have changed. In 1938, R. E. Roper, Philip Smithells' mentor, decried what he saw as the prevailing 'industrialization of movement and thought, a mass-production of parts instead of the growth of an individual whole'.[38] When Jan Eisenhardt led Canadian National Fitness Council discussions in 1945, he promoted an expansive definition of fitness that was 'spiritual, moral, mental and physical'.[39] These ideas have a genealogy through to the present. The exuberant, dangerous desires of the late 1930s to be strong and beautiful were surpassed by aspirations couched in wider dimensions of human life. These more holistic definitions would lead to later descriptions of health and fitness in terms of 'well-being'. The line connecting the period of this study, 1930s–40s, to the present, is not a straight one. What 'fitness' is and what it is for remain unsettled questions.

Meanwhile, the message that fitness is desirable or imperative remains persistent and insistent. Since the 1930s, there have been many answers to these questions, and widely divergent forms of this message. The mixture of government promotion and commercial pressure, collective purpose and individual quest remains. When the current Canadian legislation was passed in 2002, the term 'fitness' was replaced with 'physical activity', with the argument that it was preferable to refer to the activity being encouraged rather 'than to a particular end result'. But the end result always matters. And there is one line that can easily be drawn between the 1930s–40s and the present: inertia. As Lord Astor remarked in the House of Commons in 1937: thinking about other people doing exercise was almost always easier than doing it oneself.[40]

Abbreviations

AAU	Amateur Athletic Union (Canada)
ABC	Australian Broadcasting Corporation
ATL	Alexander Turnbull Library (Wellington, New Zealand)
BBC	British Broadcasting Corporation
BMA	British Medical Association
CBC	Canadian Broadcasting Corporation
CCF	Cooperative Commonwealth Federation (Canada)
CCPR	Central Council for Physical Recreation (UK)
CCRPT	Central Council of Recreative Physical Training (UK)
CRBC	Canadian Radio Broadcasting Commission
FIFA	Fédération Internationale de Football Association
HMSO	His Majesty's Stationery Office
HMV	His Master's Voice
IOC	International Olympic Commission
ILO	International Labour Organization
LCC	London County Council
MCC	Marylebone Cricket Club (UK)
NFC	National Fitness Council (UK)
NHL	National Hockey League (Canada)
NSW	New South Wales
NZRFU	New Zealand Rugby Football Union
NZUSA	New Zealand University Students Association
SCPR	Scottish Council of Physical Recreation
SPARC	Sport and Recreation New Zealand
TAB	Totalisator Agency Board (New Zealand)
UBC	University of British Columbia
WEA	Workers Educational Association
WWSA	Women's War Service Auxiliary (New Zealand)
YMCA	Young Men's Christian Association
YWCA	Young Women's Christian Association

List of Illustrations

Endnotes

Introduction

1   R51/387/5, Talks Physical Exercises File IIIa 1938–1939, Written Archives Centre, BBC, Reading.

2   Scripts for radio broadcasts, Noeline Thomson MS-Papers 8312, Alexander Turnbull Library (ATL), Wellington. Physical Welfare and Recreation Branch, *Keep Fit by Morning Exercises: Exercises Broadcast by YA stations at 7 a.m.*, Wellington, 1939, IA 1 2945 139/43, Newspaper and radio publicity, Physical Welfare and Recreation Branch, Department of Internal Affairs, Archives New Zealand, Wellington. National Fitness Council, Agency 1728 & 1732, State Records New South Wales (Sydney). See also Bill Gammage and Peter Spearritt (eds), with oral history co-ordinator Louise Douglas, *Australians 1938*, Fairfax, Syme & Weldon, Broadway, NSW, 1987, p.368.

3   Physical Training and Recreation Act 1937 (UK); Physical Welfare and Recreation Act 1937 (NZ); National Fitness Act, No.26 of 1941(Australia); An Act to establish a National Council for the purpose of promoting physical fitness (known as the National Physical Fitness Act), July 1943 (Canada). The New South Wales National Fitness scheme was introduced by an Order-in-Council of the New South Wales government. There was some interest in government-supported physical fitness campaigns in Eire, the Irish Free State, in this same period, notably in a 1938 commission recommending a programme of greater physical fitness. Relatively little action ensued and what there was, was largely limited to supporting physical education in schools: Thomas A. O'Donoghue, 'Sport, Recreation and Physical Education: The Evolution of a National Policy of Regeneration in Eire, 1926–48', *British Journal of Sports History*, 3, 2 (1986), pp.216–33.

4   The phrase used by Christopher Wilk (ed.), *Modernism, 1914–1939: Designing a New World*, V & A Publications, London, 2006.

5   Henning Eichberg (John Bale and Chris Philo, eds), *Body Cultures: Essays on Sport, Space, and Identity*, Routledge, London, 1998. It is notable that the one exception to the exclusion of relations with empire in Ross McKibbin's *Classes and Cultures: England 1918–1951*, Oxford University Press, 1998, is 'the sporting empire', Preface, p.vi.

6   Edit Mezey, 'Health and Slimming Exercises for Use in the Home', arranged and spoken by Edit Mezey, HMV Catalogue, 1938–39, Sound Archive, British Library. See also other exercise records listed in HMV Catalogues 1937–38, 1938–39. Edit Mezey was a celebrated Hungarian physical culturist. She featured in a brief newsreel item shot by Pathé on 14 April 1932 under the heading 'A little slimming a day – keeps the avoirdupois away', 4 mins, <www.britishpathe.com/record.php?id=17413>. Edit Mezey is also the voice in Ruby Grierson and Ralph Bond's film *Today We Live* (1937) in a scene showing a women's keep-fit class in a Gloucestershire village.

7   Kathy Peiss, *Hope in a Jar: The Making of America's Beauty Culture*, Harvey Holt, New York, 1998; Lois W. Banner, *American Beauty*, University of Chicago Press, 1984; Susie Johnston, 'Lighting Up: The Social History of Smoking in New Zealand, c.1920–62', MA thesis, Victoria University of Wellington, 2009; Matthew Hilton, *Smoking in British Popular Culture, 1800–2000: Perfect Pleasures*, Manchester University Press, 2000; Jarrett Rudy, *The Freedom to Smoke: Tobacco Consumption and Identity*, McGill–Queen's University Press, Montreal, 2005; Martin Pugh, '*We Danced All Night': A Social History of Britain Between the Wars*, Bodley Head, London, 2008; Jill Julius Matthews, *Dance Hall to Picture Palace: Sydney's Romance with Modernity*, Currency Press, Sydney, 2005.

8   Robert Graves and Alan Hodge, *The Long Weekend: A Social History of Great Britain, 1918–1939*, Faber, London, 1940; John Stevenson, *British Society, 1914–45*, Allen Lane, London, 1984 (cover features J. W. Tucker's 1936 painting 'Hiking'); Harvey Taylor, *A Claim on the Countryside: A History of the British Outdoor Movement*, Keele University Press, Edinburgh, 1997; Kirstie Ross, *Going Bush: New Zealanders and Nature in the Twentieth Century*, Auckland University Press, 2008; Melissa Harper, *The Ways of the Bushwalker: On Foot in Australia*, University of New South Wales Press, Sydney, 2007.

9   Patricia Vertinsky, *The Eternally Wounded Woman: Women, Doctors, and Exercise in the Late Nineteenth Century*, University of Illinois Press, Urbana, 1994; Lesley Hall, *Sex, Gender and Social Change in Britain Since 1880*, Macmillan, Basingstoke, 2000; W. F. Bynum and Roy Porter (eds), *Companion Encyclopaedia of the History of Medicine*, Routledge,

London and New York, 1993; Ana Carden-Coyne, *Reconstructing the Body: Classicism, Modernism, and the First World War*, Oxford University Press, 2009.

10 Carden-Coyne, *Reconstructing the Body*.

11 Barbara Keys, *Globalizing Sport*, Harvard University Press, Cambridge, 2006; Barbara Keys, 'The Body as a Political Space: Comparing Physical Education under Nazism and Stalinism', *German History*, 27, 3 (July 2009), pp.395–413; Shelley Baronowski, *Strength Through Joy: Consumerism and Mass Tourism in the Third Reich*, Cambridge University Press, 2004; Shelley Baronowski, 'A Family Vacation for Workers: The Strength through Joy Resort at Prora', *German History*, 25, 4 (2007), pp.539–59; Tony Collins, 'Review Article: Work, Rest and Play: Recent Trends in the History of Sport and Leisure', *Journal of Contemporary History*, 42, 2 (2007), pp.397–410; Adam Stanley, *Modernizing Tradition: Gender and Consumerism in Interwar France and Germany*, Louisiana State University Press, Baton Rouge, 2008.

12 Mark Mazower, *Dark Continent: Europe's Twentieth Century*, Vintage, New York, 1998, p.92; Alison Bashford and Philippa Levine (eds), *Oxford Handbook to the History of Eugenics*, Oxford University Press, Oxford and New York, 2010.

13 Bryan Turner, *Regulating Bodies: Essays in Medical Sociology*, Routledge, London, 1992; Kenneth Dutton, *The Perfectible Body*, Continuum, London, 1997.

14 Marshall Berman, *All That is Solid Melts into Air*, Simon & Schuster, New York, 1983.

15 Wilk (ed.), *Modernism*; Martin Daunton and Bernhard Rieger (eds), *Meanings of Modernity: Britain from the Late-Victorian Era to World War II*, Berg, Oxford and New York, 2001; Matthews, *Dance Hall and Picture Palace*; Roger Griffin, *Modernism and Fascism*, Routledge, London, 2007; Becky Conekin, Frank Mort and Chris Waters (eds), *Moments of Modernity: Reconstructing Britain 1945–1964*, Rivers Oram Press, London, 1999. Historical interest in modernity ranges broadly. For another important set of discussions on the theme, see the *American Historical Review*, 116, 3 (June 2011) featuring ten articles on 'Historians and the Question of Modernity' including Dipesh Chakrabarty's 'The Muddle of Modernity', pp.663–75.

16 Matthews, *Dance Hall and Picture Palace*.

17 They were not solely or even predominantly Freudian in origin. Mathew Thomson, *Psychological Subjects: Identity, Culture, and Health in Twentieth-century Britain*, Oxford University Press, 2006; Conekin, et al. (eds), *Moments of Modernity*; Nikolas Rose, *Inventing Our Selves: Psychology, Power and Personhood*, Cambridge University Press, 1998; Nikolas Rose, *Governing the Soul: The Shaping of the Private Self*, Routledge, London, 1990; Roy Porter (ed.), *Rewriting the Self: Histories from the Renaissance to the Present*, Routledge, London, 1997.

18 Anthony Giddens, *Modernity and Self-identity: Self and Society in the Late Modern Age*, Polity Press, Cambridge, 1991.

19 Conekin et al. (eds), *Moments of Modernity*, p.11.

20 Visit of International Advisory Committee to London, February 1939, p.1, *World Congress on Recreation and Leisure Time Proceedings*, 1939 (BL CUP.1253.c.23). See also King George VI speech launching National Fitness Campaign, London, 17 February 1938, ICL 0067783 (BBC), British Library Sound Archive (AA 1629). Christopher Lawrence and George Weisz (eds), *Greater Than the Parts: Holism in Biomedicine, 1920–1950*, Oxford University Press, 1998.

21 Philip Buckner and R. Douglas Francis (eds), *Rediscovering the British World*, University of Calgary Press, 2005; Carl Bridge and Kent Fedorowich (eds), *The British World: Diaspora, Culture and Identity*, Frank Cass, London, 2003. James Belich, *Replenishing the Earth: The Settler Revolution and the Rise of the Anglo World, 1783–1939*, Oxford University Press, Oxford and New York, 2009, makes a rather different case for the Anglo world.

22 King George VI speech, 17 February 1938; *Radio Times*, 11 February 1938, vol.58, no.750, p.62.

23 Philippa Levine, *The British Empire: Sunrise to Sunset*, Pearson Longman, Harlow, 2007; John M. MacKenzie (ed.), *Imperialism and Popular Culture*, Manchester University Press, 1986; Simon Potter, 'Webs, Networks, and Systems: Globalization and the Mass Media in the Nineteenth and Twentieth-Century British Empire', *Journal of British Studies*, 46 (July 2007), pp.621–46; Simon Potter, 'Who Listened When London Called? Reactions to the BBC Empire Service in Canada, Australia and New Zealand, 1932–1939', *Historical Journal of Film, Radio and Television*, 28, 4 (October 2008), pp.475–87; Catherine Hall (ed.), *Cultures of Empire: Colonizers in Britain and the Empire in the Nineteenth and Twentieth Centuries: A Reader*, Routledge, New York, 2000; Katie Pickles, *Female Imperialism and National Identity: Imperial Order Daughters of the Empire*, Manchester University Press,

Manchester and New York, 2002; J. A. Mangan (ed.), *Making Imperial Mentalities*, Manchester University Press, 1990; Buckner and Francis (eds), *Rediscovering the British World*; Bridge and Fedorowich (eds), *The British World*.

24 Quoted in Katharine Moore, 'The Warmth of Comradeship: The First British Empire Games and Imperial Solidarity', in J. A. Mangan (ed.), *The Cultural Bond*, Frank Cass, London, 1992, p.207.

25 See, for example, the Christmas Broadcast of Queen Elizabeth II, 25 December 2010, <www. royal.gov.uk>.

26 Secretary for the Interior, Union of South Africa to Under Secretary Department of Internal Affairs, New Zealand, 6 October 1945, IA 1 139/11/12, Archives New Zealand, Wellington.

27 H. Justin Evans, *Service to Sport: The Story of the CCPR 1935-1972*, Pelham Books in association with the Sports Council, London, 1974; Mariel Grant, 'The National Health Campaigns of 1937-1938', in Derek Fraser (ed.), *Cities, Class and Communication: Essays in Honour of Asa Briggs*, Harvester Wheatsheaf, London, 1990, pp.216-33; Mariel Grant, *Propaganda and the Role of the State in Inter-war Britain*, Clarendon Press, Oxford, 1994; Stephen G. Jones, *Sport, Politics and the Working Class: Organised Labour and Sport in Inter-war Britain*, Manchester University Press, 1988; Stephen G. Jones, 'State Intervention in Sport Between the Wars', *Journal of Contemporary History*, 22 (1987), pp.163-82; Stephen G. Jones, 'The British Workers' Sports Federation: 1923-1936', in Arnd Kruger and James Riordan (eds), *The Story of Worker Sport*, Human Kinetics, Champaign, 1996, pp.97-115; Stephen G. Jones, *Workers at Play: A Social and Economic History of Leisure, 1918-1939*, Routledge, London, 1986; Donald Macintosh, Tom Bedecki and C. E. S. Franks, *Sport and Politics in Canada: Federal Government Involvement Since 1961*, McGill-Queen's University Press, Montreal, 1988; Don Morrow, Mary Keyes, Wayne Simpson, Frank Cosentino and Ron A. Lappage, *A Concise History of Sport in Canada*, Oxford University Press, Toronto, 1989; Barbara Schrodt, 'Federal Programmes of Physical Recreation and Fitness: The Contributions of Ian Eisenhardt and BC's Pro-Rec', *Canadian Journal of Sport and Physical Education*, 15, 2 (December 1984), pp.45-61; Bruce Kidd, *The Struggle for Canadian Sport*, University of Toronto Press, 1996; Hugh D. Buchanan, 'A Critical Analysis of the 1937 Physical Welfare and Recreation Act and of Government Involvement in Recreation and Sport, 1937-1957', MA (Applied) thesis,

Victoria University of Wellington, 1978; Janet Alexander, 'Recreation: An Inappropriate Concept for Legislation?: An Examination of Two Attempts at Legislating for Recreation in New Zealand; the Physical Welfare and Recreation Act 1937, and the Recreation and Sport Act 1973', MPP research paper, Victoria University of Wellington, 1981; Caroline Daley, *Leisure and Pleasure: Reshaping and Revealing the New Zealand Body*, Auckland University Press, 2003.

28 See, for example, Mangan (ed.), *The Cultural Bond*; Keith Sandiford and Robert Stoddard (eds), *The Imperial Game*, Manchester University Press, 1998; Patrick F. McDevitt, *May the Best Man Win: Sport, Masculinity and Nationalism in Great Britain and the Empire, 1880-1935*, Palgrave Macmillan, New York, 2003; Mackenzie (ed.), *Imperialism and Popular Culture*.

29 Owen Mann, 'Confirming Tradition, Confirming Change: A Social History of the Cricket Tours to New Zealand in the 1930s', MA thesis, Victoria University of Wellington, 2011.

30 Simon Potter, *News and the British World: The Emergence of an Imperial Press System 1876-1922*, Oxford University Press, 2003; Potter, 'Webs, Networks, and Systems'.

31 Ramachandra Guha, *Corner of a Foreign Field: The Indian History of a British Sport*, Picador, London, 2002; C. L. R. James, *Beyond a Boundary*, Hutchinson, London, 1963; Keith A. Sandiford and Brian Stoddart (eds), *The Imperial Game: Cricket, Culture and Society*, Manchester University Press, Manchester and New York, 1998; Daryl Adair and Wray Vamplew, *Sport in Australian History*, Oxford University Press, Melbourne, 1997; Charlotte Macdonald, 'Ways of Belonging: Sporting Spaces in New Zealand History', in Giselle Byrnes (ed.), *The New Oxford History of New Zealand*, Oxford University Press, Melbourne, 2009.

32 James Curran and Stuart Ward, *The Unknown Nation: Australia after Empire*, Melbourne University Press, 2010; Stuart Ward (ed.), *British Culture and the End of Empire*, Manchester University Press, Manchester and New York, 2001.

33 McKibbin, *Classes and Cultures*, p.380.

34 National Fitness Council, *The National Fitness Campaign*, London, 1939, pp.3, 10.

35 Jane Lewis and Barbara Brookes, 'The Peckham Health Centre, "Pep", and the Concept of General Practice During the 1930s and 1940s', *Medical History*, 27, 2 (April 1983), pp.151-61.

36 Sandra Dawson, 'Working-class Consumers and the Campaign for Holidays with Pay', *Twentieth Century British History*, 18, 3 (2007), pp.277–305; Jones, *Workers at Play*; John Martin, *Holding the Balance: A History of the Department of Labour 1891–1995*, Canterbury University Press, Christchurch, 1996; Juliet B. Schor, *The Overworked American: The Unexpected Decline of Leisure*, Basic Books, New York, 1991.

37 Witold Rybczynski, *Waiting for the Weekend*, Viking, New York, 1991.

38 Henry William Durant, *The Problem of Leisure*, Routledge, London, 1938.

39 *Report on the World Congress for Leisure Time and Recreation Hamburg July 1936*, Prepared by the International Central Bureau of Joy and Work, Hanseatische Verlagsanstalt, Hamburg [1937]; ED 136/93 World Congress on Recreation and Leisure Time, The National Archives, London; 'First International Recreation Congress', NBKR 6/15/7, Philip Noel Baker, Papers, Churchill Archives, Churchill College, Cambridge; Victoria de Grazia, *The Culture of Consent*, Cambridge University Press, 1981, p.240.

40 de Grazia, *The Culture of Consent*.

Chapter 1: Movement is Life

1 'Movement is Life' was part of the registered trademark of the Women's League of Health and Beauty and was used on the organisation's letterhead: A. J. Cruickshank and Prunella Stack, *Movement is Life: The Intimate History of the Founder of the Women's League of Health and Beauty and of its Origin, Growth, Achievements, and Hopes for the Future*, Bell, London, 1937.

2 William (Wavell) Wakefield, Conservative MP, Swindon 1934–45, St Marylebone 1945–63. See John Reason, 'Wakefield, Wavell (William), Baron Wakefield of Kendal (1898–1983)', *Oxford Dictionary of National Biography*, Oxford University Press, first published 2004; online edn, January 2011.

3 Hansard, House of Commons Parliamentary Debates, 11 June 1937, Vol.324, p.2187. This was the third reading of the Bill. The first reading took place in March and the second in April. Chamberlain became Prime Minister on 17 May 1937, succeeding Stanley Baldwin, and one week after the coronation of George VI. See Andrew J. Crozier, 'Chamberlain, (Arthur) Neville (1869–1940)', *Oxford Dictionary of National Biography*, Oxford University Press, first published 2004; online edn, January 2008; Robert Self, *Neville Chamberlain: A Biography*, Ashgate, Aldershot, 2006.

4 Jack Williams, *Cricket and England: A Cultural and Social History of the Inter-war Years*, Frank Cass, London, 1999; Richard Holt, *Sport and the British: A History*, Oxford University Press, 1989; John Hargreaves, *Sport, Power and Culture. A Social and Historical Analysis of Popular Sports in Britain*, Polity Press, Cambridge, 1987.

5 Hansard, House of Commons Parliamentary Debates, 7 April 1937, p.207a.

6 An indicator of British admiration of German practice can be found in the HMSO's publication for the Board of Education of a pamphlet entitled *Physical Education in Germany* (HMSO, London, 1937), which was described as presenting 'The results of a recent survey of the practical steps now being taken to improve the health and physique of the German nation': HMSO, *Recreation and Physical Education for Youths and Men*, London, 1937, p.xiv.

7 Stephen G. Jones, 'State Intervention in Sport Between the Wars', *Journal of Contemporary History*, 22 (1987), pp.163–82; H. Justin Evans, *Service to Sport: The Story of the CCPR 1935–1972*, Pelham Books in association with the Sports Council, London, 1974.

8 ED 136/91, 22 July 1937, The National Archives, London.

9 Physical Training and Recreation Act 1937. The National Advisory Council first met on 1 March 1937, Captain Ellis, secretary to the committee, started work on the same day, and the National Fitness Council closed its office on 30 September 1939: ED files, The National Archives, London. See also Peter C. McIntosh, *Physical Education in England since 1800*, Bell, London, 1952, p.236.

10 Ross McKibbin, *Classes and Cultures: England 1918–1951*, Oxford University Press, 1998, p.380. Tony Mason, '"Hunger … is a Very Good Thing": Britain in the 1930s', Nick Tiratsoo (ed.), *From Blitz to Blair. A New History of Britain Since 1939*, Phoenix, London, p.7. Ina Zweiniger-Bargielowska, *Managing the Body: Beauty, Health and Fitness in Britain, 1880s–1939*, Oxford University Press, 2010, offers the most substantial recent history. The National Fitness campaign appears as the last chapter in her book. See also Richard Holt and Tony Mason, *Sport in Britain Since 1945*, Wiley-Blackwell, Oxford, 2000; Mike Huggins and Jack Williams, *Sport and the English, 1918– 1939*, Routledge, London and New York, 2006.

11 *The Observer*, 1 December 1935. In the return match in 1938, the English football team gave the Nazi salute before playing in front of a

crowd of 110,000 at Berlin's Olympic Stadium on 14 May 1938, see photograph *Illustrated London News*, featured on cover Peter J. Beck, *Scoring for Britain: International Football and International Politics, 1900–1939*, Frank Cass, London, 1999. On this occasion England beat Germany 6–3. See also Piers Brendon, *The Dark Valley: A Panorama of the 1930s*, Vintage, New York, 2002.

12 Stephen G. Jones, 'The British Workers' Sports Federation: 1923–1936', in Arnd Kruger and James Riordan (eds), *The Story of Worker Sport*, Human Kinetics, Champaign, 1996, pp.97–115; Philip Noel Baker Papers, NBKR Series 6, especially 6/54, 6/15, 6/15/7, Churchill Archives, Churchill College, Cambridge.

13 Ina Zweiniger-Bargielowska, 'The Making of a Modern Female Body: Beauty, Health and Fitness in Interwar Britain', *Women's History Review*, 20, 2 (April 2011), pp.299–317.

14 McKibbin, *Classes and Cultures*, p.379. Harvey Taylor, *A Claim on the Countryside: A History of the British Outdoor Movement*, Keele University Press, Edinburgh, 1997.

15 Cruickshank and Stack, *Movement is Life*; Prunella Stack, *Movement is Life: The Autobiography of Prunella Stack*, Harvill, London, 1973; Jill Julius Matthews, '"They had such a lot of fun": The Women's League of Health and Beauty Between the Wars', *History Workshop Journal*, 30, 1 (1990), pp.22–54; Jill Julius Matthews, 'Building the Body Beautiful', *Australian Feminist Studies*, 2, 5 (Summer 1987), pp.17–34; Jill Julius Matthews, 'Stack, Mary Meta Bagot (1883–1935)', *Oxford Dictionary of National Biography*, Oxford University Press, first published 2004; online edn, January 2008; Charlotte Macdonald, 'Body and Self: Learning to be Modern in 1920s–30s Britain', *Women's History Review*, 21, 5 (2012, forthcoming). Obituaries: Prunella Stack, *Guardian*, 2 January 2011; *Daily Mail*, 31 December 2010; 'Prunella Stack OBE 1914–2010', <www.thefitnessleague.com/media-pr/prunella-stack-obe-1914-2010>; Zweiniger-Bargielowska, *Managing the Body*; Ina Zweiniger-Bargielowska, 'Building a British Superman: Physical Culture in Interwar Britain', *Journal of Contemporary History*, 41, 4 (October 2006), pp.595–610; and Zweiniger-Bargielowska 'The Making of a Modern Female Body.

16 Sabra Milligan, *The Body and How to Keep Fit*, Premier Printing, Brighouse, 1934, p.5.

17 Christopher Wilk (ed.), *Modernism, 1914–1939: Designing a New World*, V & A Publications, London, 2006, p.249.

18 Stanley Baldwin, *A Call to the Nation: The Joint Manifesto of the Leaders of the National Government (Signed, Stanley Baldwin, J. Ramsay MacDonald, John Simon, 26th October, 1935)*, Burrup, Mathieson & Co, London, 1935; E. K. Le Fleming, *Report of the Physical Education Committee*, British Medical Association (BMA), London, 1936.

19 Cabinet minutes, Home Affairs Committee CAB 26/21, and ED 136/71, The National Archives, London.

20 'Physical Fitness: Government's Concern for the Nation', 11 November 1936, British Pathé, <www.britishpathe.com>. Sir Kingsley Wood, Conservative MP, Woolwich West 1918–43; Minister of Health, 1935–38.

21 National Fitness Council, *The National Fitness Campaign*, London, 1939, p.3 (quoting the White Paper).

22 Le Fleming, *Report of the Physical Education Committee*, p.1.

23 Mathew Thomson, *Psychological Subjects: Identity, Culture and Health in Twentieth-Century Britain*, Oxford University Press, 2006; Macdonald, 'Body and Self'. Harry Roberts' contemporary works conveyed a humanism integrating mind and body, and individual and social health: for example, see Harry Roberts, *The Practical Way to Keep Fit*, Odhams Press, London, 1939. Benjamin Gayelord Hauser, *Eat and Grow Beautiful*, Faber & Faber, London, 1936; John F. Lucy, *Be Fit and Cheerful* (based on his Radio Athlone talks), Pitman, London, 1937; R. E. Roper, *Movement and Thought*, Blackie, London, 1938; Christopher Lawrence and George Weisz (eds), *Greater Than the Parts: Holism in Biomedicine, 1920–1950*, Oxford University Press, New York and Oxford, 1998; Winston Churchill, 'Sport is the Stimulant', *News of the World*, 4 September 1938; see drafts CHAR 8/615, Churchill Archive, Churchill College, Cambridge.

24 Advertisements appear in *Recreation and Physical Fitness for Women and Girls*, p.vii, and *Recreation and Physical Fitness for Youths and Men*, p.vii.

25 *Radio Times*, 15 October 1937, broadcast on Thursday, 21 October 1937 at 4.45: Tea Time Talk, 'Making the Most of Your Looks'. Thanks to Kate Murphy, London, for this reference, and for sharing her work in progress on women in the BBC in the 1930s.

26 Andrew Whitfield, 'Stanley, Oliver Frederick George (1896–1950)', *Oxford Dictionary of National Biography*, Oxford University Press, first published 2004; online edn, January 2008. Stanley was replaced as President of

the Board of Education by the Earl Stanhope at the end of May 1937. Stanley's wife Maureen Vane-Tempest-Stewart was involved in raising funds for the Peckham Health Centre: Jane Lewis and Barbara Brookes, 'The Peckham Health Centre, "Pep", and the Concept of General Practice During the 1930s and 1940s', *Medical History*, 27, 2 (April 1983), pp.151–61.

27 Hansard, House of Commons Parliamentary Debates, 7 April 1937, p.199.

28 McIntosh, *Physical Education*, p.229. Evans also notes, regretfully, the 'meagre' representation of the physical education profession on the National Fitness Council: Evans, *Service to Sport,* pp.45–6.

29 Hansard, House of Commons Parliamentary Debates, 7 April 1937, pp.199–201.

30 Ibid., p.207. On the other hand, individualist physical culture could be dull, especially when compared with the competitive spirit in 'the thoroughly un-Marxian form' of British games with their 'spice of game and contest'.

31 Ibid., p.235

32 Ibid., pp.209–10.

33 Ibid., p.222.

34 Ibid., p.207a.

35 Ibid., p.247.

36 See Burghley's strong testimony on the point that sport transcended class divides. Competing in the Midlands, he reported seeing and meeting people from all walks of life in the shed before and after competing: Hansard, House of Commons Parliamentary Debates, 7 April 1937, pp.244–5.

37 Winston Churchill, 'Sport is the Stimulant', *News of the World*, 4 September 1938, p.12. See drafts CHAR 8/615, Churchill Archive, Churchill College, Cambridge.

38 Before becoming an MP, Bevan was involved as a local councillor in supporting the provision of playgrounds and public spaces in his south Wales home town, coal-mining Tredegar: Dai Smith, 'Bevan, Aneurin (1897–1960)', *Oxford Dictionary of National Biography*, Oxford University Press, first published 2004; online edn, January 2008; Michael Foot, *Aneurin Bevan: A Biography*, 2 volumes, Macgibbon & Kee, London, 1962–73; Dai Smith, *Aneurin Bevan and the World of South Wales*, University of Wales Press, Cardiff, 1993.

39 A reference to George Bernard Shaw's 1894 play *Arms and the Man* in which one of the main characters plays the role of the 'chocolate soldier'.

40 Hansard, House of Commons Parliamentary Debates, 7 April 1937, pp.253–8. As Minister of Health and Housing in the 1945 Labour Government, Bevan was architect of the National Health Service. In the Attlee government in 1948–49 financial difficulties meant that he had to argue for spectacles and dentures to be included in the National Health Service. To Dai Smith, one of Bevan's biographers, this was especially significant as these were 'symbolic appliances' 'to an interwar working class deprived of both': Smith, 'Bevan, Aneurin (1897–1960)'.

41 April–June 1937 Poster Services notice ED 136/91, posters issued by Central Council for Health Education, The National Archives, London. They are reproduced in Mariel Grant, *Propaganda and the Role of the State in Interwar Britain*, Clarendon Press, Oxford, 1994, p.182.

42 White Paper, Physical Training and Recreation, 1937, Cmd 5364, p.12.

43 Minutes of Cabinet Committee on Physical Training, 25 November 1936, p.5, ED 136/71, The National Archives, London.

44 Physical Recreation Committee for England and Wales, ED 136/77, 66814, The National Archives, London. Michael Maclagan, 'Bruce, Clarence Napier, Third Baron Aberdare (1885–1957)', *Oxford Dictionary of National Biography*, Oxford University Press, first published 2004; online edn, January 2008. Aberdare to PM, 5 February 1937, Aberdare to Williams, 2 February 1937, accepting invitation to chair Council, ED 136/76, The National Archives, London. In accepting the PM's invitation for the chairmanship of the National Advisory Council, Aberdare replied with some prescience. After noting that the government's announcement had 'thrilled' him at the outset, he went on to write 'The method of approach to this enormous and most important movement leads me to safeguard myself by saying that I think it must take a considerable time to find out and adjudicate on the needs of the "localities" and very long before the beneficial results appear. Psychologically I hope the nation will feel strengthened and happier in the near future.'

45 Prunella Stack (1914–2010), see endnote 15. Also 'Prunella Stack OBE 1914–2010', <www.thefitnessleague.com/media-pr/prunella-stack-obe-1914-2010>. Mrs A. J. Cruickshank, replying to an invitation to be on the Committee on Prunella's behalf (she was in Germany studying forms of physical training there), added 'May I add how deeply I and our Executive Committee appreciate the acknowledgement implied in this invitation of the work accomplished by the League. I know that Miss Stack will welcome the opportunity of further

service in the cause which she has so much at heart': A. J. Cruickshank to Baldwin, 5 February 1937, ED 136/76, The National Archives, London. On 15 October 1938 Prunella married a Scottish laird, Lord David Douglas-Hamilton; 10,000 League members turned up to see the wedding in Glasgow Cathedral, including some who had come from London in a specially hired train: Juliet Gardiner, *The Thirties: An Intimate History*, HarperPress, London, 2010, p.523.

46 Norris McWhirter, 'Cecil, David George Brownlow, Sixth Marquess of Exeter (1905–1981)', *Oxford Dictionary of National Biography*, Oxford University Press, first published 2004; online edn, October 2005. David Howell, 'Baker, Philip John Noel-, Baron Noel-Baker (1889–1982)', *Oxford Dictionary of National Biography*, Oxford University Press, first published 2004; online edn, January 2008.

47 Round won the Wimbledon singles title in June 1937: Mark Pottle, 'Round, Dorothy Edith (1909–1982)', *Oxford Dictionary of National Biography*, Oxford University Press, first published 2004; online edn, January 2011.

48 Margaret Morris (1891–1980). Margaret Morris, *My Life in Movement*, Peter Owen, London, 1969 ('reveals the author's amazing methods for growing younger'); Pam Hirsch, 'Morris, Margaret Eleanor (1891–1980)', *Oxford Dictionary of National Biography*, Oxford University Press, first published 2004; online edn, January 2008. She was in a circle of famous people of time: Picasso, G. B. Shaw, Marlene Dietrich, Suzanne Lenglen, and athletes including Jack Lovelock and hurdler Roland Harper.

49 Edward Cadogan, sometime Conservative MP, but not in Parliament in these years.

50 A group including W. McG. Eager, editor of *The Boy*, National Association of Boys' Clubs; Sir Percy Everett, Boy Scouts and Girl Guides; Captain Glynn Jones, South Wales Federation of Boys' Clubs; Mrs A. M. Grenfell, President of the YWCA; and Lady Eleanor Keane, Chairman of the National Council of Girls' Clubs, represented the social service and especially the youth side of the work. Several of these had military backgrounds: ED 136/77, The National Archives, London.

51 Sir E. Kaye Le Fleming MD, Chairman of the Council of the British Medical Association. 'He was Chairman of their Physical Education Committee and represents the Association on the Central Council of Recreative Physical Training. Knighted in New Year Honours 1937', ED 136/77, The National Archives, London. Viscount Dawson of Penn (1864–1945),

obituary, *British Medical Journal*, 17 March 1945, pp.389–92.

52 LGD to Secretary, 11 December 1936, ED 136/76, The National Archives, London.

53 Henry Pelham to P. E. Meadon, Lancashire, 22 January 1937, ED 136/77, The National Archives, London. Meadon replied with three names and Assheton was the one chosen. See also Oliver Stanley to Rt Hon Viscount Halifax, 22 January 1937: 'I am finding it rather difficult to get a really suitable woman to serve on the Grants Committee. The kind of person one wants is a knowledgeable and helpful woman, preferably one who does not live in London .... One would prefer that she should not be intimately connected with a Local Education Authority, but on the other hand, I am anxious that she should not be too closely identified with any one particular voluntary body. You might know someone in Yorkshire who would be suitable.'

54 Captain Lionel F. Ellis (c.1885–?) was appointed as secretary to the NFC. Aged 52, he had been Secretary of the National Council of Social Service since 1919. He took up the position as of 1 March 1937: ED 136/77, The National Archives, London. Ellis' military and social service background was regarded with scepticism by the physical education circle around the CCRPT: Evans, *Service to Sport*.

55 Callum G. Brown, 'Sport and the Scottish Office in the 20th Century: The Control of a Social Problem', *European Sports History Review* (1999), pp.164–82; Callum G. Brown, 'Sport and the Scottish Office in the 20th Century: The Promotion of a Social and Gender Policy', *European Sports History Review* (1999), pp.183–202; Elidh Macrae, '"Scotland for Fitness": The National Fitness Campaign and Scottish Women', *Women's History Magazine*, 62 (Spring 2010), pp.26–36. See ED 136/71, minutes of Cabinet Committee October–November 1936, where ideas were formulated for separate English, Welsh and Scottish structures. Chairman of the Scottish Grants Committee was Mr D. A. Anderson.

56 Hansard, House of Commons Parliamentary Debates, 11 June 1937, p.2177. Lees-Smith notes that athletes might give the Council physical beauty but queried whether they would have the skills to do the job.

57 Matthew Worley, *Oswald Mosley and the New Party*, Palgrave Macmillan, Basingstoke, 2010, pp.146–7, and passim. For references to Stanley as part of the YMCA, see pp.88, 126–7.

58 Press release, 27 February 1937 for publication 1 March, 'A Fitter Britain. The National Advisory Council prepares for Work', ED 136/76, The National Archives, London.

59 Janet Quigley Memo, 26 January 1937, R51/210/1, Talks Health File 1a 1932–8, Written Archive Centre (WAC), BBC. And interview notes 27 July 1937, NFC/BBC, p.2: 'Some discussion took place as to the form of talks in which the subjects they had mentioned should be handled, and it was readily agreed that it would be quite possible to sicken the public of the whole subject unless care were taken to vary the form of presentment and to employ entertaining speakers.' Evan Hughes, CBE, was appointed as Public Relations Officer for the National Fitness Council. Hughes was formerly Secretary of the National Savings Committee and for several years Director of Organisation: ED 136/91, 14 February 1938, press release, The National Archives, London. Mariel Grant has a less favourable view of the expertise deployed by the NFC and related health promotion campaigns: see Mariel Grant, 'The National Health Campaigns of 1937–1938', in Derek Fraser (ed.), *Cities, Class and Communication: Essays in Honour of Asa Briggs*, Harvester Wheatsheaf, London, 1990, pp.216–33.

60 Lord Burghley headed the NFC's crucial publicity and propaganda committee. He was, in person, a striking figure of contemporary success, power and athleticism. A winning hurdler at the 1924, 1928 and 1932 Olympics, Burghley was also known for his fair play and keen support of amateur sport. In Hudson's 1981 *Chariots of Fire*, Lord David Lindsay (played by Nigel Havers), modelled closely on Burghley, practises his technique in the park-like grounds of Elizabethan Burghley House balancing filled champagne glasses on either side of the hurdles (it was a slight exaggeration: other sources suggest it was matchboxes). But the film emphasises his attractive personality, and contrasts the aristocratic Burghley with Harold Abrahams on the one side and Eric Liddell, the devout and working class Scot, on the other. In 1937 Burghley was into his sixth year as Conservative MP for Peterborough.

61 Hansard, House of Commons Parliamentary Debates, 11 June 1937. Press Release, 'Physical Training', 30 June 1937, R51/387/4, Talks Physical Exercises File 2b, WAC BBC.

62 Ibid., p.2185.

63 Talks Director to A. C., 23 September 1929, Internal Circulating Memo, R51/387/1, Talks Physical Exercises File 1a 1925–32, WAC BBC.

64 Presentation Director to Programme Director, Memo, 7 December 1933, R51/387/2, Physical Exercises File 1b 1933–1935, WAC BBC.

65 Asa Briggs, *The Golden Age of Wireless*, Oxford University Press, London, 1965.

66 ED file 136/91 Publicity, Publicity and Propaganda Sub-committee, May–September 1938 programme plans, The National Archives, London.

67 Paul Donovan, 'Quigley, Janet Muriel Alexander (1902–1987)', *Oxford Dictionary of National Biography*, Oxford University Press, first published 2004; online edn, January 2008. Quigley had moved from the Empire Marketing Board to the BBC in 1930, first working in the Foreign Department and then in Talks. Like Phyllis Colson, she suffered life-long debility – 'a pronounced limp'.

68 Janet Quigley, memo, 26 January 1937, R51/210/1, WAC BBC. Major Gem, Organiser of Physical Training for the London County Council, Phyllis Colson and Ronald Campbell, Director of Physical Training at the University of Edinburgh, were among the speakers.

69 Janet Quigley to RDK, 8 June 1939, R32/53, WAC BBC.

70 SC 139/1/1, WAC BBC.

71 Harry Hoggan, 'How the Exercises are Put Over', SC 139/1/1, WAC BBC. Agenda No.3, Correspondence SC 19/116, WAC BBC.

72 Extracts from Listeners' Letters Recently Received, SC 139/1/1, WAC BBC.

73 'Case for Extension of Broadcasts of Physical Exercises', SC 19/116, WAC BBC. Programmes had been running for four months, from 7.35 a.m. until 7.45 a.m., on Monday, Wednesday and Friday for men, and on Tuesday, Thursday and Saturday for women. At the beginning, 8 or 9 per cent listened, which at the end dropped to 3 or 4 per cent. Of 'those listening to the exercises some 40% were actually doing them. If this proportion remains valid, it means that half a million women and nearly as many men are still doing the exercises.'

74 Memo 4 July 1940, Press Officer to Editor Radio Times, 4 July 1940, SC 139/1/1 Physical Training Publicity, WAC BBC.

75 'Physical Exercises', Listener Research Report, 21 May 1941, SC 139/1/1, WAC BBC. 'From time to time listeners to Physical Exercises, interviewed in the course of the Continuous Survey of Listening, have been asked whether they actually did the exercises or merely listened to them.' Over 17 months ... 51 per cent reported doing the exercises as well as listening (there was a low of 30 per cent in April 1941, a high of 51 per cent in March 1940); amongst women the range was 33–57 per cent (there was a high of 57 per cent in March 1940, a low of 33 per cent in June 1940). BBC research staff noted: 'All of these figures are quite probably rather inflated, for there will

always be a tendency for some people to say they do regularly do something which they think they ought to do.' Pressing the survey results further, Honorary Local Correspondents were asked to rank reasons why people who listened to exercises did not do them. Results showed marked class differences – especially on the proposition that 'People get sufficient exercise at their work' (working class = 61 per cent, middle class 36 per cent). 'People are not convinced that such exercises do them any good' (working class 18 per cent, middle class 32 per cent); more middle class people thought a reason for not doing the exercises was because the novelty of doing the exercises had worn off. For both middle and working class people, the major reason offered as to why people did not do the exercises was 'People lose so much sleep these days that they are in no mood to do exercises in the morning.' Conclusions reached by the BBC Listener Research Department were prefaced by caution that the reasons people give are not always the actual reasons why people do, or do not do things. 'A certain amount of rationalization must always be reckoned with.' 'But these answers do show that propaganda to encourage more people to join in the Physical Exercises would be up against a very widespread feeling among working class listeners that they had no need for broadcast physical exercises, and a general desire in all classes to get as much sleep as possible while it is possible. The one line in which propaganda might be effective would be in countering the loss of interest which arises simply because the novelty has worn off.'

76 'King and Queen at the Festival of Youth', newsreel, <www.britishpathe.com>. The Festival was also a fund-raising event for the King George V Jubilee Trust: Zweiniger-Bargielowska, *Managing the Body*, chapter 7.

77 *The Times*, 28 October 1937, p.13, col.b. The four films were *Strength and Beauty: Our Normal Day, Healthy Holidays, Family Fitness* and *Pennies for Health*. They are listed on the BFI database, directed by Donald Carter and narrated by E. V. Emmett. They were made to be screened as part of commercial cinema viewings and by local area committees, and distributed through various means including 'travelling cinema vans': NFC, *The National Fitness Campaign*, p.7.

78 *The Times*, 28 October 1937, p.13, col.b.

79 *Health of the Nation*, 1937, 'produced in co-operation with the Ministry of Health and the Board of Education'. See the report of the first screening on Monday 26 April in *Financial Times*, 27 April 1937, p.4. The Ministers of Education and Health were present along with most members of the NFC. 'It also deals with walking, swimming and gymnastics.' Jennifer Hargreaves, *Sporting Females: Critical Issues in the History and Sociology of Women's Sports*, Routledge, London, 1994, p.137.

80 The event was reported in *The Times* as the official opening of the operations of the National Advisory Council for Physical Training and Recreation. The event coincided with the conference of the Central Council for Health Education and was part of the launch of the Campaign for Wider Use of Health Services. Sir Kingsley Wood, Minister of Health, inaugurated the provincial campaign in connection with the new National Fitness Movement in Liverpool on 5 October 1937: *The Times*, 6 October 1937, p.11, col d.

81 Mariel Grant points to the confusion between fitness and health campaigns, with the government deliberately letting them merge, while offsetting the challenges of nutrition and 'closet conscription' by putting the two together. Healthy and fit bodies were easier – or cheaper – to deal with than sick ones: Grant, *Propaganda and the Role of the State*.

82 *The Times*, 30 September 1937, supplement.

83 Blacker to H. Brewer, 18 April 1932, quoted in Lucy Bland and Lesley Hall, 'Eugenics in Britain: The View from the Metropole', in Alison Bashford and Philippa Levine (eds), *Oxford Handbook of the History of Eugenics*, Oxford University Press, Oxford and New York, 2010, p.217.

84 'The Lord Mayor's Parade', November 1937, British Pathé newsreel footage, <www.britishpathe.com>.

85 Memo 21 October 1937, ED 136/91, The National Archives, London, notes that 'Fitness Wins' shall appear on the sweaters worn by the personnel of the NFC's exhibit in the Show – in white for the royal blue sweaters of the men, and in royal blue for the white sweaters of the women'.

86 *Evening Standard*, 9 November 1937, p.17. The Parade was widely reported, including in Wellington's *Evening Post*, where a photograph montage included the fitness groups and floats promoting Australian and New Zealand produce, 30 November 1937, p.9. The Lucas Tooth Institute was founded 1913. Sir Robert Lucas Tooth, the sole benefactor, gave £50,000 to start a Boys' Training Fund. 'In 1925 a new gymnasium was opened in Tooley Street, London, and courses were held from then onwards to qualify young men to become

instructors of physical training in boys' clubs and other youth organizations': McIntosh, *Physical Education*, p.211. See advertisement for bread in same issue, around p.11 under the heading 'Get fit – keep fit'; and the image of Miss Pamela Prior, professional champion ice skater of the world, 'To be fit is to be happy – Everyone should take part in the National Fitness Campaign.' 'All active sport demands a full store of energy. Amongst all foods, Bread stands supreme as the energy-provider and as the restorer of energy consumed.'

87 NFC Meeting, 21 February 1939, ED 113, The National Archives, London.

88 *The Times*, 13, 26 October, 10 November 1937. The text of the advertisement includes the invocation: 'The National Council of Physical Fitness, in their crusade for a healthier nation, need everybody's help. Do your part'. The more middlebrow *Radio Times*, 18 February 1938, p.33b, carries an advertisement for shoes for girls with the slogan 'National Foot Service' and in the background 'Fitness Wins': 'Fitness begins in the feet. Or we might repeat our slogan for the National Health Campaign – "Keep Fit – Keep Feet" in Start-rite Shoes. The children of a Fitter Britain will walk more, run more, jump more. And children with foot defects will get left behind.'

89 *Radio Times*, 18 February 1938, p.33b.

90 *Keep Fit*, 1937, directed by Anthony Kimmins, produced by Basil Dean, production company ATP, see <www.screenonline.org.uk/film/id/450755/index.html>, accessed 11 October 2010. The film synopsis on the George Formby website is as follows: 'Weedy barber joins Keep Fit campaign to impress pretty manicurist. He triumphs over muscular, preening rival in the boxing ring. The League of Health and Beauty was currently popular when the film was made': <www.georgeformby.co.uk/films/fit/report.htm>, accessed 11 October 2010. George Formby, 1904–61.

91 King George VI speech launching the NFC campaign, London, 17 February 1938, ICL 0067783 (BBC), British Library, Sound Archive (AA 1629). See Sarah Bradford, *The Reluctant King: The Life and Reign of George VI 1895–1952*, St Martin's Press, New York, 1989; and Denis Judd, *King George VI: 1895–1952*, Michael Joseph, London, 1982. George VI as the Duke of York already had strong associations with youth and leisure, such as the Duke of York's Camp, 1921; Patron of the Playing Fields Association; in the George V Jubilee Trust; and as patron in 1936 of the CCRPT. While he may not have had the sporty image of his golf-loving brother the Prince of Wales, he had a strong record as a supporter of welfare-oriented recreation, especially for youth. See Frank Prochaska, *Royal Bounty: The Making of a Welfare Monarchy*, Yale University Press, New Haven and London, 1995.

92 *Radio Times*, 11 February 1938, vol.58, no.750. On the cover the King is featured in full dress uniform. Inside, in the programme details, p.62, a further photograph of King George is featured, this time in casual attire – shorts, jersey, open-neck shirt – with a caption that reads, in part, 'In this picture, taken last year, His Majesty is seen enjoying the open-air life of the boys' camp he founded when he was Duke of York.'

93 HO 144/21135, The National Archives, London.

94 Press release, 'No Compulsion', 18 February 1938, ED 136/91, The National Archives, London.

95 ED 136/91, The National Archives, London. The April and May posters were produced in black and white, the June ones in full colour. They were produced and distributed by the Central Council for Health Education, 1 Thornhaugh St, Russell Square, and designed to be placed on frames formerly used by Empire Marketing Board. Edward Bawden was the likely poster artist.

The sets were developed for monthly release beginning in April 1937. Around the simple inducement 'Get Fit – Keep Fit', the series began with the foundation 'Obey the Laws of Health' (washing, eating plain food slowly and drinking plenty of water, exercise in fresh air and breathe through the nose), stepping up to more active depictions of exercise for May with a series of graphic figures playing sports under the sub-banner 'England expects every man or woman to be healthy and fit', and culminating with June's three large poster images in full colour under the heading 'National Fitness Campaign' featuring a young man and woman in everyday settings: the woman in a street ('Exercise every day – walk to work'), the man on a bicycle in the outdoors ('Exercise every week – join a club'), and the man and woman together hiking ('Enjoyment all the year round'). Hiking is depicted as an appealing activity through the suggestion of mixed sex sociability.

96 *National Fitness – The First Steps*, 25pp, HMSO, London, 1937; *In Work or Play Fitness Wins – Twenty-four Ways of Keeping Fit*, 65pp, HMSO, London, 1938: ED 136/91, The National Archives, London. The booklets were produced by the NFC, but did carry some advertising

- including from HMV records 'His Master's Voice for Brain Fitness', Ordnance Maps from Ordnance Survey, and Wright's Coal Tar Soap.

97 June 1938 memo, ED 136/91, The National Archives, London.

98 Victoria de Grazia, *The Culture of Consent: Mass Organization of Leisure in Fascist Italy*, Cambridge University Press, 1981.

99 Janet Quigley Memo, 26 January 1937, R51/210/1, Talks Health File 1a 1932-8, WAC BBC. And interview notes 27 July 1937 NFC/BBC, p.2: 'Some discussion took place as to the form of talks in which the subjects they had mentioned should be handled, and it was readily agreed that it would be quite possible to sicken the public of the whole subject unless care were taken to vary the form of presentment and to employ entertaining speakers.'

100 NFC, *The National Fitness Campaign*, p.5.

101 Ibid.

102 *Sunday Pictorial*, 21 November 1937, p.2.

103 Ibid. The article reports a number of fatalities from the outbreak.

104 Stephen G. Jones, *Workers at Play: A Social and Economic History of Leisure, 1918-1939*, Routledge, London, 1986; and 'State Intervention in Sport Between the Wars'.

105 ED 136/91. These were some of several applications received. Press release headed 'Early Morning Broadcasts'. Sixth meeting of the NFC held 14 December 1937, The National Archives, London.

106 There were 470 applications noted as having been received by June 1938: NFC Meeting minutes, 28 June 1938, ED 113/48, The National Archives, London. See also NFC, *The National Fitness Campaign*.

107 See Thierry Terret, 'Hygienization: Civic Baths and Body Cleanliness in Late Nineteenth Century France', *International Journal of the History of Sport*, 10, 3 (December 1993), pp.396-408; Rachel Winterton and Claire Parker, '*A Utilitarian Pursuit: Swimming Education in Nineteenth-Century Australia and England*', *International Journal for the History of Sport*, 26, 14 (November 2009), pp.2106-26; Claire Parker, 'An Urban Historical Perspective: Swimming a Recreational and Competitive Pursuit 1840 to 1914', PhD thesis, University of Stirling, 2003; Claire Langhamer, *Women's Leisure in England 1920-1960*, Manchester University Press, 2000; Janet Smith, *Liquid Assets: The Lidos and Open Air Swimming Pools of Britain*, English Heritage/Malavan Media, London, 2005. The Exeter Pool, designed 1937, opened 1941, was one of few

projects that was seen through to completion.

108 ED 113, The National Archives, London. Marjorie Pollard, 1899-1982, United Women's Team Games Board formed 1935: see Hargreaves, *Sporting Females*, pp.137ff. Charles Tugwell was the first organiser appointed under the NFC. Such pay differentials were not out of sync with differentials in male/female pay in the public service at the time.

109 Minutes of NFC meeting, 28 June 1938, ED 113/48. And see list of organisers and other grants in ED 136/91, The National Archives, London.

110 *The Times*, 20 May 1938, p.13 col.d. Minutes of NFC meetings, ED 113/48, The National Archives, London.

111 ED 113/39, The National Archives, London.

112 David Matless, '"The Art of Right Living": Landscape and Citizenship, 1918-1939', in Steve Pile and Nigel Thrift (eds), *Mapping the Subject: Geographies of Cultural Transformation*, Routledge, London, 1995, pp.111-13.

113 ED 113/60, and NFC Publicity file, The National Archives, London.

114 NFC minutes, ED 113/48, The National Archives, London. See also John Pemberton, 'The Boyd Orr Survey of the Nutrition of Children in Great Britain 1937-9', *History Workshop Journal*, 50 (Autumn 2000), pp.205-29; Norman Baker, 'Going to the Dogs: Hostility to Greyhound Racing in Britain: Puritanism, Socialism and Pragmatism', *Journal of Sport History*, 23, 2 (Summer 1996), pp.97-119.

115 'Excerpts from Gwen Pemberton's Diaries 1937-1939', *History Workshop Journal*, 50 (Autumn 2000), p.222.

116 King George VI's speech at the opening of the Glasgow Empire Exhibition, 3 May 1938, Sound Archive, British Library. The speech began with the declaration that 'The Exhibition is an Empire undertaking, but we do well to remember that it owes its origins and to a great extent, its execution, to the people of Scotland. It is a significant fact that the plans were being prepared at a time when this country was still under the cloud of a long industrial depression.'

117 *Scotland for Fitness*, directed by Brian Salt, G. B. Instructional Films, 1938, Scottish Screen Archive, National Library of Scotland. Initial shots pan over posters reading 'Make time to play, don't grow old before your day.'

118 Callum G. Brown, *The Death of Christian Britain: Understanding Secularisation, 1800-2000,* Routledge, London and New York, 2000; Brown, 'Sport and the Scottish Office

in the 20th Century: The Control of a Social Problem'; Brown, 'Sport and the Scottish Office in the 20ᵗʰ Century: The Promotion of a Social and Gender Policy'; Macrae, '"Scotland for Fitness"'. Macrae suggests that the Scottish campaign was less wide-ranging in the activities it made available to women than was the national fitness campaign in England. See also Fiona Skillen, 'Women and Sport in Interwar Scotland', PhD thesis, University of Glasgow, 2008 (this work was identified but has not been read by the author).

119 Major de Roemer to *The Times*, 4 August 1938, p.11, col f. See also reply by Captain Ellis (6 August), and comment by Roy Finlay (9 August). See also critical letter, *The Times* 1 August 1938.

120 *The Times*, 6 August 1938, p.11. The leader of the same day was sympathetic to Ellis.

121 See *Sport in Industry*, 1, 4 (September 1938). In the House of Commons Mr Hepworth asked the Parliamentary Secretary of the Board of Education whether he was satisfied with the present progress of the national fitness campaign: *The Times*, 20 May 1938, p.13. A perception that the campaign had faltered was also detected beyond Britain. In Sydney, C. E. W. Bean, who was a leading advocate of the local push for a government-led fitness campaign, wrote at length to another supporter, Dr J. H. L. Cumpston, Director-General of Health, on 6 June 1938 noting the lack of progress made in England. He concluded 'we hear (and the press confirms it) that their scheme has fallen very flat': Bean to Cumpston, 6 June 1938, p.2, A4135, State Records New South Wales (Sydney).

122 There were several points of complaint: grant applications were taking too long to be heard, money was taking too long to get into the hands of those eager to use it, applications were far outrunning the funds available, and those funds that had been distributed were not making enough of a difference. The tide of support with which the campaign started turned, by the late summer of 1938, to an undertow of disappointment and criticism. By then it was also true that the seriousness of the international situation was sharpening the context in which such initiatives were viewed. People were polarised about the need for preparation for war, and there was widespread distaste for anything smacking of militarism.

123 *British Medical Journal*, 13 May 1938, p.1000a.

124 CAB 23/96, p.23, The National Archives, London.

125 CAB 23/96, The National Archives, London.

This allocation was just for the capital expenditure aspect of NFC work: £341,000 had been allocated to swimming baths; £148,000 to playing fields; and £274,000 to social and recreational centres.

126 With an overwhelming demand for grant money – over £6 million in capital costs alone – applied for by the end of December 1938 (NFC, 1939, p.12), the country *had* responded to the call to do more about fitness.

127 Tony Mason described the government's fitness campaign as 'feeble': Tony Mason, '"Hunger ... is a Very Good Thing": Britain in the 1930s', in Nick Tiratsoo (ed.), *From Blitz to Blair: A New History of Britain Since 1939*, Phoenix, London, 1997, p.7. Holt and Mason, *Sport in Britain Since 1945*; Huggins and Williams, *Sport and the English*; McKibbin, *Classes and Cultures*, p.380; Zweiniger-Bargielowska, *Managing the Body*.

128 *The Times*, 6 August 1938, p.11.

129 Noel Curtis-Bennett and W. W. Wakefield had attended an earlier meeting of the World Congress in Rome in June 1938 as an official delegation: ED 136/91, The National Archives, London. In a 16 June 1938 press release from the NFC, Curtis-Bennett spoke about the development of physical recreation facilities in England and Wales; and Wakefield on 'The problem of leisure time occupation'. The objects of the conference were described as 'to illustrate the measures adopted in the various countries by public and private institutions with the aim of securing a contented and prosperous existence for the masses, strengthening at the same time the spirit of collaboration and goodwill among the peoples': ED 136/91. See also FO 395/621 British Council P 2421, 8 August 1938, Publicity Abroad for the National Fitness Councils for England and Scotland. Also ED 124/67, The National Archives, London.

130 The NFC for England and Wales were hosts to the Congress: see 'Visit of International Advisory Committee to London, February 1939', typescript, p.1, British Library Cup.1253.c.23.

131 Ley was a major figure in the Reich by the mid-to-late 1930s, and head of the labour organisation and the Kraft durch Freude. The latter named one of its especially commissioned cruise ships after him: see Shelley Baronowski, 'A Family Vacation for Workers: The Strength through Joy Resort at Prora', *German History*, 25, 4 (2007), pp.539–59.

132 As reported in Wellington, New Zealand's,

Evening Post, 28 March 1939, p.5. See also files, ED 136/93, The National Archives, London. 'Visit of International Advisory Committee to London, February 1939', British Library Cup.1253.c.23. The patron of the World Congress in Hamburg in 1936 was Rudolf Hess, then Reichminister and Deputy of the Fuhrer: *Report on the World Congress for Leisure Time and Recreation/Hamburg July 1936*, Hanseatische Verlagsanstalt, Hamburg, [1937], 732pp, British Library X.520/22711.

133 ED 136/93, The National Archives, London.

134 McIntosh, *Physical Education*, pp.234–5. *The Times*, 20 July 1939, p.13; 21 July, p.13; 22 July, p.16; 24 July, p.11; 27 July, p.15; *The Scotsman*, 21 July 1939, p.10; 24 July 1939, p.10; *The Observer*, 23 July 1939, p.19; *New York Times*, 6 August 1939. Phyllis Spafford of the Ling Assn was a member of NFC.

135 ED 113, The National Archives, London.

136 H. B. Jenkins, NFC to Mrs M. Cornell, 4 September 1939, ED 113/80, The National Archives, London.

137 Evans, *Service to Sport*, p.74.

138 ED 124/67, CCRPT's bid for continuance dated 16 October 1939 under the heading National Youth Council, The National Archives, London. See also McIntosh, *Physical Education*; Evans, *Service to Sport*, p.47 and chapter 5.

139 McIntosh attributes this to unsavoury associations of 'physical training': McIntosh, *Physical Education*, pp.229–30.

140 Melanie Oppenheimer and Nicholas Deakin (eds), *Beveridge and Voluntary Action in Britain and the Wider British World,* Manchester University Press, 2010.

141 William Beveridge, *Voluntary Action: A Report on Methods of Social Advance*, Allen & Unwin, London, 1948, p.286.

142 McKibbin, *Classes and Cultures*, chapter 9.

143 Baker, 'Going to the Dogs'.

144 Beveridge, *Voluntary Action*, p.286. I am grateful to Margaret Tennant for reminding me of this work. See also W. and J. Beveridge, *On and Off the Platform: Under the Southern Cross*, Hicks, Smith & Wright, Wellington and Melbourne, 1949; and Jose Harris, 'Voluntarism, the State, and Public–Private Partnerships in Beveridge's Social Thought', in Oppenheimer and Deakin (eds), *Beveridge*, pp.9–20, where it is noted that some staff were more critical of football pools and so on (p.17).

145 NBKR 6/15/1, 6/15/2, Noel Baker Papers, Churchill Archive, Churchill College, Cambridge.

146 'The Sporting Spirit', *Tribune*, 14 December 1945, and subsequent correspondence. The comment was first made at the time of a brief and fractious tour of England by the Soviet Dynamo football team but was also a comment on the events of the 1920s and 30s.

147 The Berlin airlift (the supply of necessities to residents of West Berlin by the United States, Britain and France in the face of the Soviet Union's blockade of the city from June 1948 to May 1949) ran from 24 June 1948 until 12 May 1949.

148 *Britain in the World of Sport: An Examination of the Factors Involved in Participation in Competitive International Sport*, Prepared and assembled by the Physical Education Department, University of Birmingham, published by Physical Education Association of Great Britain and Northern Ireland, Birmingham, 1956. The Wolfenden Committee on Sport, *Sport and the Community*, CCPR, London, 1960.

149 Denis Howell, 1923–1998. Minister of Sport 1964–70, 1974–79, Labour MP, Birmingham.

150 Established by Royal Charter on 19 September 1996, the new organisations became fully operational on 1 January 1997. See <www.uksport.gov.uk> and <www.sportengland.org>. Both bodies are responsible to the Department of Culture, Media and Sport. In 2010 UK Sport received around £100 million per year in public funds 'to lead sport in the UK to world-class success' (UK Sport's Mission). A key feature of the bid to the International Olympic Committee for hosting rights for the 2012 London Olympics was based on the claim that development of the Olympic amenities would lead to social development of an impoverished part of the city.

Chapter 2: Leisure and Democracy

1 W. F. Ingram, 'Panorama of the Playground: Physical Fitness and the "Daily Dozen"', *New Zealand Railways Magazine*, 11, 10 (January 1937), p.54.

2 Roger Robinson. 'Lovelock, John Edward', from the *Dictionary of New Zealand Biography* (DNZB), Te Ara – the Encyclopaedia of New Zealand, updated 1 September 2010, <http://www.teara.govt.nz/en/biographies/4l14/1>; Roger Robinson, 'Lovelock, John Edward (1910–1949)', *Oxford Dictionary of National Biography* (ODNB), Oxford University Press, 2004; online edn, January 2008; David Colquhoun (ed.), *As if Running on Air: The Journals of Jack Lovelock*, Craig Potton Publishing, Nelson, 2008. See also Lovelock mentioned as 'one of our most enthusiastic

supporters': Margaret Morris, *My Life in Movement*, Peter Owen, London, 1969, p.80.

3   Barry Gustafson, 'Parry, William Edward', from the *Dictionary of New Zealand Biography*, Te Ara – the Encyclopedia of New Zealand, updated 1 September 2010, <http://www.teara. govt.nz/en/biographies/3p12/1>. See also Stanley Roche, *The Red and the Gold*, Oxford University Press, Wellington, 1982, pp.157–60; Personal communication Monique Ciochetto (Parry's great-granddaughter) to author, 12 September 2011 (telephone conversation, and email); Philip Rainer, 'Company Town: An Industrial History of the Waihi Gold Mining Company Limited, 1887–1912', MA thesis, University of Auckland, 1976.

4   Physical Welfare and Recreation Act 1937, *New Zealand Statutes*, 1937.

5   Ken Alexander, 'Two World's Records for New Zealand', cover cartoon, *New Zealand Free Lance*, 19 August 1936.

6   W.E.Parry, Minister of Internal Affairs, 'The Old and New Order of Things', 17 November 1938, qMS-1629, p.1, ATL.

7   Rachel Barrowman, 'Heenan, Joseph, 1888–1951', from the *Dictionary of New Zealand Biography*, Te Ara – the Encyclopedia of New Zealand, updated 1 September 2010, <http://www.teara.govt.nz/en/biographies/4h24/1>. Scholefield was not the only librarian to have problems with readers with interests in sport. At the Timaru Public Library (established 1909), long-serving librarian Miss Culverwell was frequently having to report the theft of the sporting paper *The Referee* from the newsroom. The Bernarr Macfadden magazine *Physical Culture* and even the more upmarket *Ladies Field* were also attractive targets for lighthanded readers: see Timaru Library monthly reports, 8 December 1920, 11 April 1921, 14 November 1921, 18 November 1927, Timaru Public Library. I am indebted to Susann Liebich for these references. The demand for more sport in the popular press is also evident in the increased coverage in the populist weekly *The Truth* under editor Fred Earle. In his 8 years as sports editor, sports coverage doubled and news coverage halved. Tellingly, the scope of sports coverage also changed, shifting away from the traditional 'worker' sports of racing, boxing and billiards to encompass rugby union, golf, hockey, soccer and cricket. Dentist Bernard Freyberg contributed a swimming column, probably under the epithet 'Plunge' in the years before his military career and later appointment as Governor-General, Redmer Yska, *Truth. The Rise and Fall of the People's Paper*, Craig Potton Publishing, Nelson, 2010, pp.70–73.

8   W.H.Oliver, 'The Awakening Imagination', in W.H.Oliver with B.R.Williams (eds), *The Oxford History of New Zealand*, Oxford University Press, Wellington, 1981; Rachel Barrowman, *A Popular Vision: The Arts and the Left in New Zealand 1930–1950*, Victoria University Press, Wellington, 1991; Michael Bassett, *The Mother of all Departments: The History of the Department of Internal Affairs*, Auckland University Press in association with the Historical Branch, Department of Internal Affairs, Auckland and Wellington, 1997; Chris Hilliard, *The Bookmen's Dominion*, Auckland University Press, 2006; Caroline Daley, *Leisure and Pleasure: Reshaping and Revealing the New Zealand Body*, Auckland University Press, 2003.

9   R.A.Stothart, 'The Education of New Zealand Recreation Workers', MA thesis, Victoria University of Wellington, 1977; R.A.Stothart, 'Pegs in the Ground: Landmarks in the History of New Zealand Physical Education', *Journal of Physical Education New Zealand*, 33, 2 (September 2000), pp.5–15; Hugh D. Buchanan, 'A Critical Analysis of the 1937 Physical Welfare and Recreation Act and of Government Involvement in Recreation and Sport, 1937–1957', MA (Applied) thesis, Victoria University of Wellington, 1978; Janet Alexander, 'Recreation: An Inappropriate Concept for Legislation?: An Examination of Two Attempts at Legislating for Recreation in New Zealand: the Physical Welfare and Recreation Act 1937, and the Recreation and Sport Act 1973', MPP research paper, Victoria University of Wellington, 1981; Daley, *Leisure and Pleasure*; Pip Lynch, 'The Origins of Outdoor Recreation in New Zealand: Progressive Liberalism and Post-War Rejuvenation, 1935–1965', *New Zealand Physical Educator*, 36, 1 (May 2003), pp.63–81.

10   The 1935 ILO Convention 47 aimed for a forty-eight-hour week in industry and a longer-term commitment to a forty-hour week.

11   The eight-hour day was a precept based on a principle laid down by British socialist Robert Owen.

12   Martin, *Holding the Balance*, pp.196–202, 227–8. See also Juliet B. Schor, *The Overworked American: The Unexpected Decline of Leisure*, Basic Books, New York, 1991.

13   Martin, *Holding the Balance*, pp.196–202, 227–8. Annual Holidays Amendment Act 1945, *New Zealand Statutes*, 1945. See also 'The 1950s', www.nzhistory.net.nz/culture/the-1950s.

14   *NZPD*, 26 October 1937 (1st reading, 2nd reading 15 November 1937, *NZPD*, vol.249, p.414f).

15   Annual Report, Department of Internal Affairs, *AJHR*, 1938, H-22, p.4.

16   Heenan quoted by Buchanan, 'A Critical Analysis', p.129. Heenan was to describe 'an elasticity in the machinery of our Department to get things done with the minimum of formality'.

17   *Dominion*, 19 August 1937, editorial, p.10.

18   'Council of Sport', *Dominion*, 5 March 1937, p.12. The quotation continues: 'with the co-operation of all the different sports bodies and the co-ordination of all their activities'.

19   *Dominion*, 5 March 1937, p.12. See also 'Physical Welfare and Recreation', Statement by the Hon W. E. Parry, Minister of Internal Affairs', *AJHR*, 1944, H-22B.

20   Luckie's own efforts, over the long term, were later acknowledged when a major sports ground was named in his honour: Martin Luckie Park, Berhampore, Wellington, 1950.

21   Dr G. F. V. (Eric) Anson (1892–1969) was a long-standing member of the Hutt Valley Gun Club, and prominent member of the Hutt Valley and medical communities: *Evening Post*, 6 July 1931, p.14; obituary Basil R. Hutchinson, 'Eric Anson, anaesthetist', *New Zealand Medical Journal*, 121, 1286 (28 November 2008), at <www.nzma.org.nz>.

22   *Dominion*, 5 March 1937, p.12. The subsequent meeting was postponed from June to August.

23   Reports of Census of Sport, *New Zealand Official Yearbook*, 1925, pp.761–3, *New Zealand Official Yearbook*, 1926, pp.823–6. Official survey of the major sporting organisations revealed that rugby had 40,000 players, all male, including 12,000 schoolboys, in 670 clubs; horse racing, 25,041; tennis 19,351; bowls 15,055; then cricket, golf and athletics.

24   *Dominion*, 1 October 1937, p.3.

25   *Dominion*, 2 October 1937, p.13.

26   Annual Report, Department of Internal Affairs, *AJHR*, 1938, H-22, p.4.

27   Membership of National Council, see Annual Report, Department of Internal Affairs, *AJHR*, 1939, H-22, p.12.

28   Elizabeth Hanson, *The Politics of Social Security: The 1938 Act and Some Later Developments*, Auckland University Press, 1980; Barry Gustafson, *From the Cradle to the Grave: A Biography of Michael Joseph Savage*, Penguin, Auckland, 1986. Extensive benefits were provided 'from cradle to grave', and free medical care – a measure described as 'applied Christianity' by its supporters, 'applied lunacy' to its minority of detractors.

29   IA 1 139/20, Archives New Zealand, Wellington.

Bach had been the gym instructor at Auckland Grammar School for eight years prior to his appointment to the Physical Welfare Branch: Kirstie Ross, *Going Bush: New Zealanders and Nature in the Twentieth Century*, Auckland University Press, 2008, p.88; *Evening Post*, 20 May 1939. Helen Black returned to Australia where she took up the position as Assistant Organiser with the South Australian Fitness Council in early 1944. She was to work in South Australia National Fitness for many years and was still there in the early 1960s: Albert E. Simpson, *The National Fitness Council of South Australia: A History, South Australia Department of Recreation and Sport*, Adelaide, 1986, pp.2–5, passim. See also Buchanan, 'A Critical Analysis', p.133, fn.16.

30   Sandra Coney, *Every Girl: A Social History of Women and the YWCA in Auckland*, YWCA, Auckland, 1986; Miriam Clark, '"Be fit and add something to the person": The Sport and Physical Recreation Programme of the Wellington YWCA 1918–1939', BA (Hons) research essay in History, Victoria University of Wellington, 1993; Clare Simpson, 'Social History of the Christchurch Young Women's Christian Association, 1883–1930', MA thesis, University of Canterbury, 1984; Clare Simpson, *The One Hundred Year History of the Christchurch Young Women's Christian Association, 1883–1983*, Christchurch YWCA, Christchurch, 1983.

31   L. G. McDonald to C. Ruxton Bach, 10 February 1939; Bach to McDonald, 24 February 1939, IA 139/27, Archives New Zealand, Wellington.

32   Helen Black to Under Secretary, 17 February 1941, IA 1 139/16/4, Archives New Zealand, Wellington. Black was commenting in the application form Adams had also filled out in 1939.

33   See the kind of systematic training and qualifications of those giving instruction at the 17–31 January 1939 YWCA summer school for a course in recreational leadership in Auckland: *Auckland Star*, 19 January 1939; and YWCA materials for the course from Auckland YWCA via Sandra Coney to author. The instructors included Mrs M. Morris, 'Late of the staff of Bedford Physical Training College, England'; Miss Jeanne Harmsworth, 'Graduate of the Australian College of Physical Education'; Miss Agnes Kennedy, 'Vice President of Auckland Y.W.C.A.'; Miss Sonia Revid, 'A Russian dancer who is a trained student of the Mary Wigman School of Dancing, Berlin, and who was lately attached to the practical work of the Melbourne University Physical Training Scheme'; and Miss Elsie Bennet, 'General

secretary of the Auckland Y.W.C.A.'. Sheila Fletcher, *Women First: The Female Tradition in English Physical Education, 1880–1980*, Athlone Press, London, 1984.

34 Annual Report, Department of Internal Affairs, *AJHR*, 1940, H-22, p.7, reported 221 District Committees in existence; *AJHR*, 1939, H-22, p.13, reported 160 local committees.

35 IA 1 139/32/115, Mackenzie Country (Fairlie); IA 1 139/32/124, and IA 1 139/21/129, Greytown, Archives New Zealand, Wellington. Annual Reports, Department of Internal Affairs, *AJHR*.

36 Daley, *Leisure and Pleasure*, chapter 7, especially pp.231–7. See also *Evening Post*, 18 February 1939, p.11 and 23 February 1939, p.17.

37 IA 1 139/43 Publicity; and IA 1 139/64 Recreation Week, IA files Fitness and Recreation Weeks, Archives New Zealand, Wellington.

38 Physical Welfare Department, *Keep Fit by Morning Exercises: Exercises Broadcast by YA Stations at 7 a.m*, Wellington, 1939; T. J. Kirk-Burnand, composed and arranged, *Musical Tunes (in Simple Form): Suitable for Physical Exercises*, Physical Welfare and Recreation Branch, Department of Internal Affairs, Wellington, 1939.

39 Ross, *Going Bush*; Kirstie Ross, '"Schooled by Nature": Pakeha Tramping Between the Wars', *New Zealand Journal of History*, 35, 1 (2002), pp.51–65; Mark Pickering, *Huts*, Canterbury University Press, Christchurch, 2010, pp.243–8; John Pascoe, *Land Uplifted High*, Whitcombe & Tombs, Christchurch, 1952, pp.91–96.

40 IA 1 139/58 Group Travel, Physical Welfare Branch, Department of Internal Affairs, Archives New Zealand, Wellington. The purpose of the Group Travel scheme was described as 'to assure low-cost touring for folk of moderate means': Annual Report, Department of Internal Affairs, *AJHR*, 1947, H-22, p.8, IA 1 139/58 Group Travel Scheme, Archives New Zealand, Wellington. See also Daley, *Leisure and Pleasure*, pp.247–8; Ross, 'Signs of Landing'.

41 IA 1 139/107, Sport – Phys Ed in Australia – Visit of Miss Black – Report, Physical Welfare Branch, Archives New Zealand, Wellington.

42 Brochure and further details at IA 62/4/38, Interhouse Girls Display, Centennial Exhibition, Physical Welfare Branch, Archives New Zealand, Wellington.

43 Ibid.

44 Dennis McEldowney, 'Smithells, Philip Ashton 1910-1977', from the *Dictionary of New Zealand Biography* (DNZB), Te Ara – the Encyclopaedia of New Zealand, updated 1 September 2010, <http://www.teara. govt.nz/en/biographies/5s31/1>; Smithells Papers, ARC-0494, Hocken Library, Dunedin. R. E. Roper was the author of *Movement and Thought*, Blackie, London, 1938. See also Bruce Ross, 'Thinking the Physical: PAS, PE & Power', *Journal of Physical Education New Zealand*, 29, 4 (Summer 1996), pp.5–8 and Part II, 30, 1 (Autumn 1997), pp.3–6.

45 Rona Stephenson (Bailey), 24 December 1914-7 September 2005. Jackie Matthews, Introduction, 'A Dissenting New Zealand: She'll Never Last the Distance', and Rona Bailey, Comments, Trade Union History Project seminar, Wellington, 4 December 1993 (author's notes from seminar). A taped copy of some of the seminar proceedings is held in the Oral History Centre, ATL. See also Jan Bolwell, 'Memorial Celebration for the Life of Rona Bailey', *DANZ Quarterly*, 2 (December 2005), pp.10–11; Rona Bailey Papers, MS-Group-0901, ATL; *Dominion Post*, 29 September 2005, B7 (obituary).

46 Barrowman, *A Popular Vision*, pp.193–8.

47 *Evening Post*, 5 July 1943, p.3. When Smithells sent Rona Bailey a copy of his publication, *The Atlantic Gap* (Dunedin, 1948), he inscribed it with 'Rona, who understands, Philip, 1.5.48'. Bob Stothart, 'Obituary: Olive Smithells, 1920–2007', *New Zealand Physical Educator*, August 2007 (online source, no pagination). Smithells v Smithells, AAOM, W3265, d.1167/1943, Archives New Zealand, Wellington. My thanks to Hayley Brown for this last reference.

48 Barrowman, *A Popular Vision*.

49 Bolwell, 'Memorial Celebration'; *Dance of the Instant: The New Dance Group Wellington 1945-1947*, documentary film, produced and directed by Shirley Horrocks, Point of View Productions, Auckland, 2008. Other members of the New Dance Group were Joy Parkin, Helen Robinson (Leckie), Angela Gennings, Doff Gentry. Smithells was a non-dancing member of the group.

50 Ian McGibbon, *New Zealand and the Second World War*, Hodder Moa Beckett, Auckland, 2004; Ian McGibbon with assistance of Paul Goldstone (eds), *Oxford Companion to New Zealand Military History*, Oxford University Press, Auckland, 2000.

51 Deborah Montgomerie, *The Women's War: New Zealand Women 1939–45*, Auckland University Press, 2001.

52 See, for example, Helen Black travelling to West Coast to conduct keep-fit sessions for WWSA members: *Evening Post*, 21 April 1942, p.8.

53 *Evening Post*, 24 January 1942, p.8. See also 'Physical Fitness Wins', *Public Service Journal*, February 1942, pp.90–92.

54 Gladys Gebbie was educated at Auckland Girls' Grammar School, secretary of the Auckland Women's Cricket Association, sportswoman, Assistant Physical Director YWCA Auckland, and physical education teacher at Avonside Girls' High School before being appointed physical welfare officer. See the announcement of her and Jack Bonham's appointments as physical welfare officers in Auckland: *Auckland Star*, 4 May 1940; and photographs of the two of them in Gladys Gebbie, May 1940, IA 1 139/43, Archives New Zealand, Wellington.

55 Press report, June 1943, IA 139/7/7 Sport – Swimming-Splash Club – Auckland, Physical Welfare Branch, Archives New Zealand, Wellington.

56 Noeline Thomson to author, March 1997. Scripts for radio talks are included in Noeline Thomson Papers, MS-Papers-8312, ATL.

57 Clark, '"Be fit and add something to the person"'; YWCA Papers, MS-Group-0233, ATL; Tup Lang, 'Gisa Taglicht, 1898–1961', Charlotte Macdonald, Merimeri Penfold, Bridget Williams (eds), *The Book of New Zealand Women Ko Kui Ma Te Kaupapa*, Bridget Williams Books, Wellington, 1991, pp.648–650.

58 *Evening Post*, 5 November 1938, p.18.

59 Fiona Hall, 'New Zealand Women's Bowling Association 1948–', in Anne Else (ed.), *Women Together: A History of Women's Organisations in New Zealand: Ngā Rōpū Wāhine o Te Motu*, Daphne Brassell Associates Press/Historical Branch, Department of Internal Affairs, Wellington, 1993, pp.440–2; Noeline Thomson to author, 1992 and 31 March 1997; Noeline Thomson, in *NZ Bowler*, February/March 1997, p.41. Annual Report, Department of Internal Affairs, *AJHR,*1946, H-22, p.7, notes 'This is the Department's policy in promoting recreation in New Zealand by assisting in the establishment of new associations and new activities until such time as they are able to carry on without further assistance from the Department. In this way the New Zealand Women's Indoor Basketball Association has been established with departmental assistance, and is now carrying on as a national sporting association.'

60 *Evening Post*, 24 September 1941, p.4.

61 IA 1 139/104/25, Mercer Refreshment Rooms, Physical Welfare Branch, Archives New Zealand, Wellington. The timing of Parry's visit to Mercer is worth noting. The general election, delayed from 1941, was to be held in October 1943. There had been some tension around the coalmines in the area over regulation of wages in wartime; and more generally over the so-called furlough revolt and the commitment of troops to the Pacific as opposed to Europe. As a former miners' leader, Parry was sent to this district to campaign.

62 Charlotte Macdonald et al., 'New Zealand Marching Association', in Else (ed.), *Women Together*, pp.437–9; Charlotte Macdonald, 'Putting Bodies on the Line: Marching Spaces in Cold War Culture', in Patricia Vertinsky and John Bale (eds), *Sites of Sport: Space, Place, Experience,* Routledge, London, 2004, pp.85–100; Charlotte Macdonald, 'Moving in Unison, Dressing in Uniform: Stepping Out in Style with Marching Teams', in Bronwyn Labrum, Fiona McKergow and Stephanie Gibson (eds), *Looking Flash: Clothing in Aotearoa New Zealand*, Auckland University Press, 2007, pp.186–205; Charlotte Macdonald, 'Marching Teams and Modern Girls: Bodies and Culture in Interwar New Zealand', in Paula Birnbaum and Anna Novakov (eds), *Essays on Women's Artistic and Cultural Contributions 1919–1939: Expanded Social Roles for the New Woman Following the First World War*, Edwin Mellen Press, Lewiston, 2009, pp.23–36; Miriam Clark, '"Be fit and add something to the person": The Sport and Physical Recreation Programme of the Wellington YWCA 1918–1939', BA (Hons) research essay in History, Victoria University of Wellington, 1993.

63 Audrey Paine, 'Dunedin's Blair Atholl Marching Team: 1952 Trip: United Kingdom and Australia', *New Zealand Memories*, 88 (February–March 2011), pp.62–65. The involvement of the Central Council for Physical Recreation in the UK illustrates the continued linkage with Great Britain post-1945.

64 Tanja Bueltmann, '"Brither Scots shoulder tae shoulder": Ethnic Identity, Culture and Associationism among the Scots in New Zealand to 1930', PhD thesis, Victoria University of Wellington, 2008.

65 'Physical Welfare and Recreation', Statement by the Hon W. E. Parry, Minister of Internal Affairs, *AJHR*, 1944, H-22B, p.2

66 'Recreation Centre', *Weekly* Review, 432, National Film Unit, 1949 (documentary film); William L. Robertson, 'Lower Hutt Community Centres: Final Statement', 1950 (Hutt City Libraries online text); Ben Schrader, 'A Brave New World? Ideal Versus Reality in Post-war Naenae', *New Zealand Journal of History*, 30, 1 (April 1996), pp.61–79.

67 Annual Report, Department of Internal Affairs, *AJHR*, 1947, H-22, p.8.

68 M. P. K. Sorrenson, 'Ngata, Apirana Turupa, 1874–1950', from the *Dictionary of New Zealand Biography*, Te Ara – the Encyclopedia of New Zealand, updated 1 September 2010, <http://www.teara.govt.nz/en/biographies/3n5/1>; Monty Soutar, *Nga Tama Toa: The Price of Citizenship*, David Bateman, Auckland, 2008. For broader discussion of this context, and powerful recent interpretations of this era, see Aroha Harris, 'Dancing With the State: Maori Creative Energy and Policies of Integration, 1945–67', PhD thesis, University of Auckland, 2007, and 'Concurrent Narratives of Maori and Integration in the 1950s and 60s', *Journal of New Zealand Studies*, 6/7 (October 2007/2008), pp.139–55; Melissa Williams, '"Back-home" and Home in the City: Māori Migrations from Panguru to Auckland, 1930–1970', PhD thesis, University of Auckland, 2010. See also Michael King, 'Between Two Worlds', and Ranginui Walker, 'Maori Since 1950', in G. W. Rice (ed.), *Oxford History of New Zealand*, rev. edn, Oxford University Press, Auckland, 1992.

69 IA 1 139/2/3 Scheme for Maori recreation – general file, Archives New Zealand, Wellington.

70 Memo to Under Secretary, Department of Maori Affairs, from Assistant Under Secretary Internal Affairs, 14 July 1948, IA 1 139/2/3, Archives New Zealand, Wellington. See IA 1 139/129/13 Recreational facilities – Ratana Pa, Archives New Zealand, Wellington.

71 Heard to Under Secretary, Internal Affairs 13 November 1951, IA 1 139/2/3, Archives New Zealand, Wellington.

72 R. Sheffield, Memo, Department of Internal Affairs, 7 November 1951, IA 1 139/2/3, Scheme for Maori Recreation – general file, Physical Welfare Branch, Archives New Zealand, Wellington: 'I have done considerable social work among the Maori people. Of the 36 social recreation clubs I have formed, the majority are in Maori settlements where no other form of organised recreation except Saturday sport existed .... I coached hockey and square dancing during the past winter and have coached cricket and softball. I also conducted a Learn to Swim Week at the Maori District High School at Te Kaha, and have been to several other Maori schools introducing square dancing to the teachers.'

73 Sheffield to Under Secretary, Internal Affairs, June 1949, IA 1 139/2/3, Archives New Zealand, Wellington.

74 Ibid.

75 Sheffield had been rather more proactive in the adjacent large but sparsely populated area of the Urewera. Travelling with the local Māori chaplain, James Irwin, he spent a week touring the area providing a detailed report on the recreational facilities in the district – from traditional settlements to the new timber towns of Murupara, Kaingaroa and Te Whaiti in the Minginui valley. His survey had a wide ambit, amounting to virtually a social survey, and was pointed in identifying the lack of provision in the timber areas then being opened up with major construction projects.

76 Charlotte Macdonald, 'Ways of Belonging: Sporting Spaces in New Zealand History', in Giselle Byrnes (ed.), *The New Oxford History of New Zealand*, Oxford University Press, Melbourne, 2009, p.283.

77 Harris, 'Dancing With the State', abstract.

78 Application of Philip A. Smithells, 12 December 1946, pp.1–2, Smithells Papers, MS 1001/9, ARC-0494, Hocken Library.

79 See the picture of Smithells playing 'Homai' with children at Ratana Pā in 1943, Smithells Papers, MS-1001/45, ARC-0494, Hocken Library reproduced in Bruce Ross, 'Thinking the Physical – PAS, PE & Power', Part I, *Journal of Physical Education New Zealand*, 29, 4 (Summer 1996), pp.5–8. Part II appeared in *Journal of Physical Education New Zealand*, 30, 1 (Autumn 1997), pp.3–6.

80 Smithells, in Ross, 'Thinking the Physical', p.1; Brian Sutton-Smith, 'The Meeting of Maori and European Cultures and its effects upon the Unorganized Games of Maori Children', *Journal of the Polynesian Society*, 60, 2 & 3 (September 1951), pp.92–107; *The Ambiguity of Play*, Harvard University Press, Cambridge, 1997; Brendan Hokowhitu, 'Physical Beings: Stereotypes, Sport and the "Physical Education" of New Zealand Maori', in J. A. Mangan and A. Ritchie (eds), *Culture, Sport, Society*, Frank Cass, London, 2004, pp.192–218.

81 Robert Chapman, 'From Labour to National', in Geoffrey Rice (ed.), *The Oxford History of New Zealand*, 2nd edn, Auckland, 1992, pp.351–84.

82 Bassett, *The Mother of all Departments*; Barrowman, 'Heenan', *DNZB*.

83 David Grant, *On a Roll: A History of Gambling and Lotteries in New Zealand*, Victoria University Press, Wellington, 1994.

84 Rona Bailey, summary cv in 2006-041-123 folder, MS-Group-0901, ATL.

85 IA 1 139 Physical Welfare Branch, Archives New Zealand, Wellington. Bassett, *The Mother of All Departments*, pp.160–1.

86 Annual reports, DIA. Buchanan, 'A Critical Analysis', p.85; Alexander, 'Recreation', p.39. Final traces disappeared when the Branch

was transformed into Youth Services in 1965. One of these last officers was Lance Cross, an important figure in New Zealand basketball, later a member of the International Olympic Committee: Ron Palenski, 'Cross, Cecil Lancelot Stewart – Biography', from the *Dictionary of New Zealand Biography*, Te Ara – the Encyclopedia of New Zealand, updated 1 September 2010, <http://www.TeAra.govt.nz/en/biographies/5c47/1>.

87 Macdonald, 'The Unbalanced Parallel', in Else (ed.), *Women Together*.

88 Macdonald, 'Ways of Belonging', p.285.

89 Such ideas were reinforced by William Beveridge's emphatic statement of where the state should not be involved: see William Beveridge, *Voluntary Action: A Report on Methods of Social Advance*, Allen & Unwin, London, 1948, chapter 1; and William and Janet Beveridge, *On and Off the Platform. Under the Southern Cross*, Hicks, Smith & Wright, Wellington, 1949. I am grateful to Margaret Tennant for bringing this source to my attention.

90 Trevor Richards, *Dancing on Our Bones*, Bridget Williams Books, Wellington, 1999.

91 Bassett, *Mother of all Departments*, p.161, citing an interview with Bryan Crompton, March 1996.

92 An MA (Applied) in recreation administration was created at Victoria University of Wellington at the request of the Council for Recreation and Sport in 1977, taught by academic staff based at the university gymnasium and, from 1989, in the Faculty of Arts: Rachael Barrowman, *Victoria University of Wellington 1899–1999: A History*, Victoria University Press, Wellington, 1999, p.251. See also Buchanan, 'A Critical Analysis'; Roderick J. Simmons, 'Joe Walding and Labour's Physical Welfare Ideal: The Establishment of the Ministry of Recreation and Sport 1972–5', MA thesis, Massey University, 1998.

93 Television was broadcast in New Zealand from 1960, and by 1969 around 70 per cent of households had a set. See Margaret Tennant, *The Fabric of Welfare: Voluntary Organisations, Government and Welfare in New Zealand, 1840–2005*, Bridget Williams Books, Wellington, 2007, Part 3; and Margaret Tennant, Mike O'Brien and Jackie Sanders, *The History of the Non-profit Sector in New Zealand*, Office for the Community and Voluntary Sector, Wellington, 2008; D. C. Pitt, 'The Joiners: Associations and Leisure in New Zealand', in S. D. Webb and J. Collette (eds), *New Zealand Society: Contemporary Perspectives*, John Wiley, Sydney, pp.157–62.

94 For more on the legacy of the fresh air and sunlight campaigns and enthusiasms of the interwar decades, see Daley, *Leisure and Pleasure*; Margaret Tennant, *Children's Health, the Nation's Wealth: A History of Children's Health Camps*, Bridget Williams Books, Wellington, 1994; Nadia Gush, 'The Beauty of Health: Cora Wilding and the Sunlight League', *New Zealand Journal of History*, 43, 1 (April 2009), pp.1–17.

95 Richards, *Dancing on Our Bones*; Malcolm Templeton, *Sporting Contacts and Human Rights: New Zealand's Attitude to Race Relations in South Africa, 1921–1994,* Auckland University Press, 1998; Michael King, *The Penguin History of New Zealand*, Penguin, Auckland, 2003; Merata Mita, director, *Patu!*, Awatea Films, 1983.

96 SPARC is a Crown Entity established under the Sport and Recreation New Zealand Act 2002. See <www.sparc.org.nz>. Funding for SPARC is from two principal sources: direct Crown funding and funding supplied via the New Zealand Lottery Grants Board. In the 2010–11 years, the balance between these two income streams was approximately: 2010 $30.8m (Lottery), $58.8 (Crown); 2011 $35.2 (Lottery), $71.9m (Crown) (budget figures). The current National-led government of Prime Minster John Key has increased funding to SPARC, notably the proportion of funds targeted to High Performance Sport. In 2010–13 the budget in this output class is projected to rise from $38.3m (2010) to $53.3m (2012). The increase in the general Sport and Recreation Programmes class is projected to rise more modestly from $16.1 million to $19.3 million. Lottery funding, always an unpredictable figure (with its income dependent on lottery sales), is projected to drop for this output class. High Performance Sport has thus been made the prime priority by the government, in both the total amount of funding and in the security of the source of that funding: SPARC Statement of Intent, 2010–2013, p.22, <www.sparc.org.nz>. The period encompassed by this Statement of Intent includes the Rugby World Cup 2011, hosted by New Zealand, and the 2012 London Olympics. The goals of SPARC include New Zealand teams winning the Rugby World Cup, ten medals at the London Games (a high goal given recent performances), as well as the Silver Ferns netball team winning the World Championships in 2011 (they came second, losing out to long-term rivals Australia by one goal in double overtime) and the cricket team winning an International Cricket Council Tournament 'by 2015'.

97 See Charlotte Macdonald 'Women and Girls, Men and Boys', Te Ara: online encyclopedia of New Zealand, <www.teara.govt.nz>; Julie Park (ed.), *Ladies a Plate: Change and Continuity in the Lives of New Zealand Women*, Auckland University Press, 1991; Jock Phillips, *A Man's Country*, Penguin, Auckland, 1987; Austin Mitchell, *The Half-gallon, Quarter Acre, Pavlova Paradise*, Whitcombe & Tombs, Christchurch, 1972.

98 Clipping from *Taranaki Herald*, 25 October 1946, Pat Lawlor, 77-067-1/4, ATL.

Chapter 3: Education or Health?

1   *Sydney Morning Herald* (*SMH*), 17 December 1938, p.13. Young arrived in Sydney on the *Aorangi* on 16 December 1938.

2   'Mr Gordon Young Welcomed', *SMH*, 20 December 1938, p.12 (and the report of the welcome at the Australia Hotel by the Physical Education Advisory Committee, same paper, p.3).

3   *SMH*, 22 December 1938, p.13.

4   National Fitness Act, No.26 of 1941. The first formal measure taken by the state government of New South Wales was by Order-in-Council in 1939.

5   The main secondary works on the national fitness scheme in Australia are David Kirk, *Schooling Bodies: School Practice and Public Discourse 1880–1950*, Leicester University Press, London and Washington, 1998, which focuses almost entirely on Victoria; Imke Fischer, 'Years of Silent Control: The Influence of the Commonwealth in State Physical Education in Victoria and New South Wales', PhD thesis, University of Sydney, 2000; Imke Fischer, 'The Involvement of the Commonwealth Government in Physical Education: From Defence to National Fitness', in Richard Cashman, John O'Hara and Andrew Honey (eds), *Sport, Federation, Nation*, Walla Walla Press, Sydney, 2001, pp.16–25; A. E. Simpson, *The National Fitness Council of South Australia: A History 1939–76*, South Australia Department of Recreation and Sport, Adelaide, 1986; R. K. Gray, *The First Forty Years: The National Fitness and Community Recreation Councils of Western Australia, 1939–1978*, Department for Youth, Sport and Recreation, Perth, 1982; W. Gordon Young, 'Physical Education in Australia: A Study of the History of Physical Education in Australia and a Forecast of Future Development', MEd thesis, University of Sydney, 1962; and brief mentions in general works: Richard Cashman, *Paradise of Sport: A History of Australian Sport*, rev. ed., Walla Walla Press, Sydney, 2010; Bill Gammage and Peter Spearritt (eds), oral history co-ordinator Louise Douglas, *Australians 1938*, Fairfax, Syme & Weldon Associates, Broadway, NSW, 1987.

6   Each football code has its own very strong regional following. 'Victorian Rules', later known as 'Aussie Rules', remains the predominant football code in Victoria despite its ruling body renaming itself the Australian Football League in 1990, in a claim to national stature.

7   Cashman, *Paradise of Sport*; Daryl Adair and Wray Vamplew, *Sport in Australian History*, Oxford University Press, Melbourne, 1997.

8   Lesley Johnson, 'Wireless', in Gammage et al (eds), *Australians 1938*, p.365.

9   *Pix Magazine*, 29 January 1938–20 May 1972, a popular illustrated weekly magazine, 'with a circulation of nearly a million': Library of NSW catalogue entry, State Library New South Wales. *Pix's* photographic content often featured sporting and active bodies (only from the 1960s did this take a tabloid slant).

10 Reproduced in Johnson, 'Wireless', p.368.

11 Jill Julius Matthews, *Dance Hall and Picture Palace: Sydney's Romance with Modernity*, Currency Press, Sydney, 2005.

12 Gail Reekie, *Temptations: Sex, Selling, and the Department Store*, Allen & Unwin, St Leonards, NSW, 1993.

13 Nikola Balnave, 'Company-Sponsored Recreation in Australia: 1890–1965', *Labour History*, 85 (2003), pp.129–51; Peter Burke, 'A Social History of Workplace Australian Football 1860–1939', PhD thesis, RMIT University, 2008.

14 Grace Bros Gym photographs, Home and Away – 14253, Home and Away – 19608, Hood Collection, State Library New South Wales.

15 *The Argus*, 30 October 1939, p.8. The pageant also had a fund-raising function, with proceeds going to the Red Cross.

16 Geoff Browne, 'Weber, Ivy Lavinia (1892–1976)', *Australian Dictionary of Biography*, Vol.12, Melbourne University Press, 1990, pp.431–32. See the 'Berlei Type Indicator' in Ann Stephen, 'The Body at the Scene of Modernism', in Ann Stephen, Philip Goad and Andrew McNamara (eds), *The Untold Story of Modernism in Australia*, Miegunyah Press, Melbourne, 2008, p.52.

17 Thea Hughes led the League in Sydney from 1935. She also became a prolific writer, producing a range of popular non-fiction titles over the course of a long life. Through that time she adapted her interests in body

movement and the benefits of exercise to the changing language of the day. Her later works were classified under headings of 'self-realisation' and 'self-help'. In 1976 her *Towards Self-development* appeared, and in 1979 *Towards Social Health*, along with other titles of similar ilk and repackagings of articles that first appeared in the League magazine, *Movement*. Thea Hughes's father was the author and journalist J. Stanley Hughes (who had died by the time Thea returned to Sydney). She had a degree from the University of Sydney and worked in the university's social settlement teaching dance to girls in the club. With this background she was typical of the early leaders of the League. Australian born, she travelled to England to continue her studies in dance. While she initially enrolled with leading teachers and colleges of the day, the difficulty of getting to the top of the highly competitive world of dance to become a leading performer was very apparent. The League offered a massively popular organisation, and one where there was a crying need for trained teachers and/or those with some expertise in dance. It offered glamour and celebrity – of popular success and mass movement – as against the artistic and professional prestige of the narrower dance repertoire.

18   *SMH*, 1 October 1936, p.22, and 22 October 1936, p.26.

19   *SMH*, 22 October 1936, p.26.

20   Judith Smart, 'Feminists, Flappers and Miss Australia: Contesting the Meanings of Citizenship, Femininity and Nation in the 1920s', *Journal of Australian Studies*, 25, 71 (2001), pp.1–15; Liz Conor, *The Spectacular Modern Woman: Feminine Visibility in the 1920s*, Indiana University Press, Bloomington and Indianapolis, 2004.

21   J. R. Poynter, 'Rubinstein, Helena (1870–1965)', *Australian Dictionary of Biography*, Vol.11, Melbourne University Press, 1988, pp.475–77; Florence Graham (1884–1966), 'Elizabeth Arden', was Canadian born and lived and worked in New York, opening a store in 1909 in 5th Ave. In 1914 she expanded under her corporate name 'Elizabeth Arden', and in 1922 opened her first salon in France: Kathy Peiss, *Hope in a Jar: The Making of America's Beauty Culture*, Harvey Holt, New York, 1998.

22   Decima Norman was described by the *SMH* as 'the athletic prowess of modern woman', cited by Leonie Sandercock, 'Sport', in Gammage et al. (eds), *Australians, 1938*, p.378.

23   Bernard Apps, *The 1941 Keep Fit Book*, National Fitness Council of South Australia, 1941, p.1, Mitchell Library, State Library New South Wales.

24   Newport Summer School on Leadership, Annual Reports Recreation and Leadership Movement, p.52, A 4135, State Records New South Wales (Sydney).

25   See Recreation and Leadership annual reports, pp.44–45, A 4135, State Records New South Wales (Sydney).

26   'Building Whole Men and Whole Women: Plan for Physical Education Progressing Here', *Sunday Sun and Guardian*, 22 August 1937, detailed report on C. E. W. Bean's ideas, clipping in A4135, State Records New South Wales (Sydney).

27   *The Problem of Recreation Space in the Metropolitan Area Sydney*, Report of the National Fitness Council of New South Wales, Sydney, May 1941, pp.6–7, quoting the 1931 report, Mitchell Library, State Library New South Wales. See Official Consultative Committee of the Parks and Playgrounds Movement of New South Wales, in conjunction with the Surveyor-General, *Basic Report on the Present and Future Requirements of the Parks and Playgrounds in the Sydney Metropolitan District*, Sydney, 1932; and the 1943 sequel produced by the NSW National Fitness Council. As Bean later noted, the Parks and Playground Movement concentrated on space, while organisations such as the Recreation and Leadership Movement and individuals like Edgar Herbert concentrated on recreational teaching and activities. See C. E. W. Bean, handwritten annotation on typed circular issued by the Parks and Playground Movement, NSW, 23 June 1937, titled 'Basis for Physical Fitness Campaign'. The conference, Bean noted, 'was part of the culmination of many years thought & effort', A4135, State Records New South Wales (Sydney).

28   C. E. W Bean, 'A National Need: Real Physical Education: The Use of Leisure', *SMH*, 28 May 1938, clipping in A4135, State Records New South Wales (Sydney).

29   Gordon Young, 'Historical Outline of National Fitness and Physical Education in New South Wales', 2 January 1945, typescript, p.29, A4154, State Records New South Wales (Sydney).

30   Stephen Garton, 'Australia and New Zealand: Laboratories of Racial Science', in Alison Bashford and Philippa Levine (eds), *Oxford Handbook to the History of Eugenics*, Oxford University Press, Oxford and New York, 2010, pp.243–57; and Stephen Garton, 'Eugenics', in Graeme Davison, John Hirst and Stuart Macintyre (eds), *The Oxford Companion to*

Australian History, Oxford University Press, Melbourne, 1998, pp.226–27; see also Bashford and Levine, introduction to *Oxford Handbook to the History of Eugenics*.

31 Apps, *The 1941 Keep Fit Book*, p.1. The same page gives the following definition: 'The healthy and fit person is one whose mind is alert, whose body is strong and active, and who feels a sense of well-being.'

32 Bishop Burgmann, the Anglican bishop of Goulburn and notable social critic, was the lead speaker at the conference: Peter Hempenstall, 'Burgmann, Ernest Henry (1885–1967)', *Australian Dictionary of Biography*, Vol.13, Melbourne University Press, 1993, pp.300–1.

33 See report by Meg Johnson, physical education teacher at Emily McPherson College; and Colonel Alan Ramsay, Education, University of Melbourne, 1935: Kirk, *Schooling Bodies*.

34 Annual Report, National Council of Women of Victoria, 1936; email Judith Smart to author, 6 April 2011. My thanks to Judith Smart for this reference.

35 B. F. G. Apps, 'The National Fitness Campaign After Five Years', *New Horizons in Education*, 4, 1 (July 1944), pp.21–25. The idea that Australia lagged behind other places was one commonly expressed: see C. Harvey Sutton, 'Physical Education and National Fitness', *Australian Rhodes Review*, 4 (1939), p.62.

36 See address at the meeting by Sir Cyril Norwood, 'The New Conception of Physical Education': W. Gordon Young, 'Physical Education in Australia: A Study of the History of Physical Education in Australia and a Forecast of Future Development', MEd thesis, University of Sydney, 1962, p.108.

37 W. F. Connell, 'Browne, George Stephenson (1890–1970)', *Australian Dictionary of Biography*, Vol.13, Melbourne University Press, 1993, pp.278–80.

38 Gertrude F. Kentish, 'Duras, Fritz (1896–1965)', *Australian Dictionary of Biography*, Vol.14, Melbourne University Press, 1996, p. 61.

39 *The Argus* (Melbourne), 7 December 1938, p.7.

40 Sutton, 'Physical Education and National Fitness', p.59.

41 Like the YWCA and the YMCA, Toc H (TH) is an organisation that has Christian origins. The name is an abbreviation of Talbot House, 'Toc' signifying the letter T in the signals spelling alphabet used by the British Army in World War I. Talbot House was a soldiers' rest and recreation centre set up in Belgium in 1915.

42 Sutton, 'Physical Education and National Fitness', p.60.

43 Members of the Committee were: Harvey Sutton, C. E. W. Bean, L. C. Robson, Dr H. C. Wallace, Rev J. S. Meagher, Dr A. C. Machin, Mr Steven Lynch, Miss E. M. Lewis and Mrs S. J. Davey-Young: Young, 'Physical Education in Australia', p.113. The Committee was established on 22 December 1937.

44 Young, 'Physical Education in Australia'; Peter J. Tyler, *Humble and Obedient Servants: The Administration of New South Wales, 1901–1960*, University of New South Wales Press, Sydney, 2006.

45 38/3259 Vacancy for a Director of Physical Education, New South Wales, recommendation, 1938, A4135, State Records New South Wales (Sydney). As well as the general preference for 'British' professionals, this was also a signal that NSW sought someone who did not come from the European background of Dr Fritz Duras – there had been some protest at his appointment: see *Argus* 7 November 1936, p.20.

46 *SMH* advertisement, 1 January 1938, A4135, State Records New South Wales (Sydney). Applications closed 28 February 1938.

47 A. S. Lamb, director of physical education, McGill University, Montreal, for many years. He was born in Ballarat, Victoria, went to McGill in 1912, completed a medical degree in 1917 and was *chef de mission* for the Canadian Olympic Team 1928. He visited New Zealand and spoke on 'Recreation. Place in Education: Healthy Minds and Bodies' at a New Zealand Club luncheon, Wellington, 15 October 1934. He was escorting a party of twelve Canadian schoolboys en route to Melbourne to compete at an intra-empire public school sports meeting on 9 November: *Evening Post*, 15 October 1934, p.10. Lamb was involved in a controversial post-1928 dispute when he opposed women competing at the Olympic Games: Margaret Ann Hall, *The Girl and the Game: A History of Women's Sport in Canada*, Broadview Press, Peterborough, 2002, pp.53–54.

48 38/3259 Vacancy for a Director of Physical Education, New South Wales, recommendation, 1938, A4135, State Records New South Wales (Sydney).

49 Fischer argues that Young and the NSW appointment were more effective than what happened in Victoria: Fischer, 'Years of Silent Control'.

50 Finally pushed into action, Prime Minister Lyons and Minister of Health Stewart announced the formation of a National Fitness Council in December 1938.

51 Jim Gillespie, 'Cumpston, John Howard Lidgett (1880–1954)', in Graeme Davison, John Hirst and Stuart Macintyre (eds), *Oxford Companion to Australian History*, Oxford University Press, Melbourne, 1998, pp.166–67; Michael Roe, 'Cumpston, John Howard Lidgett (1880–1954)', *Australian Dictionary of Biography*, Vol.8, Melbourne University Press, 1981, pp.174–76; Michael Roe, *Nine Australian Progressives: Vitalism in Bourgeois Social Thought, 1890–1960*, University of Queensland Press, St Lucia, 1984.

52 Cumpston, 'National Fitness', in *Health Brings Victory: Health, Milk and National Fitness Week*, Waite & Bull, Sydney, 1941, p.55. See also Cumpston to C. E. W. Bean, 31 May 1938 and Bean to Cumpston 6 June 1938, A4135, State Records New South Wales (Sydney).

53 See the report of the Tasmanian Government Cabinet meeting bemoaning the lack of action, which finishes with the sentence: 'The link between national fitness and national defence is too obvious to require underlining': *Burra Record*, 4 April 1939, p.4.

54 Apps, 'The National Fitness Campaign After Five Years', p.21.

55 W. H. Frederick, 'Brookes, Sir Norman Everard 1877–1968', *Australian Dictionary of Biography*, Melbourne University Press, 1979.

56 Sir Frederick Stewart in a minute to Cabinet, 25 May 1939, quoted in Kirk, *Schooling Bodies*, p.123, fn 53.

57 Note Oppenheimer's very useful observation: 'The issue of Commonwealth/state/local funding and jurisdiction overlap was as complex and difficult then as it is today .... State opposition to creeping federal powers was probably a factor in the Commonwealth's reluctance to pursue both the National Fitness Council's agenda, and the community centre movement': Melanie Oppenheimer, *Volunteering: Why We Can't Survive Without It*, University of New South Wales Press, Sydney, 2008, p.58.

58 Wilf Ewens, *Gordon Young: A Man of Inspiration*, Australian Council for Health, Physical Education and Recreation, Croydon, 1994; R. I. Cashman, 'Young, William Gordon (1904–1974)', *Australian Dictionary of Biography*, Vol.16, Melbourne University Press, 2002, pp 605–6; Fischer, 'Years of Silent Control', 2000; and Fischer, 'The Involvement of the Commonwealth Government in Physical Education'. Newport Summer School on Leadership, Annual Reports Recreation and Leadership Movement, A 4135, State Records New South Wales (Sydney).

59 *Barrier Miner*, 10 October 1939, p.1.

60 Cashman, 'Young, William Gordon'. Gordon Young was appointed commissioner for softball for Australia by the Amateur Softball Association of America in 1940. Pat Young was the founding president of the New South Wales Women's Softball Association in 1947: *SMH*, 6 March 1949, p.22.

61 Links between physical welfare and physical education officers on each side of the Tasman were maintained by visits, as well as the exchange of materials, ideas and experience. Helen Black, New Zealand's first woman officer, was recruited from Australia and returned there after she left the Department of Internal Affairs in 1943. When she visited Sydney early in 1940, she brought back a large bundle of curricula materials, programme plans, and observations of schemes and discussions with colleagues in the Physical Education section of the Department of Education: IA 1 139/107, Archives New Zealand, Wellington. Gordon Young established contact with colleagues in New Zealand including inviting them to contribute to *Physical Fitness* magazine: IA 1 139/43 Newspaper and radio publicity – general file, Archives New Zealand, Wellington.

62 Helen Black to Joe Heenan, Under Secretary, Department of Internal Affairs, 12 February 1940, IA 1 139/107, Archives New Zealand, Wellington.

63 *Physical Fitness*, 1, 1 (October 1939), p.5.

64 Apps, *The 1941 Keep Fit Book*, pp.1–2.

65 Ibid., p.6.

66 *National Fitness Newsletter*, 1, 1 (October 1944), p.4.

67 'Australians Should Walk Erect', *Morning Bulletin*, 3 May 1937, p.7. See Duras' advice also in 'Sport and Spectator', *The West Australian*, 3 September 1938.

68 Sutton, 'Physical Education and National Fitness', p.57.

69 Duras, 'Sport and the Spectator', p.5. Donald Bradman (1908–2001), Australian cricketer, is widely regarded as the greatest batsman of all time. American Don Budge (1915–2000) was the dominant men's tennis player of the 1930s. In 1938 he won all four grand slams. In May 1937 Duras had made a similar appeal: 'Bradman ... is doing great work if his example urges little boys to try to become other Bradmans': *Morning Bulletin*, 3 May 1937, p.7.

70 David Walker, 'Mind and Body', in Gammage et al. (eds), *Australians 1938*, chapter 16.

71 'It seems curious that we should be establishing an organization to encourage

physical fitness, a condition which should be at once the birthright and joy of every individual. Instead of complete physical fitness being the natural and normal condition throughout life, man has so arranged the condition of his living that we find ourselves in the position of treating fitness almost as an artificial condition ... it is desirable, not only that the necessity, the benefits and the satisfaction of a state of complete physical fitness should be brought home to everybody, but that the difficulties in the way of securing this condition should be removed, and the facilities provided so that at least no person has any excuse for neglecting his duty to himself': *Physical Fitness*, 1, 3, (December 1939), p.1 editorial.

72 Robert Menzies succeeded Joe Lyons who died in 1939. The Canberra government led by Menzies passed the National Fitness Act in the winter of 1941, shortly before he came under pressure to resign from lack of support, giving way to the Labor leader, John Curtin, by the end of that year. Curtin was sworn in 7 October 1941 and remained Prime Minister until his death in 1945. The National Fitness Act (supported by all parties) did not mark the beginning of central government action, which had been inaugurated in 1939, but put the initiative on a firmer footing and increased the funding allocated. Sir Frederick Stewart, Minister of Health, introduced the Bill on 25 June 1941: 'This bill makes provision to ensure the continuity and permanence of a movement with which I have been closely associated since its inception on a Commonwealth-wide basis in 1939' (Parliamentary Debates, 1941, p.370).

73 Apps, 'The National Fitness Campaign After Five Years'.

74 Ibid., p.22.

75 Bernard Apps was employed by the South Australian National Fitness Office, then appointed to Canberra as national officer; he returned to the South Australian service and later worked at the University of Adelaide.

76 *Health Brings Victory*, p.57, Mitchell Library, State Library New South Wales.

77 Ibid., p.55.

78 *SMH*, 20 November 1942, p.7.

79 A1928 (A1928/1) National Fitness, Seventh Session of Commonwealth National Fitness Council Section III, 21/10/43 – February 1944, National Archives Australia, Canberra. Signalling the new importance of the US to the Australian and New Zealand governments, the US is also included: J. G. Lang of the Division of Physical Education, Montreal, Quebec; Dr A. S. Lamb, Honorary President, McGill

University; Joe Heenan, Under Secretary of Department of Internal Affairs and responsible for Physical Welfare Branch within that Department, New Zealand; A. A. Cole, Extension Secretary at the Central Council of Recreative Physical Training, London; John W. Studebaker, Commissioner of Education, US Office of Education, Washington DC.

80 Ibid.

81 Heather Radi, 'Swain, Edith Muriel Maitland (1880–1964)', *Australian Dictionary of Biography*, Vol.16, Melbourne University Press, 2002, pp.349–50.

82 *SMH*, 21 May 1941, p.13; and 17 December 1938, p.13. In that first notice of his arrival, Gordon Young – with an eye for his local readers – noted that his replacement at the University of Western Ontario was an Australian, Hector Kay. Hector Kay later returned to Australia.

83 *Life*, 23 January 1939, p.45. A 1948 article in *SMH*, 'Breaking World Records', 8 May 1948, p.5, described E. Harold Le Maistre as 'Lecturer-in-charge Physical Education Department', University of Sydney.

84 Kirk, *Schooling Bodies*, pp.124–5.

85 Gordon Young, 'National Fitness and the New Order', first published in the *Australian Quarterly*, March 1942, pp.2, 3, 8.

86 Stuart Macintyre, *A Concise History of Australia*, Cambridge University Press, 1999, chapter 8.

87 Apps, 'The National Fitness Campaign After Five Years', p.23.

88 Ibid.; Simpson, *The National Fitness Council of South Australia*; Gray, *The First Forty Years*; Young, 'Physical Education in Australia'; Fischer, 'Years of Silent Control'.

89 *National Fitness Newsletter*, 1, 1 (October 1944), p.1, Mitchell Library, State Library New South Wales. This was a state rather than federal publication.

90 Ibid., pp.3–4. It concludes: 'She looked at him gravely with the calm wisdom of the very young. "Hello," he said. "I'm your dad. We're going to be great friends – you and I." And he continued walking up the stairs to meet his wife.'

91 Minister for Education to Mr C. W. Burwell, November 1946, 46/NF63/5374 [November 1946], 11/19039 Precedent Book, c.1945–66, State Records New South Wales (Sydney). Maria Nugent, *Botany Bay: Where Histories Meet*, Allen & Unwin, Crows Nest, NSW, 2005, especially chapter 3 'Boomerangs for Sale: Tourism in the Birthplace of the Nation'.

92 Melissa Harper, *The Ways of the Bushwalker:*

On Foot in Australia, University of New South Wales Press, Sydney, 2007; Apps, 'The National Fitness Campaign After Five Years'; *National Fitness Newsletter*, 1, 1 (October 1944), Mitchell Library, State Library New South Wales – both make reference to youth hostelling.

93 Sharon Wall, *The Nurture of Nature: Childhood, Antimodernism, and Ontario Summer Camps, 1920–55*, University of British Columbia Press, Vancouver, 2009.

94 *SMH*, 4 April 1941, p.4. Report includes a photograph of Gordon Young and Mrs Gordon Young attending the dance to fund-raise for the National Fitness Camp at Patonga.

95 Cashman, 'Young, William Gordon (1904–1974)'; Ewens, *Gordon Young*, is the original source of these figures.

96 13/12212, 50/NF30/8370, State Records New South Wales (Sydney).

97 Gordon Young to Secretary of Education, 16 May 1950, H. S. Wyndham to Gordon Young, 30 June 1950, 50/NF27/8169 LG.BB, 11/19039, State Records New South Wales (Sydney).

98 Young, 'Physical Education in Australia'. It was to be a pattern repeated by others, eager to establish the longevity and contours of the new professional field of physical education. Having a history was useful in establishing professional status. Wilf Ewens, a student and follower of Young's, was particularly devoted to the example he had grown up with, writing both a Master's and PhD thesis on national fitness in NSW, and the administrative style of its director. In South Australia, Albert Simpson produced a history of the national fitness programme there, in which he enters the history as a protagonist part way through.

99 Fischer, 'Years of Silent Control'.

100 Kirk, *Schooling Bodies*, 1998; and David Kirk, 'Schooling Bodies through Physical Education: Insights from Social Epistemology and Curriculum History', *Studies in Philosophy and Education*, 20 (2001), pp.475–87.

101 Oppenheimer, *Volunteering*, p.55.

Chapter 4. Fitness for War and a Changed World

1 An Act to establish a National Council for the purpose of promoting physical fitness (known as the National Physical Fitness Act July 1943). This chapter relies less on the archival record. My debt to Canadian scholars is considerable, as is evident in the notes that follow.

2 See Pierre Trudeau's policy of supporting sport as a means of fostering Canadian unity in the late 1960s, as discussed in Jean Harvey, 'The Role of Sport and Recreation Policy in Fostering Citizenship: The Canadian Experience', Canadian Policy Research Networks, Ottawa, 2001.

3 The CRBC began broadcasting in 1932 and was replaced by the Canadian Broadcasting Corporation (CBC) in 1936.

4 'Installation of the President', *Canadian Medical Association Journal*, 81, 15 July 1959, pp.116–18. The Duke was pictured as making an attack on 'sub-health': Don Morrow, Mary Keyes, Wayne Simpson, Frank Cosentino and Ron Lappage, *A Concise History of Sport in Canada*, Oxford University Press, Toronto, 1989, p.326. Presidential address to the British Medical Association on Wednesday, 28 October 1959, by H. R. H. The Prince Philip, Duke of Edinburgh, *British Medical Journal*, 31 October 1959, pp. 839–40. The Duke was also serving simultaneously as President of the Canadian Medical Association. It has been understood that Dr Doris Plewes, a senior public servant in the Department of Health, supplied material for the Duke's speech: Donald Macintosh, Tom Bedecki and C. E. S. Franks, *Sport and Politics in Canada: Federal Government Involvement Since 1961*, McGill–Queen's University Press, Montreal, 1988.

5 Len Scher, *The Un-Canadians: True Stories of the Blacklist Era*, Lester, Toronto, 1992; Len Scher, director, *The Un-Canadians*, film documentary, National Film Board of Canada, 1996; Susan Markham-Starr, '"Canada Needs You": The Jan Eisenhardt Story', Paper presented to Eleventh Congress on Leisure Research, 17–20 May 1995, Canadian Association for Leisure Studies, 2005 (on-line collection); Jan Eisenhardt, 27 April 1906–26 December 2004, obituary, <www.thestar.com>, 30 December 2004; Knud Petersen, 'Jan (Øyvind) Eisenhardt', <www.danishclubmontreal.com/history>; Vancouver Parks Board, 'Jan Eisenhardt, Recreation Pioneer, Gone but Not Forgotten', <www.Vancouver.ca/PARKS/info/features/2005>. Jan Eisenhardt married Barbara Joann Ferdon in Montreal on 6 January 1948. It was the first marriage for the bride and nothing suggests it wasn't for Eisenhardt. He is described as the son of Mr O. Eisenhardt of Copenhagen, see *The Gazette, Montreal*, 7 January 1948, p.10. Jan Eisenhardt also used the name Ian Eisenhardt and is sometimes referred to by this name.

6 Barbara Keys, *Globalizing Sport*, Harvard University Press, Cambridge, 2006.

7 See Katharine Moore, '"The Warmth of

Comradeship": The First British Empire Games and Imperial Solidarity', in J. A. Mangan (ed.), *The Cultural Bond: Sport, Empire, Society*, Frank Cass, London, 1992, pp.201–12.

8   Richard P. Cavanagh, 'The Development of Canadian Sports Broadcasting 1920–78', *Canadian Journal of Communication*, 17, 3 (1992), pp.2–3.

9   This was part of a review of the Marsh Report of 1943: Harry M. Cassidy, untitled, *American Economic Review*, 33, 3 (September 1943), p.709.

10 Bruce Kidd, *The Struggle for Canadian Sport*, University of Toronto Press, 1996, p.236.

11 Arthur Stanley Lamb (1886–1958) was Director of Physical Education at McGill University from 1920 till his retirement in 1949. Citation for Dr Arthur Lamb on receipt of the R. Tait McKenzie Honour Award, 1948: Iveagh Munro, Tribute to Dr Arthur S. Lamb, 1958, both on <www.phecanada.ca>. See also Margaret Ann Hall, *The Girl and the Game: A History of Women's Sport in Canada*, Broadview Press, Peterborough, 2002, pp.53–54.

12 Quoted in Fiona A. E. McQuarrie, 'The Struggle Over Worker Leisure: An Analysis of the History of the Workers' Sports Association of Canada', *Canadian Journal of Administrative Sciences*, 27, 4 (2010), p.396. See also Bruce Kidd, 'Workers' Sport, Workers' Culture', in *The Struggle for Canadian Sport*; and James Riordan, 'The Worker Sports Movement', in James Riordan and Arnd Kruger (eds), *The International Politics of Sport in the Twentieth Century*, Spon Press, London, 1999, pp.105–20.

13 Hall, *The Girl and the Game*.

14 Kidd, *The Struggle for Canadian Sport*.

15 Ibid., pp.237–8. Morrow et al., *A Concise History of Sport in Canada*.

16 *The Times* (London), 30 June 1937, p.15, col.d.

17 Hall, *The Girl and the Game*, p.85.

18 Henning Eichberg (John Bale and Chris Philo, eds), *Body Cultures: Essays on Sport, Space, and Identity*, Routledge, London, 1998.

19 Hall, *The Girl and the Game*, pp.98–99; *Montreal Gazette*, 24 September 1935.

20 Their 1938 women's basketball team is featured in Hall, *The Girl and the Game*, p.165.

21 P. Barbara Schrodt, 'A History of Pro-Rec: The British Columbia Provincial Recreation Programme, 1934 to 1953', PhD dissertation, University of Alberta, 1979, pp.33ff.

22 Thomas Dufferin, 'Duff' Pattullo, 1873–1956. Pattullo was premier of British Columbia from 1933–41.

23 Schrodt, 'A History of Pro-Rec', pp.94ff.

24 YEC Report, 1936, quoted in Barbara Schrodt, 'Federal Programmes of Physical Recreation and Fitness: The Contributions of Ian Eisenhardt and BC's Pro-Rec', *Canadian Journal of the History of Sport and Physical Education*, 15, 2 (December 1984), p.48.

25 Schrodt, 'A History of Pro-Rec', pp.340 ff for Danish influence. See also Hans Bonde, *Gymnastics and Politics: Niels Bukh and Male Aesthetics*, Museum Tusculanum Press, Copenhagen, 2006.

26 Schrodt, 'A History of Pro-Rec', p.79.

27 Ibid., p.89.

28 Ibid., p.91.

29 See Pro-Rec records, City of Vancouver Archives, Vancouver, BC, Canada, including rich photographic record, and Barbara Schrodt collection of Pro-Rec materials at UBC Archives, University of British Columbia Library, Vancouver, Canada.

30 Schrodt, 'A History of Pro-Rec'; Schrodt, 'Federal Programmes of Physical Recreation and Fitness'.

31 Charlotte Macdonald, 'Emily's Dream: A Women's Memorial Building and a History Without Walls: Citizenship and the Politics of Public Remembrance in 1930s–40s New Zealand', in M. Lake, K. Holmes and P. Grimshaw (eds), *Women's Rights and Human Rights: International Historical Perspectives*, Macmillan, London, 2001, pp.168–83.

32 YEC Report, 1936, quoted in Schrodt, 'Federal Programmes of Physical Recreation and Fitness', p.48.

33 Schrodt, 'Federal Programmes of Physical Recreation and Fitness'.

34 Kidd, *The Struggle for Canadian Sport*, p.253.

35 National Fitness Act 1943, section 5.

36 A. S. Lamb, 'National Physical Fitness: A Duty and an Opportunity', *Canadian Welfare*, 19, 8 (1 March 1944), p.29.

37 Antonia Maioni, 'Nothing Succeeds Like the Right Kind of Failure: Postwar National Health Insurance Initiatives in Canada and the United States', *Journal of Health Politics, Policy and Law*, 20, 1 (Spring 1995), pp.5–30.

38 *House of Commons Debates: official report*, 1943, pp.5188–89.

39 Ibid.

40 Ibid., p.5189a.

41 Ibid., p.5189b.

42 Ibid., p.5191b.

43 *Debate of the Senate*, Session 1943–44, 22 July 1943, pp.372–3.

44 *House of Commons Debates: official report*, 1943, p.5361.

45 Members of National Council were: Jan
    Eisenhardt (Chairman); Dr W. C. Ross, Halifax;
    Dr Milton Grewer, Fredericton; Dr Jules
    Gilbert, Quebec City; Mr A. Burridge, Hamilton
    (Physical Director, McMaster University); Mr
    Wray Youmans, Winnipeg; Mr W. A. Wellban,
    Regina; Mr Joe H. Ross, Calgary; Mr Jerry
    Mathison, Vancouver. It was notable for
    including no women. See Lamb, 'National
    Physical Fitness', p.29; James L. Gear, 'Factors
    Influencing the Development of Government
    Sponsored Physical Fitness Programmes in
    Canada from 1850 to 1972', *Canadian Journal of
    the History of Sport and Physical Education*, 4,
    2 (1973), p.18.
46 Peter R. Elson, 'The Great White North and
    Voluntary Action: Canada's Relationship with
    Beveridge, Social Welfare and Social Justice',
    in Melanie Oppenheimer and Nicholas Deakin
    (eds), *Beveridge and Voluntary Action in Britain
    and the Wider British World*, Manchester
    University Press, 2010, p.169.
47 'Conscription', and James Struthers, 'Welfare
    State', in Gerald Hallowell (ed.), *The Oxford
    Companion to Canadian History*, Oxford
    University Press, 2004.
48 Gear, 'Factors Influencing', quoting Eisenhardt
    speaking in 1945, pp.18–19.
49 Lamb, 'National Physical Fitness', pp.27, 29.
50 The Dominion grant jumped from $10,000 in
    1943–44 to over $16,000 in 1944–45, with the
    last allocation being over $19,000 in 1952–53:
    Schrodt, 'Federal Programmes of Physical
    Recreation and Fitness', pp.54–55. The initial
    distribution of the federal grant was: BC:
    $16,015.75; Alberta: $15,590.50; Saskatchewan:
    $17,545.75; Manitoba: $14,290.00; Ontario:
    $74,173.75; Quebec: $65,248.00; New
    Brunswick: $8,957.50; Nova Scotia: $11,317.75;
    Prince Edward Island: $1,861.00: Lamb,
    'National Physical Fitness', p.27.
51 Gear, 'Factors Influencing'; Schrodt 'A History
    of Pro-Rec', and 'Federal Programmes of
    Physical Recreation and Fitness'.
52 The title of Hugh MacLennan's 1945 novel,
    Two Solitudes, has come to stand for the
    era of profound and tense distance between
    Anglophone and Francophone Canada.
53 For an assessment of the strengths and
    weaknesses of the National Physical Fitness
    Act and work of the Council, see also J.
    Thomas West, 'Physical Fitness, Sport and the
    Federal Government 1909 to 1954', *Canadian
    Journal of History of Sport and Physical Fitness*,
    4, 2 (1973), pp.26–42.
54 Shirley Tillotson, 'Citizen Participation in
    the Welfare State: An Experiment, 1945–57',
    Canadian Historical Review, 25, 4 (1994),
    pp.511–42.
55 Ibid., p.529.
56 Janice Forsyth and Michael Heine, '"A Higher
    Degree of Social Organization": Jan Eisenhardt
    and Canadian Aboriginal Sport Policy in the
    1950s', *Journal of Sport History*, 35, 2 (Summer
    2008), pp.261–77; and Janice Forsyth, 'The
    Indian Act and the (Re)shaping of Canadian
    Aboriginal Sport Practices', *International
    Journal of Canadian Studies*, 35 (Spring 2007),
    pp.95–111. What was occurring in Canada
    was part of a wider movement of postwar
    'modernisation' in citizenship for indigenous
    peoples and racial minorities: see Scott
    Simon, *Jackie Robinson and the Integration
    of Baseball*, John Wiley and Sons, Hoboken,
    2007; Marilyn Lake, *Faith: Faith Bandler, Gentle
    Activist*, Allen & Unwin, Sydney, 2003; Ranginui
    Walker, *Ka Whawhai tonu Matou: Struggle
    without End*, 2nd edn, Penguin, Auckland,
    2004; Monty Soutar, *Nga Tama Toa: The Price
    of Citizenship. C Company 28 (Maori) Battalion
    1939–1945*, David Bateman, Auckland, 2008;
    Scott Sheffield, 'Rehabilitating the Indigene:
    Post-War Reconstruction and the Image of
    the Indigenous Other in English Canada and
    New Zealand, 1943–1948', in Phillip Buckner
    and R. Douglas Francis (eds), *Rediscovering
    the British World*, University of Calgary Press,
    2005, pp.341–60; Vincent Ward, *Map of the
    Human Heart*, film, Australian Film Finance
    Corporation, 1993 (a fictional depiction but
    addressing the same theme).
57 Brian Titley, 'Indian Act', in Gerald Hallowell
    (ed.), *Oxford Companion to Canadian History*,
    Oxford University Press, 2004.
58 Forsyth and Heine, '"A Higher Degree"', p.276,
    fn.49.
59 Ibid.
60 Ibid.
61 Ibid., pp.267–8.
62 Ibid., p.268.
63 Ibid., p.270.
64 Ibid., p.271. See parallels in other former settler
    colonies, and tensions in aspirations for, and
    reactions to, modernity in this period. For
    New Zealand, see: Aroha Harris, 'Concurrent
    Narratives of Māori and Integration in the
    1950s and 60s', *Journal of New Zealand
    Studies* (2008), pp.139–55, and 'Dancing
    with the State: Maori Creative Energy and
    Policies of Integration, 1945–67', PhD thesis,
    University of Auckland, 2007; Barbara Brookes,
    'Nostalgia for "Innocent Homely Pleasures":
    The 1964 New Zealand Controversy over
    Washday at the Pa', *Gender & History*, 9,

2 (1997), pp. 242–61; Brendan Hokowhitu, '"Physical Beings": Stereotypes, Sport and the "Physical Education" of New Zealand Maori', in J. A. Mangan and A. Ritchie (eds), *Culture, Sport, Society*, Frank Cass, London, 2003, pp.192–218. For Australia, see: Richard Broome, *Aboriginal Australians: A History Since 1788*, 4th edn, Allen & Unwin, Crows Nest, NSW, 2010.

65 Forsyth and Heine, '"A Higher Degree"', p.272.

66 Ian Eisenhardt, 'The Canadian Red Man of Today', *Journal of the American Association for Health, Physical Education and Recreation*, (June 1951), pp.9–10.

67 Forsyth and Heine, '"A Higher Degree"', p.272.

68 Bruce Kidd, *Tom Longboat*, Fitzhenry & Whiteside, Markham, 1992; Resolution No.20, Confederacy of Nations, 12–14 April 1999, Ottawa, Ontario at 64.26.129.156/article. asp?id=921. The award is now administered by the Aboriginal Sports Circle, Akwesasne, Ontario, Canada: <www.aboriginalsportcircle. ca>.

69 Scher, *The Un-Canadians*, book (1992) and documentary film (1996).

70 Markham-Starr, '"Canada Needs You"'. See also Richard Cavell (ed.), *Love, Hate and Fear in Canada's Cold War*, University of Toronto Press, 2004; Gary Kinsman, Dieter K. Buse and Mercedes Steedman (eds), *Whose National Security? Canadian State Surveillance and the Creation of Enemies*, Between the Lines, Toronto, 2000. Eisenhardt Personnel File RG32, Series C2, Historical Personnel Files, Volume 1408, File 1906.04.24, pts 1 and 2, Library and Archives Canada (the author has not, however, been granted permission to access the file at the time of writing).

71 Hon Paul Martin, minister responsible through most of the Council's life, Memo of meeting with sports officials and the Minister of National Health and Welfare, September 1949, Public Archives of Canada, quoted by West, 'Physical Fitness', p.41.

72 William Beveridge, *Voluntary Action: A Report on Methods of Social Advance*, Allen & Unwin, London, 1948; Elson, 'The Great White North and Voluntary Action'.

73 Quoted in Deborah McPhail, 'What to Do With the "tubby hubby"? Obesity, the Crisis of Masculinity, and the Nuclear Family in Early Cold War Canada', *Antipode*, 41, 5 (November 2009), p.1021.

74 Ibid.

75 Ibid., pp. 1026–7. The author's parents had copies of these booklets on the shelves of their New Zealand home in the late 1960s.

76 Mackenzie King's Liberals were re-elected in the 1945 general election on the back of the universal Family Allowances scheme, the Veterans' Charter and promises for a secure future. But with the return of prosperity and successful resumption of peacetime life and work, hunger for continued state extension and an ambitious programme of social security ebbed from its 1943–45 high point. The popularity of the CCF leftwing party also receded post-1945, taking the heat off the government.

77 See West, 'Physical Fitness'.

78 Schrodt, 'Federal Programmes of Physical Recreation and Fitness', p.55.

79 J. T. Bryden and E. Hardy, 'Abolish the National Physical Fitness Undertaking?', *Effective Government*, 16 (November 1951), pp.1–5.

80 Blair Fraser, 'Backstage Ottawa', *MacLean's*, 1 August 1954, p.51, quoted in West, 'Physical Fitness', p.42.

81 'Installation of the President', *Canadian Medical Association Journal*, 81 (15 July 1959), pp.116–17.

82 Cavanagh, 'The Development of Canadian Sports Broadcasting'. It is estimated that by 1956, 60 per cent of Canadian homes had a television set.

83 A substantial report by the Canadian Sports Advisory Council setting out 'Problems Arising from Physical Fitness Deficiencies in Canada' had been completed in 1958 and also forms an important precursor to the 1961 legislation: Morrow et al., *A Concise History of Sport in Canada*, p.326.

84 An Act to Promote Physical Activity and Sport (LS-429E), 2002, Background, Government of Canada, <http://dsp-psd.pwgsc.gc.ca/ Collection-R/LoPBdP/LS/371/371c54-e.htm>.

85 Morrow et al., *A Concise History of Sport in Canada*; Macintosh et al., *Sport and Politics in Canada*, especially chapter 2; Kidd, *The Struggle for Canadian Sport*.

86 Phillip Buckner (ed.), *Canada and the End of Empire*, UBC Press, Vancouver and Toronto, 2005; Phillip Buckner (ed.), *Canada and the British Empire*, Oxford History of the British Empire Companion Series, Oxford University Press, 2008.

87 'Installation of the President', *Canadian Medical Association Journal*, 81, 15 July 1959, pp.116–18. See chapter 1 for an account of the speech: King George VI speech launching the National Fitness Campaign, London, 17 February 1938, ICL 0067783 (BBC), British Library, Sound Archive (AA 1629).

Chapter 5: Healthy Bodies, States and Modernity

1   Philip A. Smithells, *The Atlantic Gap: The Case for Better Understanding in Physical Education*, Dunedin, 1948, p.15.

2   Antonia Maioni, 'Nothing Succeeds Like the Right Kind of Failure: Postwar National Health Insurance Initiatives in Canada and the United States', *Journal of Health Politics, Policy and Law*, 20, 1 (Spring 1995), pp.5–30; Matthew Worley, *Oswald Mosley and the New Party*, Palgrave Macmillan, Basingstoke, 2010, p.11.

3   The modern exposition of citizenship owes much to T. H. Marshall, although he may not recognise this particular elaboration of his model: T. H. Marshall, *Citizenship and Social Class and Other Essays*, Cambridge University Press, 1950. There has been much subsequent discussion of his ideas. For a useful consideration, see Martin Bulmer and Anthony M. Rees (eds), *Citizenship Today: The Contemporary Relevance of T. H. Marshall*, University College of London Press, 1996.

4   See advertisements for butter by Australian and New Zealand producers in NFC booklets, discussed in Chapter 2. Catherine Hall and Sonya O. Rose (eds), *At Home with the Empire: Metropolitan Culture and the Imperial World*, Cambridge University Press, 2006.

5   Les Cleveland, 'What They Liked: Movies and Modernity Downunder', *Journal of Popular Culture*, 36, 4 (2003), pp.756–79.

6   David Cannadine, 'Empire', in *History in Our Time*, Yale University Press, New Haven and London, 1998, p.154 (first published in *Past & Present*, 147, May 1995).

7   See, for example, the terms on which cricket teams toured New Zealand in the 1930s, and the highly asymmetrical relations between playing 'nations': Owen Mann, 'Confirming Tradition, Confirming Change: A Social History of the Cricket Tours to New Zealand in the 1930s', MA thesis, Victoria University of Wellington, 2011; K. Sandiford and B. Stoddart (eds), *The Imperial Game: Cricket, Culture and Society*, Manchester University Press, 1999; Jack Williams, *Cricket and England: A Cultural and Social History of the Inter-war Years*, Frank Cass, London, 2003.

8   See Susann Liebich, 'Reading Communities and Networks', PhD in progress, Victoria University of Wellington, 2011, for more on the Home Reading Union.

9   Kristine Alexander, 'The Girl Guide Movement and Imperial Internationalism During the 1920s and 1930s', *Journal of the History of Childhood and Youth*, 2, 1 (2009), pp.37–63.

10 Martin Daunton and Bernhard Reiger (eds), *Meanings of Modernity: Britain from the Late-Victorian Era to World War II*, Berg, Oxford and New York, 2001, p.15.

11 The Statute of Westminster applied immediately to Canada. Australia and New Zealand had to adopt it by separate legislation, which they did in 1942 and 1947, respectively. While Australia and New Zealand were more reticent about the formal step, they welcomed the greater recognition of the distinctive character and stature of their governments and societies within the broader imperial family, and especially as 'first equal' Dominions.

12 *Imperial Conference, 1937, Summary of Proceedings*, Cmd 5482, p.46.

13 The words of Mackenzie King, Prime Minister of Canada, *Imperial Conference, 1937, Summary of Proceedings*, p.50.

14 Sarah Bradford, *The Reluctant King: The Life and Reign of George VI 1895-1952*, St Martins Press, New York, 1990, p.215.

15 Joan Tumblety, 'Medicine in History and Society', short abstract, c.2010, <www.soton. ac.uk/history/docs/medical.../tumblety_ research.pdf>.

16 Ian Tyrell, *Transnational Nation: United States History in Global Perspective Since 1879*, Palgrave Macmillan, Basingstoke, 2007; James Belich, *Replenishing the Earth: The Settler Revolution and the Rise of the Anglo World, 1783-1939*, Oxford University Press, Oxford and New York, 2009.

17 Smithells, 'The Atlantic Gap', is a testimony to the divergent traditions, practices and absence of shared knowledge between the US, and Britain, New Zealand and Australia. The 'gap' was less profound with Canada.

18 Ross McKibbin, *Classes and Cultures: England 1918-1951*, Oxford University Press, 1998.

19 Peter J. Beck, 'Confronting George Orwell: Philip Noel-Baker on International Sport, Particularly the Olympic Movement, as Peacemaker', *European Sports History Review*, 5 (2003), pp.187–207; George Orwell, 'The Sporting Spirit', *Tribune*, 14 December 1945.

20 James Curran and Stuart Ward, *The Unknown Nation: Australia After Empire*, Melbourne University Press, 2010.

21 Christmas Broadcast 2010, <www.royal.gov. uk>.

22 Prochaska makes the case for 'the welfare monarchy', and his argument could be extended for the twentieth century to the 'the modern sporting monarchy': see Frank Prochaska, *Royal Bounty: The Making of a Welfare Monarchy*, Yale University Press, New

Haven & London, 1995.

23 Juliet B. Schor, *The Overworked American: The Unexpected Decline of Leisure*, Basic Books, New York, 1991.

24 Margaret Tennant, *The Fabric of Welfare: Voluntary Organisations, Government and Welfare in New Zealand, 1840–2005*, Bridget Williams Books, Wellington, 2007.

25 McKibbin, *Class and Cultures*.

26 William Beveridge, *Voluntary Action: A Report on Methods of Social Advance*, Allen & Unwin, London, 1948, p.10. See also Frank Prochaska, *The Voluntary Impulse: Philanthropy in Modern Britain*, Faber & Faber, London, 1988; Melanie Oppenheimer and Nicholas Deakin (eds), *Beveridge and Voluntary Action in the Wider British World*, Manchester University Press, 2010.

27 See, for example, *The Future of Voluntary Organisations: Report of the Wolfenden Committee*, Croom Helm, London, 1978; Bagehot, 'Lost in the Woods', *The Economist*, 5 February 2011, p.58; 'No Such Thing', and 'Platoons Under Siege', *The Economist*, 12 February 2011, pp.14, 63–64; *The Economist* 1 October 2011, p.20 (David Cameron's government condemned for wasting 'time and political capital on the dud theme of the "Big Society" and naïve waffle about voluntarism').

28 Ana Carden-Coyne, *Reconstructing the Body: Classicism, Modernism, and the First World War*, Oxford University Press, 2009.

29 Advertisement in National Fitness Council, *In Work and Play Fitness Wins*, London, 1938, p.59.

30 See Roger Griffin, *Modernism and Fascism: The Sense of a Beginning under Mussolini and Hitler*, Palgrave Macmillan, Basingstoke, 2007; Kevin Passmore, *Fascism: A Very Short Introduction*, Oxford University Press, 2002; Philip Morgan, *Fascism in Europe, 1919–1945*, Routledge, London, 2002.

31 Susan Sontag, 'Fascinating Fascism', in *Under the Sign of Saturn*, Vintage Books, New York, 1981, pp.73–108 (first published in *New York Review of Books*, 6 February 1975); and Ray Müller's film 'The Wonderful Horrible Life of Leni Riefenstahl'.

32 Alison Light, *Forever England: Femininity, Literature, and Conservatism Between the Wars*, Routledge, London, 1991; Sharon Wall, *The Nurture of Nature: Childhood, Antimodernism, and Ontario Summer Camps, 1920–55*, University of British Columbia Press, Vancouver, 2009

33 Adrian Bingham, *Gender: Modernity and the Popular Press in Inter-war Britain*,

Clarendon at Oxford University Press, 2004; Jill Julius Matthews, *Dance Hall to Picture Palace: Sydney's Romance with Modernity*, Currency Press, Sydney, 2005; Carden-Coyne, *Reconstructing the Body*; Daunton and Rieger (eds), *Meanings of Modernity*.

34 See, for example, *Scotland for Fitness, film, 1938*; David Matless,'"The Art of Right Living": Landscape and Citizenship, 1918–1939', in Steve Pile and Nigel Thrift (eds), *Mapping the Subject: Geographies of Cultural Transformation*, Routledge, London, 1995, pp.93–122; John Lowerson, 'Battles for the Countryside', in F. Gloversmith (ed.), *Class, Culture and Social Change: A New View of the 1930s*, Harvester, Brighton, 1980, pp.258–80; Harvey Taylor, *A Claim on the Countryside: A History of the British Outdoor Movement*, Keele University Press, Edinburgh, 1997; Kirstie Ross, *Going Bush: New Zealanders and Nature in the Twentieth Century,* Auckland University Press, 2008; and Kirstie Ross, '"Schooled by Nature": Pakeha Tramping Between the Wars', New Zealand Journal of History, 35, 1 (2002), pp.51–65.

35 Colin Tatz, *The Obstacle Race. Aborigines in Sport*, UNSW Press, Syndey, 1995; Kathryn M. Hunter, 'Rough Riding: Aboriginal Participation in Rodeos and Travelling Shows to the 1950s', *Aboriginal History*, 32 (2008), pp.82–96.

36 John F. Kennedy, 'The Soft American', *Sports Illustrated*, 26 December 1960, pp.16–25.

37 Christine Halse, 'Bio-Citizenship: Virtue Discourses and the Birth of the Bio-citizen', in Jan Wright and Valerie Harwood (eds), *Biopolitics and the 'Obesity Epidemic': Governing Bodies*, Routledge, New York and London, 2009, pp.44–59.

38 R.E. Roper, *Movement and Thought*, Blackie Press, London, 1938, p.162.

39 James L. Gear, 'Factors Influencing the Development of Government Sponsored Physical Fitness Programmes in Canada from 1850 to 1972', *Canadian Journal of the History of Sport and Physical Education*, 4, 2 (1973), pp.1–25, quoting Eisenhardt, 1945, pp.18–19.

40 See Sport England's calculations: only 7 million Britons play sport on a regular basis, 16.6 per cent of the current population, and their target is to get an additional 1 million active: Sport England, 2009–2010 annual report. SPARC's vision: 'Everyone. Every day. Enjoying and excelling through sport and recreation': <www.sparc.org.nz>.

Bibliography

PRIMARY SOURCES

National Archives, London (formerly Public Record Office)

ED 113/20 Finance

ED 113/25 Policy

ED 113/35 Devon and Cornwall Area Committee (Exeter covered swimming bath, 1938–41)

ED 113/39 Northamptonshire, Leicestershire and Rutland Area Committee

ED 113/40 Nottinghamshire and Derby Area Committee

ED 113/45, 46, 47 Grants Committee Minutes

ED 113/48 Minutes, National Advisory Committee, 3 May 1937–2 May 1939

ED 113/49 Minutes, Sub-committees, National Advisory Council

ED 113/50 Sub Committees

ED 113/56 Amateur Boxing Association

ED 113/60 London/British Maccabi Association

ED 113/69 National Amateur Rowing Association, 1937–39

ED 113/70 National Amateur Wrestling Association, 1938–39

ED 113/77 Slough Social Centre

ED 113/80 Women's Amateur Athletic Association

ED 113/81 Women's League of Health and Beauty, Welsh League of Youth

ED 113/82 Women Team Games Board (Marjorie Pollard), 1937–40

ED 124/67 Central Council of Physical Recreation Grant, 16 October 1939

ED 136/1 Central Council of Recreative Physical Training, 1936–38

ED 136/71 National Government Scheme

ED 136/74 Misc. correspondence, attitudes of various bodies to government plans

ED 136/75 Misc. minutes and correspondence

ED 136/76 National Advisory Council constitution; invitations to members and replies

ED 136/77 Grants Committee, appointment of members

ED 136/81 Comment on items in The Times, 16 May 1939

ED 136/88 General

ED 136/91 Publicity

ED 136/93 World Congress on Recreation and Leisure Time

ED 136/94 Future policy regarding National Fitness Council, 1939

BT 60/47/3 Glasgow Empire Exhibition

BT 60/47/7 Glasgow Empire Exhibition

CAB 23/96 Minutes, Cabinet Meeting, 14 December 1938

CAB 26/21 Home Affairs Committee, Physical Training and Recreation Bill, Memo by President of the Board of Education and the Secretary of State for Scotland, 4 March 1937 (Draft Bill)

CB 1/1 National Playing Fields Association, Inaugural meeting, Royal Albert Hall, 8 July 1925, Report of Proceedings

HO 144/21135 National Fitness Council – Royal Title (my thanks to Sarah Davis/Home Office for providing access to this file)

MAF 48/727 Access to Mountains Act 1939

MAF 48/728 Access to Mountains Act 1939, Correspondence

F 32/6 Forestry Commission, Correspondence 1924–39 (Access to Mountains Act 1939)

FO 370 + FO 371 London Olympics 1948 (Various sub-files, spans 1945–48)

FO 395/621 British Council (includes item P2421 8 August 1938 Publicity Abroad for the National Fitness Councils for England and Scotland)

CAB 124/767 London Olympics

FO 938/205 1948 Olympics

HLG 71/1698 Ministry of Health, Access to Mountains, c.1945–47

Churchill Archives, Churchill College, Cambridge

Philip Noel Baker Papers, NBKR

Series 1 Constituency Papers

1/116 Correspondence re White Paper on Education

Series 2 Labour Party

2/33 Correspondence and Papers on Labour's Foreign Policy 1936

2/34 Papers and Cuttings re 'Unity' campaign

2/44 Correspondence re Labour Party Foreign Policy 1938–41

Series 3 British Domestic Affairs

3/106 Papers re National Health Campaign 1939–41

3/107 Papers of Central Council of Physical Recreation

3/108 Pamphlets on aspects of health 1943–46

3/110 Correspondence, Reports, Printed Handouts re Health and National Health Service Bill

3/112 Memo on British Propaganda in Germany, 1939

Series 4 International Affairs

4/465 Correspondence, Minutes and Reports of League of Nations concerning trafficking in women and children, 1921–3

Series 6 Sport

6/2 Athletics 1938–50

6/2/1

6/2/2 Athletic Friends' Correspondence 1949–50

6/3 Ascent of Everest and Athletics

6/3/1 PJNB Personal Athletics 1938 to 1949

6/3/2

6/4 National Advisory Council for Physical Training (National Fitness Council)

6/4/1 Magazines and programmes

6/4/2 National Advisory Council for Physical Training. Parliamentary Papers

6/15 Olympics and sport in general, 1925–48

6/15/1 1948 Olympics

6/15/2 British Olympic Association

6/15/3 Athletics Achilles

6/15/4 Athletics AAA

6/15/5 Sports Fellowship

6/15/6 Inter Varsity Athletics Board

6/15/7 Athletics, British Workers' Sports Association

6/15/8 Olympic Games clippings and correspondence

6/54/1 Athletics, Olympic Games 1936, Correspondence

6/54/2 Athletics, Olympic Games 1936, Press cuttings, memoranda and articles

6/54/3 Olympics in Germany, 1935–36

6/54/4 Sport 1924

Series 8 Speeches and Broadcasts

8/7/2 Speeches on sports, athletics and rural amenities, 1927–43

8/7/3 Speeches to youth groups

8/16/1 Speeches to Labour Women's Meetings 1928–39

8/61/4 Speeches on sport, 1943–50

Series 9 Correspondence

9/65 Personal correspondence, 1932–34, 1938–40

9/93

9/93/1

Series 11 Miscellaneous

11/4 Pocket diaries

Winston Churchill Papers, CHAR

8/615 Literary: News of the World articles by WSC 2 May '38–Sep '38

BBC Written Archives Centre, Reading

R16/519 Education: General Surveys – Physical Training 1943

R16/390 Education: General Schools Council: Scottish Physical Training Committee 1938–42

R28/119 News Ministry of Health File 1 1927–54

R32/53 Parliamentary Questions Physical Exercises 1937–39

R34/514 Policy Physical Exercises for Schools 1936–43

R51/387/1 Talks Physical Exercises File 1a 1925–32

R51/387/2 Talks Physical Exercises File 1b 1933–35

R51/387/3 Talks Physical Exercises File 2a March–November 1936

R51/387/4 Talks Physical Exercises File 2b December 1936–37

R51/387/5 Talks Physical Exercises File IIIa 1938–39

R51/387/6 Talks Physical Exercise File IIIb January–March 1940

R51/387/7 Talks Physical Exercises File Iva April–May 1940

R51/387/1 Talks Physical Exercises Files IVb and V June 1940–56

R51/338 Talks National Fitness Council 1937–39

R51/210/1 Talks Health File 1a 1932–38

R51/210/2 Talks Health File 1b 1938–40

R51/210/3 Talks Health File 2a 1942

R51/210/4 Talks Health File 2b 1943–44

R51/210/5 Talks Health File 3 1945–46

R51/210/6 Talks Health File 4a 1947–49

SC19/115/1 Physical Training VI

SC19/115/2 Physical Training VIII

SC19/116 Programme Arrangements (Glasgow) Physical Training – Central Council of Recreative Physical Training Minutes

SC 139/1/1 Physical Training Publicity

T14/78 TV Obs Alexandra Park Women's League of Health and Beauty 1937–38

T14/1336 TV Obs Wembley – Stadium: International Festival of Sport and Physical Training 1938

T32/273 TV Talks Physical Training Series 1937

T32/419 TV Talks Ministry of Health 1937–67 Scripts Only Index Cards

Archives New Zealand, Wellington

IA 1 139 Physical Welfare Branch

IA 1 139/2/3 Scheme for Maori recreation – general file

IA 1 139/7/7 Sport-Swimming – Splash Club – Auckland

IA 1 139/11/12 Correspondence, South African government

IA 1 139/16/4 Application by Miss D. Adams for Physical Welfare Officer February 1941

IA 1 139/20 Suggested appointment Mr C. R. Bach

IA 1 139/27 Scholarships University of Southern California, 1939

IA 1 139/32 Physical Fitness Week

IA 1 139/32/1 Radio broadcasts

IA 1 139/32/115 Mackenzie Country (Fairlie)

IA 1 139/32/124 Greytown

IA 1 139/43 Sport – Fitness and Rec – Newspaper and radio publicity, General file, 8 November 1938–25 June 1952

IA 1 139/43/2 Sport – Propaganda and publicity – Preparation of radio talks, 1939–51

IA 1 139/43/11 Women's Radio Session

IA 1 139/58 Group Travel Scheme

IA 1 139/64 Recreation Week, 1939, General file

IA 1 139/73/48 Chinese Sports Meeting and association, Wellington

IA 1 139/74/34 Sport – Waikato area officer – Staff arrangements

IA 1 139/90 Napier Business Girls' Interhouse Carnival

IA 1 139/90/1 National Interhouse Association Activities

IA 1 139/90/2 New Zealand Interhouse Girls Association

IA 1 139/90/4 Girls Recreation Council – general file

IA 1 139/104/25 Mercer Refreshment Rooms, 1943

IA 1 139/104/31 Sport – Auckland Area Officer – Radiant Health Clubs

IA 1 139/107 Sport – Phys Ed in Australia – Visit of Miss Black – Report, 1940

IA 1 139/21/129 Sport – District Committee – Greytown

IA 1 139/21/139 Greytown District Committee

IA 62, 4/38 Inter-house Girls Display, Centennial Exhibition 1940

AAOM W3265 Supreme Court, Wellington

Alexander Turnbull Library, Wellington

Rona Bailey Papers, MS-Group-0901

J. W. Heenan Papers, MS-Papers-1132

Hutt County Council, MS-Papers-1293-119/12

National Dance Archive of New Zealand, PA1-q-547 (92-002 Collection)

Pat Lawlor, Papers, 77-067-1/4

Parry, William Edward 1878–1952, 'The old and new order of things' by the Hon W. E. Parry, Minister of Internal Affairs, 17 November 1939, qMS-1629

R. A. Stothart Papers, MS-Papers-9096

Noeline Thomson Papers, MS-Papers 8312

YWCA Papers, MS-Group-0233

Hocken Library, University of Otago, Dunedin

Smithells Papers, MS 1001/1-40, ARC-0494

Family Collection

W. E. Parry, Papers, Memorabilia, Photograph Albums, Ciochetto Family, Auckland and Waipawa

State Records New South Wales, Sydney

Agency No. 1728

Series No. 15323 Minutes of the meetings of the National Fitness Council, and Series No. 15322 Minutes of meetings of the [National Fitness Council] Executive Committee, bound in same volume.

National Fitness Council, Policy Book, 11/19038

Bound selection of documents relating to National Fitness Council 1939–59

National Fitness Council, Precedent Book, c.1945–66, 11/19039

National Fitness Correspondence files

13/12206, 45/2/571

13/12206, 45/6N/605

13/12212, 50/NF30/8370

13/12209

13/12214, 51/NF3/8661 Commonwealth Posture Survey

44/6/11 Australian High Commission

5/5430 Sunday Sport, 1916-31

Accession A4135: Materials relating to National Fitness Council, New South Wales

Accession A4154: Materials relating to National Fitness Council, New South Wales

State Library New South Wales (Mitchell Library Collection), Sydney

Clark, F. Le Gros (ed.), *National Fitness: A Brief Essay on Contemporary Britain*, Macmillan, London, 1938

Health Brings Victory: Health, Milk and National Fitness Week, Sydney, 1941

National Fitness Newsletter, 1, 1 (October 1944)

The Problem of Recreation Space in the Metropolitan Area Sydney. Report of the National Fitness Council of New South Wales, May 1941, Sydney, 1941

National Archives of Australia, Canberra
Department of Health

A1928 (A1928/1) National Fitness, Seventh Session of Commonwealth National Fitness Council Section III, 21/10/43 – February 1944

A4639 (A4639/1) Fourth Menzies Ministry, Folders of Cabinet Submissions Commonwealth National Fitness Council – Appointment of Members

A9753 (A9753/1) National Fitness Council Articles and misc papers, 1945–46

A9753 (A9753/1) Victorian National Fitness Council – Minutes (duplicate copies) and Reports and Addresses

A9753 (A9753/1). 27. Victorian National Fitness Council – Minutes (duplicate copies), and Reports and Addresses

A11625 (A11625/1) Tasmania National Fitness Council

Australian War Memorial, Canberra
C.E.W.Bean Collection

AWM 38, 3DRL 6673/429 Papers Relating to National Fitness Council, New South Wales

AWM 27, 370/21 Correspondence with Dr J.H.L. Cumpston

City of Vancouver Archives, Vancouver
Pro-Rec photographs

Vancouver Women's Building Ltd. Year Book, 1922, Pam 1922-18

Vancouver Women's Building, Diary and Directory, 1943, Pam 1943-41

Newspapers and Periodicals
The Argus (Melbourne) 1936–1939
Barrier Miner (Broken Hill, New South Wales) 1939
Berliner Illustrite Zeitung (Berlin), 1936
Burra Record (Burra, South Australia) 1939
Dominion (Wellington) 1937
Dominion Post (Wellington) 2005
The Economist (London) 2011
Evening Post (Wellington) 1931–44
Evening Standard (London) 1937
Financial Times (London) 1937
The Gazette, Montreal (Montreal) 1948
Guardian (London) 2011
Morning Bulletin (Rockhampton, Queensland) 1937
The New Zealand Free Lance (Wellington) 1935–36
Physical Fitness (State Council for Physical Fitness, Sydney) 1939–40
Pix (Sydney) 1938–72
The Press (Christchurch) 2008

Radio Times (London) 1937–38
Sport in Industry (National Council of Sport in Industry and Commerce, London) 1938
Sun-Herald (Sydney) 1974
Sunday Pictorial (London) 1937
Sunday Sun and Guardian (Sydney) 1937
Sydney Morning Herald 1935–38
The Times (London) 1937–38
The West Australian (Perth) 1938

Government Parliamentary Papers
Appendices to the Journal of House of Representatives (AJHR) New Zealand
AJHR, H-22, Annual Reports, Department of Internal Affairs, 1935–60
Debates, House of Commons, Canada, 1943
Debates, Parliament of the Commonwealth of Australia, vol.167, 1941
Hansard, House of Commons Parliamentary Debates, 1937
Imperial Conference, 1937, Summary of Proceedings, Cmd 5482
New Zealand Parliamentary Debates, 1934–37
White Paper, *Physical Training and Recreation*, 1937, Cmd 5364 (UK)

Legislation
Australia
National Fitness Act, No.26 of 1941

Canada
An Act to establish a National Council for the purpose of promoting physical fitness (known as the National Physical Fitness Act), July 1943
Fitness and Amateur Sport Act 1961
An Act to Promote Physical Activity and Sport (LS-429E) 2002

New Zealand
Physical Welfare and Recreation Act 1937
Annual Holidays Amendment Act 1945 (9 Geo VI 1945 No. 20)
Recreation and Sport Act 1973
Sport, Fitness, and Leisure Act 1987 (no. 13)
Sport and Recreation New Zealand Act 2002 (no. 38)

UK
Physical Welfare and Recreation Act (1 Geo VI 1937 No.14)
Recreation and Sport Act 1973 (1973 No.36)
The Recreation and Sport Act 1987 (1987, No.13)

Films

A Little Slimming a Day – Keeps the Avoirdupois Away, Eve's Film Review, 14 April 1932

Barnett, Charles, *Health of the Nation*, National Progress Film Company, 1937

British Pathé <www.britishpathe.com>

Carter, Donald, *Strength and Beauty: Family Fitness*, Gaumont-British Instructional, 1937

___, *Strength and Beauty: Healthy Holidays*, Gaumont-British Instructional, 1937

___, *Strength and Beauty: Our Normal Day*, Gaumont-British Instructional, 1937

___, *Strength and Beauty: Pennies for Health*, Gaumont-British Instructional, 1937

Forlong, Michael, *Rhythm and Movement*, National Film Unit, Wellington, 1948

Grierson, Ruby and Ralph Bond, *Today We Live*, Strand Film Company, 1937

Horrocks, Shirley, *Dance of the Instant: The New Dance Group Wellington 1945–1947*, Point of View Productions, 2009

How to Drown, National Film Unit, Archives New Zealand, 1951

Hudson, Hugh, *Chariots of Fire*, Enigma Productions, 1981

If War Should Come, GPO Film Unit, 1939

Jennings, Humphrey, *Spare Time*, GPO Film Unit, 1939

Keep Fit, directed by Anthony Kimmins, producer Basil Dean, production company ATP, 1937, see <www.screenonline.org.uk/film/id/450755/index.html>, accessed 11 October 2010, <www.georgeformby.co.uk/films/fit/report.htm>, accessed 11 October 2010

King and Queen at the Festival of Youth, Pathé Gazette, 1937

Kimmins, Anthony, *Keep Fit*, ATP, 1937

Land of Promise: The British Documentary Movement 1930–1950, British Film Institute, 2008

'Making the Singlets', *Weekly Review*, 431, National Film Unit, 1949, RV701, Archives New Zealand [for 1950 Empire Games]

Physical Fitness: Government's Concern for the Nation, Pathé Gazette, 1936

'Recreation Centre', *Weekly Review*, 432, National Film Unit, RV701 1949

Rhythm and Movement, National Film Unit, 1948, Archives New Zealand

Scher, Len, *The Un-Canadians: True Stories of the Blacklist Era*, Film Board of Canada, 1996

Scotland for Fitness, directed by Brian Salt, G.B. Instructional Films, 1938, Scottish Screen Archive, National Library of Scotland

Screen Online <www.screenonline.org.uk>

Ward, Vincent, *Map of the Human Heart*, Australian Film Finance Corporation, 1993

Audio

King George VI speech launching the National Fitness Campaign, London, 17 February 1938, ICL 0067783 (BBC) AA1629, Sound Archive, British Library

King George VI speech opening Glasgow Empire Exhibition, May 1938, Sound Archive, British Library

Mezey, Edit, 'Health and Slimming Exercises for Use in the Home', arranged and spoken by Edit Mezey, HMV Catalogue, 1938–39, Sound Archive, British Library

Books and Articles – Primary

Apps, B. F. G., *The 1941 Keep Fit Book*, National Fitness Council of South Australia, 1941

___, 'The National Fitness Campaign After Five Years', *New Horizons in Education*, 4, 1 (July 1944), pp.21–25

Ashton, Beatrice, 'An Interview with Gisa Taglicht', *YWCA Review* [New Zealand], Vol.15 (1948), pp.2–4

Baldwin, Stanley, *A Call to the Nation: The Joint Manifesto of the Leaders of the National Government (Signed, Stanley Baldwin, J. Ramsay MacDonald, John Simon, 26th October, 1935)*, Burrup, Mathieson & Co, London, 1935

Beveridge, William, *Voluntary Action: A Report on Methods of Social Advance*, Allen & Unwin, London, 1948

Britain in the World of Sport: An Examination of the Factors Involved in Participation in Competitive International Sport, Prepared and assembled by the Physical Education Department, University of Birmingham, published by Physical Education Association of Great Britain and Northern Ireland, Birmingham, 1956

Bryden, J. T. and E. Hardy, 'Abolish the National Physical Fitness Undertaking?', *Effective Government*, 16 (November 1951), pp.1–5

Cassidy, Harry M., Untitled review, *American Economic Review*, 33, 3 (September 1943), pp.709–12.

Churchill, Winston, 'Sport is a Stimulant in our Workaday World', *News of the World*, 5 June 1938, p.12

Cruickshank, A. J. and Prunella Stack, *Movement is Life: The Intimate History of the Founder of the Women's League of Health and Beauty and of its Origin, Growth, Achievements, and Hopes for the Future*, Bell, London, 1937

Durant, Henry, *The Problem of Leisure*, Routledge, London, 1938

Eisenhardt, Ian, 'The Canadian Red Man of Today', *Journal of the American Association for Health, Physical Education and Recreation*, June 1951; pp.9–10

Greig, B. D. A. (ed.), *Tararua Story: Published in Commemoration of the Silver Jubilee of the Tararua Tramping Club, 1919–1944*, Tararua Tramping Club Inc., Wellington, 1946

Hauser, Bengamin Gayelor, *Eat and Grow Beautiful*, Faber & Faber, London, 1936

Health Brings Victory: Health, Milk and National Fitness Week, Waite & Bull, Sydney, 1941

Hodges, Frank, *Industrial Welfare: Its Place in our National Life Being a Speech Delivered at the Third Annual Conference of Welfare Supervisors at Balliol College on September 20ᵗʰ 1922*, published by Industrial Welfare Society, London, 1922

In Work or Play Fitness Wins – Twenty-four Ways of Keeping Fit, HMSO, London, 1938

Ingram, W. F., 'Panorama of the Playground: Physical Fitness and the "Daily Dozen"', *New Zealand Railways Magazine*, 11, 10 (January 1937), p.54

'Installation of the President', *Canadian Medical Association Journal*, 81 (15 July, 1959), pp.116–18

Kennedy, John F., 'Sport on the New Frontier: The Soft American', *Sports Illustrated*, 26 December 1960, pp.16–25

Lamb, A. S., 'National Physical Fitness: A Duty and an Opportunity', *Canadian Welfare*, 19, 8 (1 March 1944), pp.27–30

Le Fleming, E. K., *Report of the Physical Education Committee*, British Medical Association, London, 1936

Lucy, John F., *Keep Fit & Cheerful*, Pitman, London, 1937

'Margaret Morris Movement of Dancing and Physical Culture', *The New Zealand Girl*, April 1937, p.3

McMillan, David Gervan, *A National Health Service: New Zealand of Tomorrow*, NZ Worker, Wellington, 1934

Milligan, Sabra, *The Body and How to Keep Fit*, Premier Printing, Brighouse, 1934

Morris, Margaret, *Basic Physical Training*, W. Heinemann Ltd, London, 1937

___, *My Life in Movement,* Peter Owen, London, 1969

National Fitness – The First Steps, HMSO, London, 1937

Physical Education in Germany, pamphlet 109, Board of Education, HMSO, 1937

Physical Welfare and Recreation Branch, *Keep Fit by Morning Exercises: Exercises Broadcast by YA Stations at 7 a.m.,* Wellington, 1939

'Presidential Address to the British Medical Association', 28 October 1959, by H. R. H. The Prince Philip, Duke of Edinburgh, *British Medical Journal* (31 October 1959), pp.839–40

Recreation and Physical Fitness for Women and Girls, HMSO, London, 1937

Recreation and Physical Fitness for Youths and Men, HMSO, London, 1937

Report on the World Congress for Leisure Time and Recreation/Hamburg July 1936, Prepared by the International Central Bureau of Joy and Work, Hanseatische Verlagsanstalt, Hamburg, [1937]

Roberts, Harry, *The Practical Way to Keep Fit*, Odhams Press, London, 1939

Roper, R. E., *Movement and Thought*, Blackie, London, 1938

Russell, Bertrand, 'Philip Noel-Baker: A Tribute by Earl Russell', *International Relations*, 2, 1 (1960), pp.1–2

Smithells, Philip, 'Playing Down the Games', *Journal of Education,* 88, 1049 (December 1956), pp.517–19

___, *The Atlantic Gap: The Case for Better Understanding in Physical Education,* Dunedin, 1948

Sport and the Community: Report of the Wolfenden Committee on Sport, Central Council of Physical Recreation, London, 1961

Stack, Prunella, *Movement is Life: The Autobiography of Prunella Stack*, Harvill, London, 1973

Story, L. M., 'This "Keep Fit" Business', *The New Zealand Girl*, June 1939, pp.2–3

Sutton, C. Harvey, 'Physical Education and National Fitness', *Australian Rhodes Review*, 4 (1939), pp.56–62

'The Leisure of the Younger Worker', *International Labor Review*, 9, 6 (June 1924), pp.829–35

The National Fitness Campaign, National Fitness Council, London, 1939

Young, Gordon, 'National Fitness and the New Order', *Australian Quarterly,* 14, 1 (March 1942), pp.19–26

SECONDARY SOURCES

Books and Articles

Adair, Daryl and Wray Vamplew, *Sport in Australian History*, Oxford University Press, Melbourne, 1997

Alexander, Kristine, 'The Girl Guide Movement and Imperial Internationalism During the 1920s and

1930s', *Journal of the History of Childhood and Youth*, 2, 1 (2009), pp.37–63

Arnold, Trevor C., *Status and Influence of Sport and Physical Recreational Activities in British Columbia During the Depression and World War II*, University of British Columbia Press, Vancouver, 1973

Atkinson, Neill, *Trainland: How Railways Made New Zealand*, Random House, Auckland, 2007

Baker, Norman, 'Going to the Dogs: Hostility to Greyhound Racing in Britain: Puritanism, Socialism and Pragmatism', *Journal of Sport History*, 23, 2 (Summer 1996), pp.97–119

Balnave, Nikola, 'Company-sponsored Recreation in Australia: 1890–1965', *Labour History*, 85 (November 2003), pp.129–51

Banner, Lois W., *American Beauty*, University of Chicago Press, 1984

Baronowski, Shelley, 'A Family Vacation for Workers: The Strength through Joy Resort at Prora', *German History*, 25, 4 (2007), pp.539–59

___, *Strength Through Joy: Consumerism and Mass Tourism in the Third Reich*, Cambridge University Press, 2004

Barrowman, Rachel, *A Popular Vision: The Arts and the Left in New Zealand, 1930–1950*, Victoria University Press, Wellington, 1991

___, 'Heenan, Joseph, 1888–1951', from the *Dictionary of New Zealand Biography*, Te Ara – the Encyclopaedia of New Zealand, updated 1 September 2010, http://www.teara.govt.nz/en/biographies/4h24/1

___, *Victoria University of Wellington, 1899–1999: A History*, Victoria University Press, Wellington, 1999

Bashford, Alison and Philippa Levine (eds), *The Oxford Handbook to the History of Eugenics*, Oxford University Press, Oxford and New York, 2010

Bassett, Michael, *The Mother of All Departments: The History of the Department of Internal Affairs*, Auckland University Press in association with the Historical Branch, Department of Internal Affairs, Auckland, 1997

Bassett, Michael and Michael King, *Tomorrow Comes the Song: A Life of Peter Fraser*, Penguin, Auckland, 2001

Beaglehole, T. H., *A Life of J. C. Beaglehole*, Victoria University Press, Wellington, 2007

Beasley, A. W., 'Gillies, Alexander – Biography', from the *Dictionary of New Zealand Biography*, Te Ara – the Encyclopedia of New Zealand, updated 1 September 2010, http://www.teara.govt.nz/en/biographies/5g10/1

Beck, Peter, 'Britain and the Cold War's "Cultural Olympics": Responding to the Political Drive of Soviet Sport, 1945–58', *Contemporary British History*, 19, 2 (June 2005), pp.169–85

___, 'Confronting George Orwell: Philip Noel-Baker on International Sport, Particularly the Olympic Movement, as Peacemaker', *European Sports History Review*, 5 (2003), pp.187–207

___, *Scoring for Britain: International Football and International Politics, 1900–1939*, Frank Cass, London, 1999

Belich, James, *Paradise Reforged: A History of the New Zealanders, 1880–2000*, Penguin, Auckland, 2002

___, *Replenishing the Earth: The Settler Revolution and the Rise of the Anglo World, 1783–1939*, Oxford University Press, Oxford and New York, 2009

Beloff, Michael, 'Bennett, Sir Henry Honywood Curtis (1879–1936)', *Oxford Dictionary of National Biography*, Oxford University Press, first published 2004; online edn, January 2008

Berman, Marshall, *All That is Solid Melts into Air: The Experience of Modernity*, Simon and Schuster, New York, 1982

Beveridge, W. and J., *On and Off the Platform: Under the Southern Cross*, Hicks, Smith & Wright, Wellington and Melbourne, 1949

Bingham, Adrian, *Gender: Modernity and the Popular Press in Inter-war Britain*, Clarendon at Oxford University Press, 2004

Bloomfield, Anne, 'Drill and Dance as Symbols of Imperialism', in J. A. Mangan (ed.), *Making Imperial Mentalities*, Manchester University Press, 1990, pp. 74–96.

Bolwell, Jan, 'Memorial Celebration for the Life of Rona Bailey', *DANZ Quarterly*, 2 (December 2005), pp.10–11

Bonde, Han, *Gymnastics and Politics: Niels Bukh and Male Aesthetics*, Museum Tusculanum Press, Copenhagen, 2006

Bourdieu, Pierre, *Distinction*, English translation, Routledge, London, 1984

Bourke, Joanna, *Dismembering the Male: Men's Bodies, Britain and the Great War*, Reaktion Books, London, 1996

Boydell, Christine, 'Fashioning Identities: Gender, Class and the Self', *Journal of Contemporary History*, 39, 1 (January 2004), pp.137–46

Bradford, Sarah, *The Reluctant King: The Life and Reign of George VI 1895-1952*, St Martin's Press, New York, 1989

Branson, Noreen and Margot Heinemann, *Britain in the Nineteen Thirties*, Weidenfeld & Nicholson, London, 1971

Brendon, Piers, *The Dark Valley: A Panorama of the 1930s*, Vintage, New York, 2002

Breward, Christopher and Caroline Evans (eds), *Fashion and Modernity*, Berg, Oxford and New York, 2005

Bridge, Carl and Kent Fedorowich (eds), *The British World: Diaspora, Culture and Identity*, Frank Cass, London, 2003

Briggs, Asa, *The Golden Age of Wireless*, Oxford University Press, London, 1965

Britton, Sarah, '"Come and see the Empire by the all red route": Anti-imperialism and Exhibitions in Interwar Britain', *History Workshop Journal*, 69, 1 (Spring 2010), pp.68–89

Brookes, Barbara, 'Nostalgia for "Innocent Homely Pleasures": The 1964 New Zealand Controversy over *Washday at the Pa*', *Gender & History*, 9, 2 (1997), pp. 242–61

Broome, Richard, *Aboriginal Australians: A History Since 1788*, 4th edn, Allen & Unwin, Crows Nest, NSW, 2010

Brown, Callum G., 'Sport and the Scottish Office in the 20th Century: The Control of a Social Problem', *European Sports History Review* (1999), pp.164–82

___, 'Sport and the Scottish Office in the 20th Century: The Promotion of a Social and Gender Policy', *European Sports History Review* (1999), pp.183–202

___, *The Death of Christian Britain: Understanding Secularisation, 1800–2000*, Routledge, London and New York, 2000

Browne, Elspeth, 'Cuthbert Browne, Grace Johnston (1900–1988)', *Australian Dictionary of Biography*, Vol.17, Melbourne University Press, 1990, pp.288–9

Browne, Geoff, 'Weber, Ivy Lavinia (1892–1976)', *Australian Dictionary of Biography*, Vol.12, Melbourne University Press, 1990, pp.431–32

Buckner, Philip and R. Douglas Francis (eds), *Rediscovering the British World*, University of Calgary Press, 2005

Bulmer, Martin and Anthony M. Rees (eds), *Citizenship Today: The Contemporary Relevance of T. H. Marshall*, University College of London Press, 1996

Burman, Barbara and Carole Turbin, 'Material Strategies Engendered', *Gender & History*, 14, 3 (November 2002), pp.371–70

Campion, Edith, 'Maria Dronke, 1904–1987', in Charlotte Macdonald, Merimeri Penfold and Bridget Williams (eds), *The Book of New Zealand Women*, Bridget Williams Books, Wellington, 1991, pp.193–95

Cannadine, David, 'Empire', in *History in Our Time*, Yale University Press, New Haven and London, 1998, pp. 48–58 (first published in *Past & Present*, 147, May 1995)

Canning, Kathleen, *Gender History in Practice: Historical Perspectives on Bodies, Class and Citizenship*, Cornell University Press, Ithaca, 2006

___, 'The Body as Method? Reflections on the Place of the Body in Gender History', *Gender & History*, 11, 3 (November 1999), pp.499–513

Carden-Coyne, Ana, *Reconstructing the Body: Classicism, Modernism, and the First World War*, Oxford University Press, 2009

Cashman, R. I., 'Young, William Gordon (1904–1974)', *Australian Dictionary of Biography*, Vol.16, Melbourne University Press, 2002, pp.605–6

Cashman, Richard, *Paradise of Sport: A History of Australian Sport*, rev. ed., Walla Walla Press, Sydney, 2010

Cavanagh, Richard P., 'The Development of Canadian Sports Broadcasting 1920–78', *Canadian Journal of Communication*, 17, 3 (1992)

Cavell, Richard (ed.), *Love, Hate and Fear in Canada's Cold War*, University of Toronto Press, 2004

Chakrabarty, Dipesh, 'The Muddle of Modernity', *American Historical Review*, 116, 3 (June 2011), pp.663–75

Chapman, Robert, 'From Labour to National', in Geoffrey Rice (ed.), *The Oxford History of New Zealand*, 2nd edn, Auckland, 1992, pp.351–84

Clarke, Peter, *Hope and Glory: Britain 1900–1990*, Penguin, London, 1996

Clarsen, Georgine, *Eat My Dust: Early Women Motorists*, The John Hopkins University Press, Baltimore, 2008

Cleveland, Les, 'What They Liked: Movies and Modernity Downunder', *Journal of Popular Culture*, 36, 4 (2003), pp.756–79

Collins, Tony, 'Review Article: Work, Rest and Play: Recent Trends in the History of Sport and Leisure', *Journal of Contemporary History*, 42, 2 (2007), pp.397–410

Colquhoun, David (ed.), *As if Running on Air: The Journals of Jack Lovelock*, Craig Potton Publishing, Nelson, 2008

Conekin, Becky E., '"Magazines are essentially about the here and now. And this was wartime": British Vogue's Responses to the Second World War', in Philippa Levine and Susan Grayzel (eds), *Gender, Labour, War and Empire: Essays on Modern Britain*, Palgrave Macmillan, Basingstoke, 2009, pp.116–38

Conekin, Becky, Frank Mort and Chris Waters (eds), *Moments of Modernity: Reconstructing Britain 1945-1964*, Rivers Oram Press, London, 1999

Coney, Sandra, Every Girl: A Social History of Women and the YWCA in Auckland 1885–1985, YWCA, Auckland, 1986

Connell, Sean, 'Gender and the Car in Interwar Britain', in Moira Donald and Linda Hurcombe (eds), Gender and Material Culture in Historical Perspective, Palgrave MacMillan, Basingstoke, 2000, pp.175–91

Connell, W. F., 'Browne, George Stephenson (1890–1970)', Australian Dictionary of Biography, Vol.13, Melbourne University Press, 1993, pp.278–80

Conor, Liz, The Spectacular Modern Woman: Feminine Visibility in the Twenties, Indiana University Press, Bloomington, 2004

Constantine, Stephen (ed.), Emigrants and Empire: British Settlement in the Dominions Between the Wars, Manchester University Press, 1990

Corner, Margaret, No Easy Victory: Towards Equal Pay for Women in the Government Service 1890–1960, New Zealand Public Service Association and Dan Long Trust, Wellington, 1988

Crawford, John and James Watson, '"The most appeasing line": New Zealand and Nazi Germany, 1935–40', Journal of Imperial and Commonwealth History, 38, 1 (March 2010), pp.75–97

Crozier, Andrew J., 'Chamberlain, (Arthur) Neville (1869–1940)', Oxford Dictionary of National Biography, Oxford University Press, first published 2004; online edn, January 2008

Curran, James and Stuart Ward, The Unknown Nation: Australia After Empire, Melbourne University Press, 2010

Daley, Caroline, Leisure and Pleasure: Reshaping and Revealing the New Zealand Body, Auckland University Press, 2003

___, 'The Body Builder and Beauty Contests', Journal of Australian Studies, 25, 71 (2001), pp.55–66

Daunton, Martin and Bernhard Rieger (eds), Meanings of Modernity: Britain from the Late-Victorian Era to World War II, Berg, Oxford and New York, 2001

Dawson, Sandra, 'Working-class Consumers and the Campaign for Holidays with Pay', Twentieth Century British History, 18, 3 (2007), pp.277–305

Day, Patrick, The Radio Years: History of Broadcasting in New Zealand, Auckland University Press, 1994

de Grazia, Victoria, How Fascism Ruled Women: Italy 1920–45, University of California Press, Berkeley, 1992

___, The Culture of Consent: Mass Organization of Leisure in Fascist Italy, Cambridge University Press, 1981

Deacon, Desley and Joy Damousi (eds), Talking and Listening in the Age of Modernity, ANU Press, Canberra, 2007

Dennis, Jonathan, Irihapeti Ramsden and Patricia Grace (eds), The Silent Migration: Ngati Poneke Young Maori Club 1937–1948, Huia Publishing, Wellington, 2002

Dirlik, Arif, 'The Ideological Foundations of the New Life Movement: A Study in Counter Revolution', Journal of Asian Studies, 34, 4 (August 1975), pp.945–80

Donovan, Paul, 'Quigley, Janet Muriel Alexander (1902–1987)', Oxford Dictionary of National Biography, Oxford University Press, first published 2004; online edn, January 2008

Dow, Derek, 'Hercus, Charles Ernest – Biography', from the Dictionary of New Zealand Biography, Te Ara – the Encyclopedia of New Zealand, updated 1 September 2010, http://www.teara.govt.nz/en/biographies/4h28/1

___, Safeguarding the Public Health, Victoria University Press, Wellington, 1995

Dutton, David, Neville Chamberlain, Arnold, London, 2000

Dutton, Kenneth, The Perfectible Body, Continuum, London, 1997

Eichberg, Henning (John Bale and Chris Philo, eds), Body Cultures: Essays on Sport, Space, and Identity, Routledge, London, 1998

Eley, Geoff, A Crooked Line: From Cultural History to the History of Society, University of Michigan Press, Ann Arbor, 2005

Elson, Peter F., 'The Great White North and Voluntary Action: Canada's Relationship with Beveridge, Social Welfare, and Social Justice', in Melanie Oppenheimer and Nicholas Deakin (eds), Beveridge and Voluntary Action in Britain and the Wider British World, Manchester University Press, 2010, pp.166–186

Erdozain, Dominic, The Problem of Pleasure: Sport, Recreation and the Crisis of Victorian Religion, Boydell Press, Woodbridge, 2010

Evans, H. Justin, Service to Sport: The Story of the CCPR 1935–1972, Pelham Books in association with the Sports Council, London, 1974

Ewens, Wilf, Gordon Young: A Man of Inspiration, Australian Council for Health, Physical Education and Recreation, Croydon, 1994

Felski, Rita, The Gender of Modernity, Harvard University Press, Cambridge, 1995

Fields, Jill, '"Fighting the corsetless evil": Shaping Corsets and Culture, 1900–1930', Journal of Social History, 33, 2 (Winter 1999), pp.355–84

Fischer, Imke, 'The Involvement of the Commonwealth Government in Physical Education: From Defence to National Fitness', in R. Cashman, J. O'Hara and A. Honey (eds), *Sport, Federation, Nation*, Walla Walla Press, Sydney, 2001, pp.16–25

Fitzgerald, Robert, *British Labour Management and Industrial Welfare 1846–1939*, Croom Helm, London, 1988

Fletcher, Sheila, *Women First: The Female Tradition in English Physical Education, 1880–1980*, Athlone Press, London, 1984

Foot, Michael, *Aneurin Bevan: A Biography*, 2 volumes, Macgibbon & Kee, London, 1962–73

Forsyth, Janice, 'The Indian Act and the (Re) shaping of Canadian Aboriginal Sport Practices', *International Journal of Canadian Studies*, 35 (Spring 2007), pp.95–111

Forsyth, Janice and Michael Heine, '"A Higher Degree of Social Organization": Jan Eisenhardt and Canadian Aboriginal Sport Policy in the 1950s', *Journal of Sport History*, 35, 2 (Summer 2008), pp.261–77

Frederick, W. H., 'Brookes, Sir Norman Everard 1877–1968', *Australian Dictionary of Biography*, Melbourne University Press, 1979

Fry, Ruth, '"Don't let down the side": Physical Education in the Curriculum for New Zealand Schoolgirls, 1900–1945', in Barbara Brookes, Charlotte Macdonald and Margaret Tennant (eds), *Women in History*, Allen & Unwin, Wellington, 1986, pp.101–18

Fusco, Caroline, 'Cultural Landscapes of Purification: Sports Spaces and Discourses of Whiteness', *Sociology of Sport Journal*, 22, 3 (September 2005), pp.283–310

Gammage, Bill and Peter Spearritt (eds), with oral history co-ordinator Louise Douglas, *Australians 1938*, Fairfax, Syme & Weldon, Broadway, NSW, 1987

Gardiner, Juliet, *The Thirties: An Intimate History*, HarperPress, London, 2010

Garton, Stephen, 'Eugenics', in Graeme Davison, John Hirst and Stuart Macintyre (eds), *The Oxford Companion to Australian History*, Oxford University Press, Melbourne, 1998, pp.228–9

___, 'Eugenics in Australia and New Zealand: Laboratories of Racial Science', in Alison Bashford and Philippa Levine (eds), *The Oxford Handbook of the History of Eugenics*, Oxford University Press, Oxford and New York, 2010, pp.243–44

Gear, James L., 'Factors Influencing the Development of Government Sponsored Physical Fitness Programmes in Canada from 1850 to 1972', *Canadian Journal of the History of Sport and Physical Education*, 4, 2 (1973), pp.1–25

Gibbons, Stella, *Cold Comfort Farm*, Longman, London, 1932

Giddens, Anthony, *Modernity and Self-identity*, Polity, Cambridge, 1991

Gilbert, Martin, *Britain Between the Wars*, Longmans, London, 1964

Gillespie, Jim, 'Cumpston, John Howard Lidgett (1880–1954)', in Graeme Davison, John Hirst and Stuart Macintyre (eds), *Oxford Companion to Australian History*, Oxford University Press, Melbourne, 1998, pp.167

Godber, George, *The Health Service: Past, Present, Future*, Athlone Press, London, 1975

Gori, Gigliola, 'A Glittering Icon of Fascist Femininity: Trebisonda "Ondina" Valla', *International Journal of the History of Sport*, 18, 1 (March 2001), pp.173–95

___, *Italian Fascism and the Female Body*, Routledge, London, 2004

Government Schools of New South Wales 1848–2003, Department of Education and Training, 2003

Grant, David, *On a Roll: A History of Gambling and Lotteries in New Zealand*, Victoria University Press, Wellington, 1994

Grant, Mariel, *Propaganda and the Role of the State in Inter-war Britain*, Clarendon Press, Oxford, 1994

___, 'The National Health Campaigns of 1937–1938', in Derek Fraser (ed.), *Cities, Class and Communication: Essays in Honour of Asa Briggs*, Harvester Wheatsheaf, London, 1990, pp.216–33

Graves, Robert and Alan Hodge, *The Long Weekend: A Social History of Great Britain 1918–1939*, Faber, London, 1940

Gray, R. K., *The First Forty Years: The National Fitness and Community Recreation Councils of Western Australia, 1939–1978*, Department for Youth, Sport and Recreation, Perth, 1982

Griffin, Roger, *Modernism and Fascism: The Sense of a Beginning under Mussolini and Hitler*, Palgrave Macmillan, Basingstoke, 2007

Grundlingh, Albert, '"Gone to the dogs": The Cultural Politics of Gambling – The Rise and Fall of British Greyhound Racing on the Witwatersrand, 1932–1949', in Lance Van Sittert and Sandra Swart (eds), *Canis Africanis: A Dog History of Southern Africa*, Brill, Leiden, 2008, pp.217–34

Guha, Ramachandra, *Corner of a Foreign Field: The Indian History of a British Sport*, Picador, London, 2002

Gush, Nadia, 'The Beauty of Health: Cora Wilding and the Sunlight League', *New Zealand Journal of History*, 43, 1 (2009), pp.1–17

Gustafson, Barry, 'Parry, William Edward – Biography', from the *Dictionary of New Zealand Biography*, Te Ara – the Encyclopedia of New Zealand, updated 1 September 2010, http://www.teara.govt.nz/en/biographies/3p12/1

Hall, Catherine (ed.), *Cultures of Empire: Colonizers in Britain and the Empire in the Nineteenth and Twentieth Centuries: A Reader*, Routledge, New York, 2000

Hall, Catherine and Sonya O. Rose (eds), *At Home with the Empire: Metropolitan Culture and the Imperial World*, Cambridge University Press, 2006

Hall, Fiona, 'New Zealand Women's Bowling Association 1948–', in Anne Else (ed.), *Women Together: A History of Women's Organisations in New Zealand: Ngā Rōpū Wāhine o Te Motu*, Daphne Brasell Associates Press/Historical Branch, Department of Internal Affairs, Wellington, 1993, pp.440–2

Hall, Lesley, *Sex, Gender and Social Change in Britain Since 1880*, Macmillan, Basingstoke, 2000

Hall, Margaret Ann, *The Girl and the Game: A History of Women's Sport in Canada*, Broadview Press, Peterborough, 2002

Hallowell, Gerald (ed.), *The Oxford Companion to Canadian History*, Oxford University Press, 2004

Halse, Christine, 'Bio-citizenship: Virtue Discourses and the Birth of the Bio-citizen', in Jan Wright and Valerie Harwood (eds), *Biopolitics and the 'Obesity Epidemic': Governing Bodies*, Routledge, New York and London, 2009, pp.45–59

Hansen, Peter H., 'Modern Mountains', in Martin Daunton and Bernhard Rieger (eds), *Meanings of Modernity: Britain from the Late-Victorian Era to World War II*, Berg, Oxford and New York, 2001, pp.185–202

Hanson, Elizabeth, *The Politics of Social Security: The 1938 Act and Some Later Developments*, Auckland University Press, 1980

Hargreaves, Jennifer, *Sporting Females: Critical Issues in the History and Sociology of Women's Sports*, Routledge, London, 1994

Hargreaves, Jennifer and Patricia Vertinsky (eds), *Physical Culture, Power and the Body*, Routledge, London, 2007

Hargreaves, John, *Sport, Power and Culture: A Social and Historical Analysis of Popular Sports in Britain*, Polity Press, Cambridge, 1987

Harper, Melissa, *The Ways of the Bushwalker: On Foot in Australia*, University of New South Wales Press, Sydney, 2007

Harris, Aroha, 'Concurrent Narratives of Māori and Integration in the 1950s and 60s', *Journal of New Zealand Studies* (2008), pp.139–55

___, *Hikoi: Forty Years of Maori Protest*, Huia Publishing, Wellington, 2004

Harris, Jose, 'Voluntarism, the State, and Public–Private Partnerships in Beveridge's Social Thought', in Melanie Oppenheimer and Nicholas Deakin (eds), *Beveridge and Voluntary Action in the Wider British World*, Manchester University Press, 2010, pp.9–20

Harvey, Jean, 'The Role of Sport and Recreation Policy in Fostering Citizenship: The Canadian Experience', Canadian Policy Research Networks, Ottawa, 2001

Hau, Michael, *The Cult of Health and Beauty in Germany: A Social History, 1890–1930*, University of Chicago Press, 2003

Hempenstall, Peter, 'Burgmann, Ernest Henry (1885–1967)', *Australian Dictionary of Biography*, Vol.13, Melbourne University Press, 1993, pp.300–1

Heydon, Susan, 'McMillan, David Gervan – Biography' from the *Dictionary of New Zealand Biography*, Te Ara – the Encyclopedia of New Zealand, updated 1 September 2010, http://www.teara.govt.nz/en/biographies/4m25/1

Higgs, Edward, 'Leisure and the State: The History of Popular Culture as Reflected in the Public Records', *History Workshop Journal*, 15, 1 (Spring 1983), pp.141–50

Hilliard, Chris, *The Bookmen's Dominion*, Auckland University Press, 2006

Hilton, Matthew, *Smoking in British Popular Culture, 1800–2000: Perfect Pleasures*, Manchester University Press, 2000

Hirsch, Pam, 'Morris, Margaret Eleanor (1891–1980)' *Oxford Dictionary of National Biography*, Oxford University Press, first published 2004; online edn, January 2008

Hokowhitu, Brendan, 'Physical Beings: Stereotypes, Sport and the "Physical Education" of New Zealand Maori', in J. A. Mangan and A. Ritchie (eds), *Culture, Sport, Society*, Frank Cass, London, 2004, pp.192–218

Holt, Richard, *Sport and the British: A History*, Oxford University Press, 1989

Holt, Richard and Tony Mason, *Sport in Britain Since 1945*, Wiley-Blackwell, Oxford, 2000

Howell, David, 'Baker, Philip John Noel-, Baron Noel-Baker (1889–1982)', *Oxford Dictionary of National Biography*, Oxford University Press, first published 2004; online edn, January 2008

Huggins, Mike and Jack Williams, *Sport and the*

English, 1918–1939, Routledge, London and New York, 2006

Hughes, Thea Stanley, *Towards Self-development*, self-published, Sydney, 1976

___, *Towards Social Health*, Movement Publications, London and Sydney, 1979

Hunter, Kathryn M., 'Rough Riding: Aboriginal Participation in Rodeos and Travelling Shows to the 1950s', *Aboriginal History*, 32 (2008), pp.82–96

Inglis, K. S., 'Bean Charles Edwin Woodrow (1879–1968)', *Australian Dictionary of Biography*, Vol.7, Melbourne University Press, 1979, pp.226–29

Jackson Lears, T. J., 'From Salvation to Self-realisation: Advertising and the Therapeutic Roots of the Consumer Culture, 1800–1930', in Richard Wightman Fox and T. J. Jackson Lears (eds), *The Culture of Consumption: Critical Essays in American History, 1880–1980*, Pantheon, New York, 1983, pp.3–38, 213–18

James, C. L. R., *Beyond a Boundary*, Hutchinson, London, 1963

Johnson, Lesley, 'Wireless', in Bill Gammage and Peter Spearritt (eds), and oral history co-ordinator Louise Douglas, *Australians 1938*, Fairfax, Syme & Weldon Associates, Broadway, NSW, 1987, pp.365–72

Jones, Stephen G., *Sport, Politics and the Working Class: Organised Labour and Sport in Inter-war Britain*, Manchester University Press, 1988

___, 'State Intervention in Sport Between the Wars', *Journal of Contemporary History*, 22 (1987), pp.163–82

___, 'The British Workers' Sports Federation: 1923–1936', in Arnd Kruger and James Riordan (eds), *The Story of Worker Sport*, Human Kinetics, Champaign, 1996, pp.97–115

___, *Workers at Play: A Social and Economic History of Leisure, 1918–1939*, Routledge, London, 1986

Judd, Denis, *King George VI: 1895–1952*, Michael Joseph, London, 1982

Judt, Tony, *Postwar: A History of Europe Since 1945*, Penguin, New York, 2005

Kenny, Nicolas, 'From Body and Home to Nation and World: The Varying Scales of Transnational Urbanism in Montreal and Brussels at the Turn of the Twentieth Century', *Urban History*, 36, 3 (July 2009), pp.223–42

Kentish, Gertrude F., 'Duras, Fritz (1896–1965)', *Australian Dictionary of Biography*, Vol.14, Melbourne University Press, 1996, p.61

Keys, Barbara, *Globalizing Sport*, Harvard University Press, Cambridge, 2006

___, 'The Body as a Political Space: Comparing Physical Education under Nazism and Stalinism', *German History*, 27, 3 (July 2009), pp.395–413

Kidd, Bruce, *The Struggle for Canadian Sport*, University of Toronto Press, 1996

___, *Tom Longboat*, Fitzhenry & Whiteside, Markham, 2004

King, Michael, 'Between Two Worlds', in G. W. Rice (ed.), *Oxford History of New Zealand*, 2nd edn, Oxford University Press, Auckland, 1992

___, *The Penguin History of New Zealand*, Penguin, Auckland, 2003

Kingsley Kent, Susan, *Making Peace: The Reconstruction of Gender in Interwar Britain*, Princeton University Press, New Jersey, 1993

Kinsman, Gary, Dieter K. Buse and Mercedes Steedman (eds), *Whose National Security? Canadian State Surveillance and the Creation of Enemies*, Between the Lines, Toronto, 2000

Kirk, David, *Schooling Bodies: School Practice and Public Discourse 1880–1950*, Leicester University Press, London and Washington, 1998

___, 'Schooling Bodies through Physical Education: Insights from Social Epistemology and Curriculum History', *Studies in Philosophy and Education*, 20 (2001), pp.475–87

Kirkham, Pat, 'Fashioning the Feminine: Dress, Appearance and Femininity in Wartime Britain', in Christine Gledhill and Gillian Swanson (eds), *Nationalising Femininity: Culture, Sexuality and British Cinema in the Second World War*, Manchester University Press, 1996, pp.152–74.

Knott, John, 'Speed, Modernity and the Motor Car: The Making of the 1909 Motor Traffic Act in New South Wales', *Australian Historical Studies*, 26, 103 (October 1994), pp.221–41

___, '"The Conquering Car": Technology, Symbolism and the Motorisation of Australia before World War II', *Australian Historical Studies*, 31, 114, (April 2000), pp.1–26

Kracauer, Siegfried, *The Mass Ornament: Weimar Essays*, Harvard University Press, Cambridge, 1995

Kruger, Arnd, 'Strength Through Joy: The Culture of Consent Under Fascism, Nazism and Francoism', in James Riordan and Arnd Kruger (eds), *The International Politics of Sport in the Twentieth Century*, Spon Press, London, 1999, pp.67–89

Kruger, Arnd and James Riordan (eds), *The Story of Worker Sport*, Human Kinetics, Champaign, 1996, pp.1–25

Labrum, Bronwyn, Fiona McKergow and Stephanie Gibson (eds), *Looking Flash: Clothing in Aotearoa New Zealand*, Auckland University Press, 2007

Lake, M., K. Holmes and P. Grimshaw (eds), Women's Rights and Human Rights: International Historical Perspectives, Macmillan, Basingstoke, 2001

Lake, Marilyn, *Faith: Faith Bandler, Gentle Activist*, Allen & Unwin, Sydney, 2003

Lake, Marilyn and Henry Reynolds, *Drawing the Global Colour Line: White Men's Countries and the Question of Racial Equality*, Melbourne University Publishing, Carlton, 2008

Lang, Tup, 'Gisa Taglicht, ?1898-1981', in Charlotte Macdonald, Merimeri Penfold and Bridget Williams (eds), *The Book of New Zealand Women*, Bridget Williams Books, Wellington, 1991, pp.648-50

Langhamer, Claire, *Women's Leisure in England 1920-1960*, Manchester University Press, 2000

Lawrence, Christopher and George Weisz (eds), *Greater than the Parts: Holism in Biomedicine, 1920-1950*, Oxford University Press, New York and Oxford, 1998

Levine, Philippa, *The British Empire: Sunrise to Sunset*, Pearson Longman, Harlow, 2007

Lewis, Jane and Barbara Brookes, 'The Peckham Health Centre, "Pep", and the Concept of General Practice During the 1930s and 1940s', *Medical History*, 27, 2 (April 1983), pp.151-61

Light, Alison, *Forever England: Femininity, Literature, and Conservatism Between the Wars*, Routledge, London, 1991

Lowerson, John, 'Battles for the Countryside', in F. Gloversmith (ed.), *Class, Culture and Social Change: A New View of the 1930s*, Harvester, Brighton, 1980, pp.258-80

____, 'Starting from Your Own Past?: The Serious Business of Leisure History', *Journal of Contemporary History*, 36, 3 (July 2001), pp.517-29

Lynch, Pip, 'The Origins of Outdoor Education in New Zealand: Progressive Liberalism and Post-war Rejuvenation, 1935-1965', *New Zealand Physical Educator*, 36, 1 (May 2003), pp.63-81

Macdonald, Charlotte, 'Body and Self: Learning to be Modern in 1920s-30s Britain', *Women's History Review*, 21, 5, 2012 (forthcoming)

____, 'Emily's Dream: A Women's Memorial Building and a History Without Walls. Citizenship and the Politics of Public Remembrance in 1930s-40s New Zealand', in M. Lake, K. Holmes and P. Grimshaw (eds), *Women's Rights and Human Rights: International Historical Perspectives*, Macmillan, London, 2001, pp.168-83

____, 'Marching Teams and Modern Girls: Bodies and Culture in Interwar New Zealand', in Paula Birnbaum and Anna Novakov (eds), *Essays on Women's Artistic and Cultural Contributions 1919-1939: Expanded Social Roles for the New Woman Following the First World War*, Edwin Mellen Press, Lewiston, 2009, pp.23-36

____, 'Moving in Unison, Dressing in Uniform: Stepping Out in Style With Marching Teams', in Bronwyn Labrum, Fiona McKergow and Stephanie Gibson (eds), *Looking Flash: Clothing in Aotearoa New Zealand*, Auckland University Press, 2007, pp.186-205

____, 'Putting Bodies on the Line: Marching Spaces in Cold War Culture', in Patricia Vertinsky and John Bale (eds), *Sites of Sport: Space, Place, Experience*, Routledge, London, 2004, pp.85-100

____, 'The Unbalanced Parallel', in Anne Else (ed.), *Women Together: A History of Women's Organisations in New Zealand: Ngā Rōpū Wāhine o Te Motu*, Daphne Brasell Associates Press/ Historical Branch, Department of Internal Affairs, Wellington, 1993, pp.402-16

____, 'Ways of Belonging: Sporting Spaces in New Zealand History', in Giselle Byrnes (ed.), *The New Oxford History of New Zealand*, Oxford University Press, Melbourne, 2009, pp.269-96

____, 'Women and Girls, Men and Boys', *Te Ara: online encyclopedia of New Zealand*, <www.teara.govt.nz>

Macintosh, Donald, Tom Bedecki and C. E. S. Franks, *Sport and Politics in Canada: Federal Government Involvement Since 1961*, McGill-Queen's University Press, Montreal, 1988

Macintyre, Stuart, *A Concise History of Australia*, Cambridge University Press, 1999

MacKenzie, John M. (ed.), *Imperialism and Popular Culture*, Manchester University Press, 1986

____, '"In touch with the infinite": The BBC and the Empire, 1923-53', in John M. MacKenzie (ed.), *Imperialism and Popular Culture*, Manchester University Press, 1986, pp.165-91

Maclagan, Michael, 'Bruce, Clarence Napier, Third Baron Aberdare (1885-1957)', *Oxford Dictionary of National Biography*, Oxford University Press, first published 2004; online edn, January 2008

Maclean, Chris, *John Pascoe*, Craig Potton Publishing in association with the Whitcombe Press, Nelson, 2003

Macrae, Elidh, '"Scotland for Fitness": The National Fitness Campaign and Scottish Women', *Women's History Magazine*, 62 (Spring 2010), pp.26-36

Maioni, Antonia, 'Nothing Succeeds Like the Right Kind of Failure: Postwar National Health Insurance Initiatives in Canada and the United States', *Journal of Health Politics, Policy and*

Law, 20, 1 (Spring 1995), pp.5–30

Mandell, Richard D., *The Nazi Olympics*, MacMillan, New York, 1971 (reissued University of Illinois Press, Urbana, 1987)

Mangan, J. A. (ed.), *Making Imperial Mentalities*, Manchester University Press, 1990

___ (ed.), *Shaping the Superman: Fascist Body as Political Icon – Aryan Fascism*, Frank Cass, London, 1999

___ (ed.), *The Cultural Bond: Sport, Empire, Society*, Frank Cass, London, 1992

Markham-Starr, Susan, '"Canada Needs You": The Jan Eisenhardt Story', paper presented to Eleventh Congress on Leisure Research, 17–20 May 1995, Canadian Association for Leisure Studies, 2005

Marshall, T. H., *Citizenship and Social Class and Other Essays*, Cambridge University Press, 1950

Martin, John, *Holding the Balance: A History of the Department of Labour 1891–1995*, Canterbury University Press, Christchurch, 1996

Mason, Tony, '"Hunger ... is a very good thing": Britain in the 1930s', in Nick Tiratsoo (ed.), *From Blitz to Blair: A New History of Britain Since 1939*, Weidenfeld & Nicolson, London, 1997, pp.1–24

Matless, David, '"The Art of Right Living": Landscape and Citizenship, 1918–1939', in Steve Pile and Nigel Thrift (eds), *Mapping the Subject: Geographies of Cultural Transformation*, Routledge, London, 1995, pp.93–122

Matthews, Jill Julius, 'Building the Body Beautiful', *Australian Feminist Studies*, 2, 5 (Summer 1987), pp.17–34

___, *Dance Hall to Picture Palace: Sydney's Romance with Modernity*, Currency Press, Sydney, 2005

___, '"They had such a lot of fun": The Women's League of Health and Beauty Between the Wars', *History Workshop Journal*, 30, 1 (1990), pp.22–54

Mazower, Mark, *Dark Continent: Europe's Twentieth Century*, Vintage, New York, 1998

McClure, Margaret, *The Wonder Country: Making New Zealand Tourism*, Auckland University Press, 2004

McEldowney, Dennis, 'Smithells, Philip Ashton 1910–1977', from the *Dictionary of New Zealand Biography* (DNZB), Te Ara – the Encyclopaedia of New Zealand, updated 1 September 2010, <http://www.teara.govt.nz/en/biographies/5s31/1>

McGibbon, Ian, 'Berendsen, Carl August', from the *Dictionary of New Zealand Biography*, Te Ara – the Encyclopedia of New Zealand, updated 1 September 2010, http://www.teara.govt.nz/en/biographies/4b25

McGibbon, Ian, with assistance of Paul Goldstone (eds), *The Oxford Companion to New Zealand Military History*, Oxford University Press, Auckland, 2000

McIntosh, Peter C., *Physical Education in England since 1800*, Bell, London, 1952 (rev and enlarged edn, 1968)

McIntyre, W. David, *New Zealand Prepares for War: Defence Policy, 1919–1939*, Canterbury University Press, Christchurch, 1988

McKibbin, Ross, *Classes and Cultures: England 1918–1951*, Oxford University Press, 1998

McMillan, N. A. C., 'Blomfield, Meynell Strathmore – Biography', from the *Dictionary of New Zealand Biography*, Te Ara – the Encyclopedia of New Zealand, updated 1 September 2010, http://www.teara.govt.nz/en/biographies/4b40/1

McPhail, Deborah, 'What to do with the "tubby hubby"? Obesity, the Crisis of Masculinity, and the Nuclear Family in Early Cold War Canada', *Antipode*, 41, 5 (November 2009), pp.1021–50

McQuarrie, Fiona A. E., 'The Struggle Over Worker Leisure: An Analysis of the History of the Workers' Sports Association of Canada', *Canadian Journal of Administrative Sciences*, 27, 4 (2010), pp.391–402

McWhirter, Norris, 'Cecil, David George Brownlow, Sixth Marquess of Exeter (1905–1981)', *Oxford Dictionary of National Biography*, Oxford University Press, first published 2004; online edn, October 2005

Metge, Joan, *A New Maori Migration: Urban and Rural Relations in Northern New Zealand*, Athlone Press, London, 1964

Mitchell, Austin, *The Half-gallon, Quarter Acre, Pavlova Paradise*, Whitcombe & Tombs, Christchurch, 1972

Moore, Katharine, '"The Warmth of Comradeship": The First British Empire Games and Imperial Solidarity', in J. A. Mangan (ed.), *The Cultural Bond*, Frank Cass, London, 1992, pp.201–8

Morgan, Philip, *Fascism in Europe, 1919–1945*, Routledge, London, 2002

Morrow, Don, Mary Keyes, Wayne Simpson, Frank Cosentino and Ron A. Lappage, *A Concise History of Sport in Canada*, Oxford University Press, Toronto, 1989

Mowat, Charles Loch, *Britain Between the Wars 1918–1940*, Methuen, London, 1955

Nelson, Mariah Burton, *The Stronger Women Get, the More Men Love Football: Sexism and the American Culture of Sports*, Harcourt Brace, New York, 1994

Nugent, Maria, *Botany Bay: Where Histories Meet*, Allen & Unwin, Crows Nest, NSW, 2005

Nye, Robert, 'Degeneration, Neurasthenia and the Culture of Sport in *belle époque* France', *Journal of Contemporary History*, 17, 1 (1982), pp.51–68

O'Donoghue, Thomas A., 'Sport, Recreation and Physical Education: The Evolution of a National Policy of Regeneration in Eire, 1926–48', *British Journal of Sports History*, 3, 2 (1986), pp.216–33

Ofer, Inbal, 'Am I that Body? Seccion Femenina de la Fet and the Struggle for the Institution of Physical Education and Competitive Sports for Women in Franco's Spain', *Journal of Social History*, 39, 4 (Summer 2006), pp.989–1010

O'Hagan, Sean, *The Pride of Southern Rebels: On the Occasion of the Otago Rugby Football Union Centenary, 1881–1981*, Pilgrims South Press, Dunedin, 1981

Oliver, W. H. with B. R. Williams (eds), *The Oxford History of New Zealand*, Oxford University Press, Wellington, 1981

Oppenheimer, Melanie, *Volunteering: Why We Can't Survive Without It*, University of New South Wales Press, Sydney, 2008

Oppenheimer, Melanie and Nicholas Deakin (eds), *Beveridge and Voluntary Action in the Wider British World*, Manchester University Press, 2010

Orange, Claudia, *The Treaty of Waitangi*, Allen & Unwin, Wellington, 1987

Orwell, George, *Books v. Cigarettes*, Penguin, Great Ideas Collection, London, 2008

Palenski, Ron, 'Cross, Cecil Lancelot Stewart – Biography', from the *Dictionary of New Zealand Biography*, Te Ara – the Encyclopedia of New Zealand, updated 1 September 2010, http://www.teara.govt.nz/en/biographies/5c47/1

Park, Julie (ed.), *Ladies a Plate: Change and Continuity in the Lives of New Zealand Women*, Auckland University Press, 1991

Pascoe, John, *Land Uplifted High*, Whitcombe & Tombs, Christchurch, 1952

Passmore, Kevin, *Fascism: A Very Short Introduction*, Oxford University Press, 2002

Paulicelli, Eugenia, *Fashion Under Fascism: Beyond the Black Shirt*, Berg, Oxford, 2004

Paulicelli, Eugenia and Hazel Clark (eds), *The Fabric of Cultures: Fashion, Identity and Globalization*, Routledge, Oxford, 2009

Peiss, Kathy, *Hope in a Jar: The Making of America's Beauty Culture*, Harvey Holt, New York, 1998

Pemberton, John, 'The Boyd Orr Survey of the Nutrition of Children in Great Britain 1937–9', *History Workshop Journal*, 50 (Autumn 2000), pp.205–29

Phillips, Jock, *A Man's Country*, Penguin, Auckland, 1987

Pickering, Mark, *Huts*, Canterbury University Press, Christchurch, 2010

Pickles, Katie, *Female Imperialism and National Identity: Imperial Order Daughters of the Empire*, Manchester University Press, Manchester and New York, 2002

Pitt, D. C., 'The Joiners: Associations and Leisure in New Zealand', in S. D. Webb and J. Collette (eds), *New Zealand Society: Contemporary Perspectives*, John Wiley, Sydney, pp.157–62.

Porter, Roy (ed.), *Rewriting the Self: Histories from the Renaissance to the Present*, Routledge, London, 1997

Potter, Simon, *News and the British World: The Emergence of an Imperial Press System 1876–1922*, Oxford University Press, 2003

___, 'Webs, Networks, and Systems: Globalization and the Mass Media in the Nineteenth and Twentieth-Century British Empire', *Journal of British Studies*, 46 (July 2007), pp.621–46

___, 'Who Listened When London Called? Reactions to the BBC Empire Service in Canada, Australia and New Zealand, 1932–1939', *Historical Journal of Film, Radio and Television*, 28, 4 (October 2008), pp.475–87

Pottle, Mark, 'Round, Dorothy Edith (1909–1982)', *Oxford Dictionary of National Biography*, first published 2004; online edn, January 2011

Poynter, J. R., 'Rubinstein, Helena (1870–1965)', *Australian Dictionary of Biography*, Vol.11, Melbourne University Press, 1988, pp.475–77

Prochaska, Frank, *Royal Bounty: The Making of a Welfare Monarchy*, Yale University Press, New Haven and London, 1995

___, *The Voluntary Impulse: Philanthropy in Modern Britain*, Faber & Faber, London, 1988

Proctor, Tammy, *On My Honour: Guides and Scouts in Interwar Britain*, American Philosophical Society, Philadelphia, 2002

___, '(Uni)Forming Interwar Youth: Girl Guides and Boy Scouts in Britain, 1908–1939', *History Workshop Journal*, 45 (Spring 1998), pp.103–34

Pugh, Martin, 'Britain and its Empire', in R. J. B. Bosworth (ed.), *The Oxford Handbook of Fascism*, Oxford University Press, 2009, pp.489–506.

___, 'We danced all night': A Social History of Britain Between the Wars*, The Bodley Head, London, 2008

Radi, Heather, 'Swain, Edith Muriel Maitland (1880–1964)', *Australian Dictionary of Biography*, Vol.16, Melbourne University Press, 2002, pp.349–50

Reekie, Gail, *Temptations: Sex, Selling, and the*

Department Store, Allen & Unwin, St Leonards, NSW, 1993

Richards, Trevor, *Dancing on Our Bones: New Zealand, South Africa, Rugby and Racism*, Bridget Williams Books, Wellington, 1999

Rieger, Bernard, *Technology and the Culture of Modernity in Britain and Germany, 1890-1945*, Cambridge University Press, 2009

Riordan, James and Arnd Kruger (eds), *The International Politics of Sport in the Twentieth Century*, Spon Press, London, 1999

Robinson, Roger, 'Lovelock, John Edward – Biography', from the *Dictionary of New Zealand Biography*, Te Ara – the Encyclopaedia of New Zealand, updated 1 September 2010, http://www.teara.govt.nz/en/biographies/4l14/1

___, 'Lovelock, John Edward (1910-1949)', *Oxford Dictionary of National Biography*, Oxford University Press, first published 2004; online edn, January 2008

Roche, Stanley, *The Red and the Gold*, Oxford University Press, Wellington, 1982

Roe, Michael, 'Cumpston, John Howard Lidgett (1880-1954)', *Australian Dictionary of Biography*, Vol.8, Melbourne University Press, 1981, pp.174-76

___, *Nine Australian Progressives: Vitalism in Bourgeois Social Thought, 1890-1960*, University of Queensland Press, St Lucia, 1984

Rose, Nikolas, *Governing the Soul: The Shaping of the Private Self*, Routledge, London, 1990

___, *Inventing Our Selves: Psychology, Power and Personhood*, Cambridge University Press, 1998

Rose, Sonya, *Which People's War? National Identity and Citizenship in Wartime Britain 1939-1945*, Oxford University Press, 2003

Ross, Bruce, 'Thinking the Physical: PAS, PE & Power', *Journal of Physical Education New Zealand*, Part I, 29, 4 (Summer 1996), pp.5-8, and Part II, 30, 1 (Autumn 1997), pp.3-6

Ross, Kirstie, *Going Bush: New Zealanders and Nature in the Twentieth Century*, Auckland University Press, 2008

___, '"Schooled by Nature": Pakeha Tramping Between the Wars', *New Zealand Journal of History*, 35, 1 (2002), pp.51-65

Rudy, Jarrett, *The Freedom to Smoke: Tobacco Consumption and Identity*, McGill-Queen's University Press, Montreal, 2005

Rybczynski, Witold, *Waiting for the Weekend*, Viking, New York, 1991

Sandercock, Leonie, 'Sport', in Bill Gammage and Peter Spearritt (eds), and oral history co-ordinator Louise Douglas, *Australians 1938*, Fairfax, Syme & Weldon Associates, Broadway, NSW, 1987, pp.373-89

Sandiford, Keith A. and Brian Stoddart (eds), *The Imperial Game: Cricket, Culture and Society*, Manchester University Press, Manchester and New York, 1998

Scher, Len, *The Un-Canadians: True Stories of the Blacklist Era*, Lester, Toronto, 1992

Schiller, Kay and Christopher Young, 'The History and Historiography of Sport in Germany: Social, Cultural and Political Perspectives', *German History*, 27, 3 (July 2009), pp.313-30

Schmidt, Christine, 'Undressing Kellerman, Uncovering Broadhurst: The Modern Woman and "Un-Australia"', *Fashion Theory: The Journal of Dress and Body Culture*, 13, 4 (December 2009), pp.481-97

Schor, Juliet B., *The Overworked American: The Unexpected Decline of Leisure*, Basic Books, New York, 1991

Schrader, Ben, 'A Brave New World? Ideal Versus Reality in Post-war Naenae', *New Zealand Journal of History*, 30, 1 (April 1996), pp.61-79

Schrodt, Barbara, 'Federal Programmes of Physical Recreation and Fitness: The Contributions of Ian Esienhardt and BC's Pro-Rec', *Canadian Journal of Sport and Physical Education*, 15, 2 (December 1984), pp.45-61

Self, Robert, *Neville Chamberlain: A Biography*, Ashgate, Aldershot, 2006

Sheffield, Scott, 'Rehabilitating the Indigene: Post-War Reconstruction and the Image of the Indigenous Other in English Canada and New Zealand, 1943-1948', in Phillip Alfred Buckner and R. Douglas Francis (eds), *Rediscovering the British World*, University of Calgary Press, 2005, pp.341-60

Simon, Scott, *Jackie Robinson and the Integration of Baseball*, John Wiley, Hoboken, 2007

Simpson, Albert E., *The National Fitness Council of South Australia: A History 1939-76*, South Australia Department of Recreation and Sport, Adelaide, 1986

Simpson, Clare, *The One Hundred Year History of the Christchurch Young Women's Christian Association, 1883-1983*, Christchurch YWCA, 1983

Small, R.B., 'The Pioneers of Physical Education in Scotland', in J.A. Mangan and R.B. Small (eds), *Sport, Culture, Society: International Historical and Sociological Perspectives: Proceedings of the VIII Commonwealth and International Conference on Sport, Physical Education, Dance, Recreation, and Health: Conference '86 Glasgow, 18-23 July*, Spon, London, 1986, pp.60-67

Smart, Judith, 'Feminists, Flappers and Miss Australia: Contesting the Meanings of

Citizenship, Femininity and Nation in the 1920s', *Journal of Australian Studies*, 25, 71 (2001), pp.1–15

Smith, Dai, *Aneurin Bevan and the World of South Wales*, University of Wales Press, Cardiff, 1993

___, 'Bevan, Aneurin (1897–1960)', *Oxford Dictionary of National Biography*, Oxford University Press, first published 2004; online edn, January 2008

Smith, Janet, *Liquid Assets: The Lidos and Open Air Swimming Pools of Britain*, English Heritage/Malavan Media, London, 2005

Smith, Max, *Champion Blokes: 44 Great New Zealand Sports Men Then and Now*, Whitcombe and Tombs, Christchurch, 1964

Sontag, Susan, *Under the Sign of Saturn*, Vintage Books, New York, 1981

Sorrenson, M. P. K., 'Ngata, Apirana Turupa, 1874–1950', from the *Dictionary of New Zealand Biography*, Te Ara – the Encyclopedia of New Zealand, updated 1 September 2010, http://www.teara.govt.nz/en/biographies/3n5/1

Soutar, Monty, *Nga Tama Toa: The Price of Citizenship: C Company 28 (Maori) Battalion 1939–1945*, David Bateman, Auckland, 2008

Spence, Jonathan D., 'The Question of Pearl Buck', *The New York Review of Books*, 57 (15),14 October 2010, pp.51–53

Stanley, Adam, *Modernizing Tradition: Gender and Consumerism in Interwar France and Germany*, Louisiana State University Press, Baton Rouge, 2008

Steedman, Carolyn, 'McMillan, Margaret (1860–1931)', *Oxford Dictionary of National Biography*, Oxford University Press, first published 2004; online edn, January 2008

Stenhouse, John, 'Religion and Society', in Giselle Byrnes (ed.), *The New Oxford History of New Zealand*, Oxford University Press, Melbourne, 2009, chapter 14

Stephen, Ann, Philip Goad and Andrew McNamara (eds), *The Untold Story of Modernism in Australia*, Miegunyah Press, Melbourne, 2008

Stevenson, John, *British Society 1914–45*, Allen Lane, London, 1984

Stoddart, B. and K. Sandiford (eds), *The Imperial Game: Cricket, Culture and Society*, Manchester University Press, 1999

Stothart, R. A., 'Pegs in the Ground: Landmarks in the History of New Zealand's Physical Education', *Journal of Physical Education New Zealand*, 33, 2 (September 2000), pp.5–15

Sutton-Smith, Brian, 'The Meeting of Maori and European Cultures and its effects upon the Unorganised Games of Maori Children', *Journal of the Polynesian Society*, 60, 2 & 3 (September 1951), pp.92–107

___, *The Ambiguity of Play*, Harvard University Press, Cambridge, 1997

Taylor, Harvey, *A Claim on the Countryside: A History of the British Outdoor Movement*, Keele University Press, Edinburgh, 1997

Templeton, Malcolm, *Sporting Contacts and Human Rights: New Zealand's Attitude to Race Relations in South Africa, 1921–1994*, Auckland University Press, 1998

Tennant, Margaret, *Children's Health, the Nation's Wealth: A History of Children's Health Camps*, Bridget Williams Books, Wellington, 1994

___, *The Fabric of Welfare: Voluntary Organisations, Government and Welfare in New Zealand, 1840–2005*, Bridget Williams Books, Wellington, 2007

Tennant, Margaret, Mike O'Brien and Jackie Sanders, *The History of the Non-profit Sector in New Zealand*, Office for the Community and Voluntary Sector, Wellington, 2008

Terret, Thierry, 'Hygienization: Civic Baths and Body Cleanliness in Late Nineteenth Century France', *International Journal of the History of Sport*, 10, 3 (December 1993), pp.396–408

Thompson, Lynne, '"The Golden Thread of Empire": Women's Popular Education in the Lancashire Federation of Women's Institutes 1920–39', *Journal of Educational Administration and History*, 28, 1 (1996), pp.42–57

Thompson, Paul, *New Zealand: A Century of Images*, Te Papa Press, Wellington, 1998

Thomson, Mathew, *Psychological Subjects: Identity, Culture and Health in Twentieth-Century Britain*, Oxford University Press, 2006

Tillotson, Shirley, 'Citizen Participation in the Welfare State: An Experiment, 1945–57', *Canadian Historical Review*, 25, 4 (1994), pp.511–42

Titley, Brian, 'Indian Act', in Gerald Hallowell (ed.), *Oxford Companion to Canadian History*, Oxford University Press, 2004

Toepfer, Karl Eric, *Empire of Ecstasy: Nudity and Movement in German Body Culture, 1910–35*, University of California Press, Berkeley, 1997

Tumblety, Joan, 'Medicine in History and Society', short abstract, c.2010, <www.soton.ac.uk/history/docs/medical.../tumblety_research.pdf>

Turner, Bryan, *Regulating Bodies: Essays in Medical Sociology*, Routledge, London, 1992

Tyler, Peter J., *Humble and Obedient Servants: The Administration of New South Wales, 1901–1960*, University of New South Wales Press, Sydney, 2006

Tyrell, Ian, *Transnational Nation: United States History in Global Perspective Since 1879*, Palgrave Macmillan, Basingstoke, 2007

Vertinsky, Patricia, *The Eternally Wounded Woman: Women, Doctors, and Exercise in the Late Nineteenth Century*, University of Illinois Press, Urbana, 1994

Vials, Chris, 'The Popular Front in the American Century: Life Magazine, Margaret Bourke-White, and Consumer Realism, 1936–1941', *American Periodicals*, 16, 1 (2006), p.74

Walker, D. R., 'Sutton, Harvey (1882–1963)', *Australian Dictionary of Biography*, Vol.12, Melbourne University Press, 1990, pp.143–44

Walker, David, 'Mind and Body', in Bill Gammage and Peter Spearritt (eds), with oral history co-ordinator Louise Douglas, *Australians 1938*, Fairfax, Syme & Weldon, Broadway, NSW, 1987, chapter 16

Walker, Ranginui, *Ka Whawhai Tonu Matou: Struggle without End*, 2nd edn, Penguin, Auckland, 2004

___, 'Maori People since 1950', in G. W. Rice (ed.), *Oxford History of New Zealand*, 2nd edn, Oxford University Press, Auckland, 1992, chapter 19

Wall, Sharon, 'Making Modern Childhood, the Natural Way: Psychology, Mental Hygiene and Progressive Education at Ontario Summer Camps, 1920–1955', *Historical Studies in Education*, 20, 2 (Fall 2008), pp.73–110

___, *The Nurture of Nature: Childhood, Antimodernism, and Ontario Summer Camps, 1920–55*, University of British Columbia Press, Vancouver, 2009

Walvin, James, *Leisure and Society, 1830–1950*, Longman, London, 1978

Ward, Stuart (ed.), *British Culture and the End of Empire*, Manchester University Press, Manchester and New York, 2001

Weber, Eugen, 'Gymnastics and Sports in Fin-de-Siécle France: Opium of the Classes?', *American Historical Review*, 76, 1 (February 1971), pp.70–99

Webster, Charles, 'Healthy or Hungry Thirties?', *History Workshop*, 13 (Spring 1982), pp.110–29

___, *Problems of Health Care the National Health Service before 1957*, The Health Services Since the War, Vol.1, HMSO, London, 1988

West, J. Thomas, 'Physical Fitness, Sport and the Federal Government 1909 to 1954', *Canadian Journal of History of Sport and Physical Fitness*, 4, 2 (1973), pp.26–42

Whitehead, Sarah, '"A territory of such varied picturesqueness": Gerard Carrington and the Beginnings of the Christchurch Tramping Club', *Records of the Canterbury Museum*, 24 (2010), pp.15–26

Whitfield, Andrew, 'Stanley, Oliver Frederick George (1896–1950)', *Oxford Dictionary of National Biography*, Oxford University Press, first published 2004; online edn, January 2008

Wilk, Christopher (ed.), *Modernism, 1914–1939: Designing a New World*, V & A Publications, London, 2006

Williams, Jack, *Cricket and England: A Cultural and Social History of the Inter-war Years*, Frank Cass, London, 2003

Williams, John Alexander, *Turning to Nature in Germany: Hiking, Nudism, and Conservation, 1900–1940*, Stanford University Press, 2007

Wilson, Elizabeth, *Adorned in Dreams: Fashion and Modernity*, rev edn, Rutgers University Press, New Brunswick, 2003

___, 'Fashion and Modernity', in C. Breward and C. Evans (eds), *Fashion and Modernity*, Berg, Oxford and New York, 2005, pp.9–14

Winship, Janice, 'Women's Magazines: Times of War and Management of the Self in *Woman's Own*', in Christine Gledhill and Gillian Swanson (eds), *Nationalising Femininity: Culture, Sexuality and British Cinema in the Second World War*, Manchester University Press, 1996, pp.127–39

Winterton, Rachel and Claire Parker, 'A Utilitarian Pursuit: Swimming Education in Nineteenth-Century Australia and England', *International Journal for the History of Sport*, 26, 14 (November 2009), pp.2106–26

Worley, Matthew, *Oswald Mosley and the New Party*, Palgrave Macmillan, Basingstoke, 2010

Wosh, Peter J., 'Sound Minds and Unsound Bodies: Massachusetts Schools and Mandatory Physical Training', *The New England Quarterly*, 55, 1 (March 1982), pp.39–60

Wright, Jan and Valerie Harwood (eds), *Biopolitics and the 'Obesity Epidemic': Governing Bodies*, Routledge, New York and London, 2009

Zweiniger-Bargielowska, Ina, 'Building a British Superman: Physical Culture in Interwar Britain', *Journal of Contemporary History*, 41, 4 (October 2006), pp.595–610

___, *Managing the Body: Beauty, Health and Fitness in Britain, 1880s–1939*, Oxford University Press, 2010

___, 'The Making of a Modern Female Body: Beauty, Health and Fitness in Interwar Britain', *Women's History Review*, 20, 2 (April 2011), pp.299–317

Theses and Unpublished Papers

Alexander, Janet, 'Recreation: An Inappropriate Concept for Legislation?: An Examination of Two Attempts at Legislating for Recreation in New Zealand: the Physical Welfare and Recreation Act 1937, and the Recreation and Sport Act 1973', MPP research paper, Victoria University of Wellington, 1981

Bailey, Rona, Comments, 'A Dissenting New Zealand: She'll Never Last the Distance', Trade Union History Project seminar, Wellington, 4 December 1993

Buchanan, Hugh D., 'A Critical Analysis of the 1937 Physical Welfare and Recreation Act and of Government Involvement in Recreation and Sport, 1937–1957', MA (Applied) thesis, Victoria University of Wellington, 1978

Bueltmann, Tanja, '"Brither Scots shoulder tae shoulder": Ethnic Identity, Culture and Associationism Among the Scots in New Zealand to 1930', PhD thesis, Victoria University of Wellington, 2008

Burke, Peter, 'A Social History of Workplace Australian Football, 1860–1939', PhD thesis, RMIT University, 2008

Clark, Miriam, '"Be fit and add something to the person": The Sport and Physical Recreation Programme of the Wellington YWCA 1918–1939', BA (Hons) research essay in History, Victoria University of Wellington, 1993

Clements, Samantha R., 'Feminism, Citizenship and Social Activity: The Role and Importance of Local Women's Organizations, Nottingham 1918–1969', PhD thesis, University of Nottingham, 2008

Ewens, Wilfred Wallace, 'Gordon Young: The Passing of an Era', PhD thesis, University of Oregon, 1973

Fischer, Imke, 'Years of Silent Control: The Influence of the Commonwealth in State Physical Education in Victoria and New South Wales', PhD thesis, University of Sydney, 2000

Fry, Margot, 'A Servant of Many Masters: A History of the National Film Unit of New Zealand, 1941 to 1976', MA thesis, Victoria University of Wellington, 1995

Gush, Nadia, 'Cultural Fields of the Canterbury Plains: Women and Cultural Citizenship in Canterbury c.1890–1940', PhD thesis, Victoria University of Wellington, 2007

Harris, Aroha, 'Dancing with the State: Maori Creative Energy and Policies of Integration, 1945–67', PhD thesis, University of Auckland, 2007

Johnston, Susie, 'Lighting Up: The Social History of Smoking in New Zealand, c.1920–62', MA thesis, Victoria University of Wellington, 2009

Liebich, Susann, 'Connected Readers: Reading Practices and Communities across the British World, c.1890–1930', PhD in progress, Victoria University of Wellington, 2011

Lynch, Anthony, 'Otago 17 – Southland 11: A Social History of Otago Rugby in the 1940s', BA (Hons), University of Otago, 1984

Macdonald, Charlotte, 'Bodies, Nations, Empire: Sports and Fitness Campaigns in 1930s Britain and New Zealand', Victoria University of Wellington presentation, March 2004

____, 'Getting Fat, Fit and Healthy: Why Was it So Difficult? Health and Fitness Campaigns in Interwar Britain and New Zealand', Health and History Conference, University of Auckland, February 2005

____, 'National Fitness: Joy and Work in the Empire', presented at New Zealand Historical Association Conference, Otago, November 2003

Mann, Owen, 'Confirming Tradition, Confirming Change: A Social History of the Cricket Tours to New Zealand in the 1930s', MA thesis, Victoria University of Wellington, 2011

Matthews, Jackie, Introduction, 'A Dissenting New Zealand: She'll Never Last the Distance', Trade Union History Project seminar, Wellington, 4 December 1993

McMillan, David Gervan, 'A Study on Poor-family Dietary (Investigation of food Supply Per Day and Review of Statistics)', Preventive Medicine dissertation, University of Otago, 1927

Parker, Claire, 'An Urban Historical Perspective: Swimming as a Recreational and Competitive Pursuit 1840 to 1914', PhD thesis, University of Stirling, 2003

Rainer, Philip, 'Company Town: An Industrial History of the Waihi Gold Mining Company Limited, 1887–1912', MA thesis, University of Auckland, 1976

Ross, Kirstie, 'Signs of Landing. Pakeha Outdoor Recreation and the Cultural Colonisation of New Zealand', MA thesis, University of Auckland, 1999

Schrodt, P. Barbara, 'A History of Pro-Rec: The British Columbia Provincial Recreation Programme, 1934 to 1953', PhD dissertation, University of Alberta, 1979

Simmons, Roderick J., 'Joe Walding and Labour's Physical Welfare Ideal: The Establishment of the Ministry of Recreation and Sport 1972–5', MA thesis, Massey University, 1998

Skillen, Fiona, 'Women and Sport in Interwar Scotland', PhD thesis, University of Glasgow, 2008

Stothart, R. A., 'The Education of New Zealand Recreation Workers', MA thesis, Victoria University of Wellington, 1977

Stowe, Deborah, 'John Pascoe's Photography of the New Zealand Home Front During the Second World War: An Historical Analysis', MA thesis, Victoria University of Wellington, 2006

Williams, Melissa, '"Back-home" and Home in the City: Māori Migrations from Panguru to Auckland, 1930–1970', PhD thesis, University of Auckland, 2010

Woods, Megan, 'Integrating the Nation: Gendering Maori Urbanisation and Integration, 1942–1969', PhD thesis, University of Canterbury, 2002

Young, W. Gordon, 'Physical Education in Australia: A Study of the History of Physical Education in Australia and a Forecast of Future Development', MEd thesis, University of Sydney, 1962

Index